The New Complete
MEDICAL
and HEALTH
ENCYCLOPEDIA

The New Complete
MEDICAL
and HEALTH
ENCYCLOPEDIA

EDITED BY
Richard J. Wagman, M.D., F.A.C.P.

Assistant Clinical Professor of Medicine
Downstate Medical Center
New York, New York

AND BY
the Ferguson Editorial Staff

Volume Three

FERGUSON PUBLISHING COMPANY/CHICAGO

Editor

Richard J. Wagman, M.D.,
F.A.C.P.
Assistant Clinical Professor of
    Medicine
Downstate Medical Center
New York, New York

Contributors to The New Complete Medical and Health Encyclopedia

Consultant in Surgery

N. Henry Moss, M.D., F.A.C.S.
Associate Clinical Professor of
    Surgery
Temple University Health Sciences
    Center and Albert Einstein
    Medical Center;
Past President, American Medical
    Writers Association;
Past President, New York Academy
    of Sciences

Consultant in Gynecology

Douglass S. Thompson, M.D.
Clinical Professor of Obstetrics and
    Gynecology and Clinical Associate
    Professor of Community Medicine
University of Pittsburgh School of
    Medicine

Consultant in Pediatrics

Charles H. Bauer, M.D.
Clinical Associate Professor of
    Pediatrics and Chief of Pediatric
    Gastroenterology
The New York Hospital-Cornell
    Medical Center
New York, New York

Consultants in Psychiatry

Julian J. Clark, M.D.
Assistant Professor of Psychiatry
                and
Rita W. Clark, M.D.
Clinical Assistant Professor of
    Psychiatry
Downstate Medical Center

Consulting Editor

Kenneth N. Anderson
Formerly Editor
Today's Health

Bruce O. Berg, M.D.
Associate Professor
Departments of Neurology and
    Pediatrics
Director, Child Neurology
University of California
San Francisco, California

D. Jeanne Collins
Assistant Professor
College of Allied Health Professions
University of Kentucky
Lexington, Kentucky

Anthony A. Davis
Vice President and Education
    Consultant
Metropolitan X-Ray and Medical
    Sales, Inc.
Olney, Maryland

Peter A. Dickinson
Editor Emeritus
Harvest Years/Retirement Living

Gordon K. Farley, M.D.
Associate Professor of Child
    Psychiatry
Director, Day Care Center
University of Colorado Medical
    Center

Arthur Fisher
Group Editor
Science and Engineering
Popular Science

Edmund H. Harvey, Jr.
Editor
Science World

Helene MacLean
Medical writer

Ben Patrusky
Science writer

Stanley E. Weiss, M.D.
Assistant Attending Physician, Renal
    Service
Beth Israel Hospital and Medical
    Center, New York

Jeffrey S. Willner, M.D.
Attending Radiologist
Southampton Hospital
Southampton, New York

Contents

Volume III

21

Skin and Hair

Not many people have perfectly proportioned faces and bodies, but practically anyone, at any age, can present an attractive appearance if skin is healthy-looking and glowing and hair is clean and shining. Healthy skin and hair can be achieved through good health habits, cleanliness, and personal grooming. Expensive skin-and-hair products may boost self-confidence, but they are a poor substitute for proper diet, exercise, enough sleep, and soap and water or cleansing creams.

The condition of skin and hair reflects a person's physical and emotional health. Of course, general appearance is determined not only by what is going on inside the body but also by outward circumstances, such as extremes of temperature or the use of harsh soaps. Appearance can also be altered temporarily by cosmetics and permanently by surgery.

The Skin

The skin is one of the most important organs of the body. It serves as protection against infection by germs and shields delicate underlying tissue against injury. Approximately one-third of the bloodstream flows through the skin, and as the blood vessels contract or relax in response to heat and cold, the skin acts as a thermostat that helps control body temperature. The two million sweat glands in the skin also regulate body temperature through the evaporation of perspiration. The many delicate nerve endings in the skin make it a sense organ responsive not only to heat and cold but also to pleasure, pain, and pressure.

Certain cells in the skin produce a protective pigmentation that determines its color and guards against overexposure to the ultraviolet rays of the sun. By absorption and elimination, the skin helps regulate the body's chemical and fluid balance. One of the miracles of the skin is that it constantly renews itself.

Structure of the Skin

The skin is made up of two layers. The outer layer, or *epidermis,* has a surface of horny, nonliving cells that form the body's protective envelope. These cells are constantly being shed and replaced by new ones, which are made in the lower or inner layer of the epidermis.

Underneath the epidermis is the *dermis,* the thicker part of the skin. It contains blood vessels, nerves, and connective tissue. The sweat glands are located in the dermis, and they collect fluid containing water, salt, and waste products from the blood. This fluid is sent through tiny canals that end in pores on the skin's surface.

The oil, or *sebaceous,* glands that secrete the oil that lubricates the surface of the skin and hair are also located in the dermis. They are most often associated with hair *follicles.*

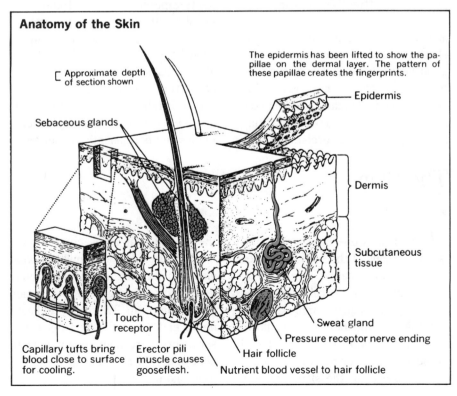

Anatomy of the Skin

The epidermis has been lifted to show the papillae on the dermal layer. The pattern of these papillae creates the fingerprints.

⌐ Approximate depth of section shown

Epidermis

Sebaceous glands

Dermis

Subcutaneous tissue

Touch receptor

Sweat gland

Pressure receptor nerve ending

Capillary tufts bring blood close to surface for cooling.

Erector pili muscle causes gooseflesh.

Hair follicle

Nutrient blood vessel to hair follicle

Hair follicles and oil glands are found over most of the body, with the exception of the palms of the hands and the soles of the feet.

The layer of fatty tissue below the dermis, called *subcutaneous* tissue, acts as an insulator against heat and cold and as a shock absorber against injury.

Skin Color

The basic skin color of each person is determined at birth, and is a part of his heritage that cannot be changed.

Melanin

There are four pigments in the normal skin that affect its color: melanin, oxygenated hemoglobin, reduced hemoglobin, and various carotenes. Of these, *melanin* is the most powerful. The cells that produce it are the same in all races, but there is wide variation in the amount produced, and wide variation in its color, which ranges from black to light tan. Every adult has about 60,000 melanin-producing cells in each square inch of skin.

Melanin cells also affect eye color. When the cells are deep in the eye, the color produced is blue or green. When they are close to the surface, the eye is brown. An *albino,* a person with no melanin, has eyes that appear pink, because the stronger pigment that ordinarily masks the blood vessels is lacking.

Hemoglobin

The pigment that gives blood its color, called *hemoglobin,* has the next greatest effect on skin color. When it is combined with oxygen, a bright red is the result, and this in turn produces the rosy complexion associated with good health in light-skinned people. When such people suffer from reduced hemoglobin because of anemia, they appear to be excessively pale. A concentration of reduced hemoglobin gives the skin a bluish appearance. Because hemoglobin has a weaker coloring effect than the melanin that determines basic skin color, these variations are more visible in lighter-skinned individuals.

Carotenes

The weakest pigments in the skin are the *carotenes*. These produce a yellowish tone that is increased by eating excessive amounts of carrots and oranges. In people with black or brown skin, excess carotene is usually masked by the melanin pigment.

Aging Skin

Skin appearance is affected by both internal and external factors. A baby's skin has a silken quality because it has not yet begun to show the effects of continued exposure to sun and wind. The skin problems associated with adolescence reflect the many glandular changes that occur during the transition to adulthood. As the years pass, the skin becomes the most obvious indicator of aging.

Heredity, general health, and exposure to the elements are some of the factors that contribute to aging skin. Because people with darker skin have built-in protection against the ravages of the sun, their skin usually has a younger appearance than that of lighter-skinned people of comparable age.

In general, the skin of an older person is characterized by wrinkles and shininess. It feels thinner when pinched because it has lost its elasticity and part of the underlying fat that gives firmness to a younger skin.

Constant exposure to sunlight is now thought to play a more important role in the visible aging of skin than the aging process itself. Such exposure also appears to be directly related to the greater frequency of skin cancer among farmers, sailors, and others who spend most of their working hours out of doors.

Care of the Skin

Healthy, normal skin should be washed regularly with mild soap and warm water to remove grease, perspiration, and accumulated dirt. For those with a limited water supply or inadequate bath and shower facilities, sponge baths are a good substitute if the sponge or washcloth is thoroughly rinsed as various parts of the body are washed. Many people feel that a shower is a much more efficient way of getting clean than a bath, since the bath water becomes the receptacle for the dirt washed from the body, instead of its being rinsed away.

No matter what method is used, all soap should be thoroughly rinsed off the skin after washing. Unless specifically prescribed by a physician, medicated or germicidal soaps should not be used, since they may be an irritant. Skin should be dried with a fluffy towel, and bath towels should never be shared. Hands should be washed several times a day, and fingernails kept clean.

Facial skin requires special care because of its constant exposure. The face should be cleaned in the morning and before bedtime. Some people may prefer to use a cleansing cream rather than soap and water. Everyone should avoid massaging soap into the skin, because this may cause drying.

Dry and Oily Skin

Both heredity and environment account for the wide variation in the amount of oil and perspiration secreted by the glands of different people. Also, the same person's skin may be oily in one part of the body and dry in another. Skin on the nose and chin tends to be the oiliest.

Dry Skin

This condition is the result of loss of water from the outer surface of the epidermis and its insufficient replacement from the tissues below. Some causes of the moisture loss are too frequent use of soap and detergents, and constant exposure to dry air. Anyone spending a great deal of time in air-conditioned surroundings in which the humidity has been greatly lowered is likely to suffer from dry skin.

To correct the condition, the use of soap and water should be kept to a minimum for those parts of the body where the skin is dry. Cleansing creams or lotions containing lanolin should be used on the face, hands, elbows, and wherever else necessary. If tub baths are taken, a bath oil can be used in the water or applied to the skin after drying. Baby oil is just as effective and much cheaper than glamorously packaged and overadvertised products. Baby oil or a protective lotion should also be used on any parts of the body exposed to direct sunlight for any extended length of time. Applying oil to the skin will not, however, prevent wrinkles.

Oily Skin

The amount of oil that comes to the surface of the skin through the sebaceous glands is the result not only of heredity but also of temperature and emotional state. In warm weather, when the skin perspires more freely, the oil spreads like a film on the surface moisture. Nonoily foundation lotions can be helpful in keeping the oil spread to a minimum, and so can frequent washing with soap and water. When washing is inconvenient during the day, cleansing pads packaged to fit in pocket or purse are a quick and efficient solution for both men and women.

Too much friction from complexion brushes, rough washcloths, or harsh soaps may irritate rather than improve an oily skin condition.

Deodorants and Antiperspirants

Sweat glands are present almost everywhere in the skin except for the lips and a few other areas. Most of them give off the extremely dilute salt water known as sweat, or perspiration. Their purpose is to cool the body by evaporation of water. Body odors are not produced by perspiration itself but by the bacterial activity that takes place in the perspiration. The activity is most intense in warm, moist parts of the body from which perspiration cannot evaporate quickly, such as the underarm area.

Deodorants

The basic means of keeping this type of bacterial growth under control is through personal cleanliness of both skin and clothing. Deodorant soaps containing antiseptic chemicals are now available. Though they do not kill bacteria, they do reduce the speed with which they multiply.

Underarm deodorants also help to eliminate the odor. They are not meant to stop the flow of perspiration but rather to slow down bacterial growth and mask body odors with their own scent. Such deodorants should be applied immediately after bathing. They are usually more effective if the underarm area is shaved, since the hair in this unexposed area collects perspiration and encourages bacterial growth.

Antiperspirants

Antiperspirants differ from deodorants in that they not only affect the rate of bacterial growth but also reduce the amount of perspiration that reaches the skin surface. Because the action of the chemical salts they contain is cumulative, they seem to be more effective with repeated use. Antiperspirants come under the category of drugs, and their contents must be printed on the container. Deodorants are considered cosmetics, and may or may not name their contents on the package.

No matter what the nature of the advertising claim, neither type of product completely stops the flow of perspiration, nor would it be desirable to do so. Effectiveness of the various brands differs from one person to another. Some may produce a mild allergic reaction; others might be too weak to do a good job. It is practical to experiment with a few different brands, using them under similar conditions, to find the type that works best for you.

Creams and Cosmetics

The bewildering number of creams and cosmetics on the market and the exaggerated claims of some of their advertising can be reduced to a few simple facts. Beauty preparations should be judged by the user on their merits rather than on their claims.

Cold Creams and Cleansing Creams

These two products are essentially the same. They are designed to remove accumulated skin secretions, dirt, and grime, and should be promptly removed from the skin with a soft towel or tissue.

Lubricating Creams and Lotions

Also called night creams, moisturizing creams, and conditioning creams, these products are supposed to prevent the loss of moisture from the skin and promote its smoothness. They are usually left on overnight or for an extended length of time. Anyone with dry skin will find it helpful to apply a moisturizer under foundation cream. This will help keep the skin from drying out even further, and protect it against the effects of air-conditioning.

Vanishing Creams and Foundation Creams

These products also serve the purpose of providing the skin with moisture, but are meant to be applied immediately before putting on makeup.

Rejuvenating Creams

There is no scientific proof that any of the "royal jelly," "secret formula," or "hormone" creams produce a marked improvement on aging skin. They cannot eliminate wrinkles, nor can they regenerate skin tissue.

Medicated Creams and Lotions

These products should not be used except on the advice of a physician, since they may cause or aggravate skin disorders of various kinds.

Lipsticks

Lipsticks contain lanolin, a mixture of oil and wax, a coloring dye, and pigment, as well as perfume. Any of these substances can cause an allergic reaction in individual cases, but such reactions are uncommon. Sometimes the reaction is caused by the staining dye, in which case a "nonpermanent" lipstick should be used.

Cosmetics and the Sensitive Skin

Anyone with a cosmetic problem resulting from sensitive skin should consult a *dermatologist,* a physician specializing in the skin and its diseases. Cosmetic companies will inform a physician of the ingredients in their products, and he or she can then recommend a brand that will agree with the patient's specific skin problems. The physician may also recommend a special nonallergenic preparation.

Eye Makeup

Eye-liner and mascara brushes and pencils—and lipsticks, for that matter—can carry infection and should never be borrowed or lent. *Hypoallergenic* makeup, which is specially made for those who get allergic reactions to regular eye makeup, is available.

Suntanning Creams and Lotions

Growing awareness that exposure to the sun may cause skin cancer (see "Skin Cancer" in Ch. 18, *Cancer*) has led to a demand for a variety of skin creams and lotions. The preparations protect the skin or speed the tanning process. Many of the "sunblocks" and "sunscreens" keep the ultraviolet radiation in sunlight from reaching the skin. They are adapted to six basic skin types, ranging from type 1, which burns easily and never tans, to types 5 and 6, which never burn and usually tan well.

Skin lotions and creams are rated according to a "sun protection factor" (SPF). Among the basic ratings are SPF 4, providing "moderate protection;" SPF 8, a "maximal" sunscreen; and SPF 15, with "ultra" protection. Other ratings range up to SPF 50. Some medical authorities question the need for sunscreens rated higher than 15 or 20. Food and Drug Administration ratings go only to SPF 15. Many newer sunscreens are greaseless, hypoallergenic, waterproof, or PABA-free. PABA, or para-aminobenzoic acid, is a sunscreen chemical that can irritate skin and stain clothing.

Sunscreen ratings indicate, in theory, how long the user can stay in the sun without burning. A lotion or cream with a rating of SPF 2 should allow users to remain exposed twice as long as they could with no protection at all. The Skin Cancer Foundation believes that persons who burn in the sun should uniformly wear an SPF 15 protective preparation.

Persons who want suntans have many products from which to choose. "Tanning accelerators" in lotion form speed up the tanning process. A pocket-sized "sun exposure meter" operated electronically alerts the user when overexposure may be taking place. The meter is programmed with the individual's skin type and SPF.

Tanning Pills

Case-studies have proven that tanning pills can cause serious medical problems, possibly resulting in death. Ailments include aplastic anemia (a decrease in the production of red blood cells), orange skin, headaches, weight loss, easy bruising, and increased fatigue. Treatment involves blood transfusion therapy. Physicians believe that the ingredient canthaxanthin is responsible for the disorders.

This drug is not approved as a prescription or an over-the-counter preparation by the Federal Drug Administration. Ultimately, this product serves no purpose, and it is best to avoid using it.

Hair

Hair originates in tiny sacs or follicles deep in the dermis layer of skin tissue. The part of the hair below the skin surface is the root; the part above is the shaft. Hair follicles are closely connected to the sebaceous glands, which secrete oil to the scalp and give hair its natural sheen. Hair grows from the root outward, pushing the shaft farther from the scalp.

Texture

Each individual hair is made up of nonliving cells that contain a tough protein called *keratin*. Hair texture differs from one part of the body to another. It also differs between the sexes, among individuals, and among the different races.

If an individual hair is oval in cross-section, it is curly along its length. If the cross-section is round, the hair is straight. Thick, wiry hair is usually triangular or kidney-shaped. The fineness or coarseness of hair texture is related to its natural color.

Curling

Anyone using a home permanent preparation should follow the instructions with great care: improper mixing, application, or exposure time could result in serious damage to the hair.

Electric curling irons are not safe, because they may cause pinpoint burns in the scalp that are hardly noticeable at the time but may lead to permanent small areas of baldness. The danger can be minimized, however, if instructions for use are followed exactly. It is especially important that the iron not be hot enough to singe the hair. Setting lotions used with rollers or clips have a tendency to dull the hair unless they are completely brushed out.

Straightening

The least harmful as well as the least effective way of straightening the hair temporarily is the use of pomades. They are usually considered unsatisfactory by women because they are too greasy, but are often used by men with short, unruly hair. Heat-pressing the hair with a metal comb is longer-lasting but can cause substantial damage by burning the scalp. The practice of ironing the hair should be discouraged, since it causes dryness and brittleness, with resultant breakage. Chemical straighteners should be used with great care, since they may cause serious burns. Special efforts must be made to protect the eyes from contact with these products.

Hair Color

In the same way that melanin colors the skin, it also determines hair color. The less melanin, the lighter the hair. As each hair loses its melanin pigment, it gradually turns gray, then white. It is assumed that the age at which hair begins to gray is an inherited characteristic and therefore can't be postponed or prevented by eating special foods, by taking vitamins, or by the external application of creams. The only way to recolor gray hair is by the use of a chemical dye.

Dyes and Tints

Anyone wishing to make a radical change in hair color should consult a trained and reliable hairdresser. Trying to turn black hair bright red or dark red hair to blond with a home preparation can sometimes end up with unwanted purplish or greenish results. When tints or dyes are used at home to lighten or darken the hair color by one or two shades, instructions accompanying the product must be followed carefully. Anyone with a tendency to contract contact dermatitis should make a patch test on the skin to check on possible allergic reactions. Hair should be tinted or dyed no more often than once a month.

Dye Stripping

The only safe way to get rid of an unwanted dye color that has been used on the hair is to let it grow out. The technique known as stripping takes all color from the hair and reduces it to a dangerously weak mass. It is then redyed its natural color. Such a procedure should never be undertaken by anyone except a trained beautician, if at all.

Bleaching

Hydrogen peroxide is mixed with a hair lightener to prebleach hair before applying blond tints. Bleaching with peroxide alone can cause more damage to the hair than dyeing or tinting it with a reliable commercial preparation, because it causes dryness, brittleness, and breakage.

General Hair Care

Properly cared for hair usually looks clean, shiny, and alive. Unfortunately, too many people mask the natural good looks of their hair with unnecessary sprays and "beauty" preparations.

Washing the Hair

Hair should be washed about once a week—more often if it tends to be oily. The claims made by shampoo manufacturers need not always be taken too seriously, since most shampoos contain nothing more than soap or detergent and a perfuming agent. No shampoo can restore the natural oils to the hair at the same time that it washes it. A castile shampoo is good for dry hair, and one containing tincture of green soap is good for oily hair.

Thorough rinsing is essential to eliminate any soap deposit. If the local water is hard, a detergent shampoo can be rinsed off more easily than one containing soap.

Drying the Hair

Drying the hair in sunlight or under a heat-controlled dryer is more satisfactory than trying to rub it dry with a towel. Gentle brushing during drying reactivates the natural oils that give hair its shine. Brushing in general is excellent for the appearance of the hair. Be sure to wash both brush and comb as often as the hair is washed.

Hair pomades should be avoided or used sparingly, since they are sometimes so heavy that they clog the pores of the scalp. A little bit of olive oil or baby oil can be rubbed into dry hair after shampooing. This is also good for babies' hair.

There is no scientific evidence that creme rinses, protein rinses, or beer rinses accomplish anything for the hair other than making it somewhat more manageable if it is naturally fine and flyaway.

Dandruff

Simple dandruff is a condition in which the scalp begins to itch and flake a few days after the hair has been washed. There is no evidence that the problem is related to germ infection.

Oiliness and persistent dandruff may appear not only on the scalp but also on the sides of the nose or the chest. In such cases, a dermatologist should be consulted. Both light and serious cases often respond well to prescription medicines containing tars. These preparations control the dandruff, but there is no known cure for it.

Nits

Head lice sometimes infect adults as well as children. These tiny parasites usually live on the part of the scalp near the nape of the neck, and when they bite, they cause itching. They attach their eggs, which are called *nits,* to the shaft of the hair, and when they are plentiful, they can be seen by a trained eye as tiny, silvery-white ovals. This condition is highly contagious and can be passed from one head to another by way of combs, brushes, hats, head scarfs, and towels. A physician can be consulted for information on effective ways of eliminating nits—usually by the application of chemicals and the use of a fine-tooth comb.

Baldness

Under the normal circumstances of combing, brushing, and shampooing, a person loses anywhere from 25 to 100 hairs a day. Because new hairs start growing each day, the loss and replacement usually balance each other. When the loss rate is greater than the replacement rate, thinning and baldness are the result.

The medical name for baldness is *alopecia,* the most common form of which is *male pattern baldness.* Dr. Eugene Van Scott, Professor of Dermatology of Temple University's Health Sciences Center, sums up the opinion of medical authorities on the three factors responsible for this type of baldness: sex, age, and heredity. Unfortunately, these are three factors over which medical science has no control.

Two drugs have been approved for regrowing hair: minoxidil and finasteride. Minoxidil, a topical solution, is available over the counter and is sold under the brand name Rogaine and as a generic drug. Approximately 25 percent of men and 20 percent of women using it experience some hair growth. Finasteride, a pill marketed as Prope-

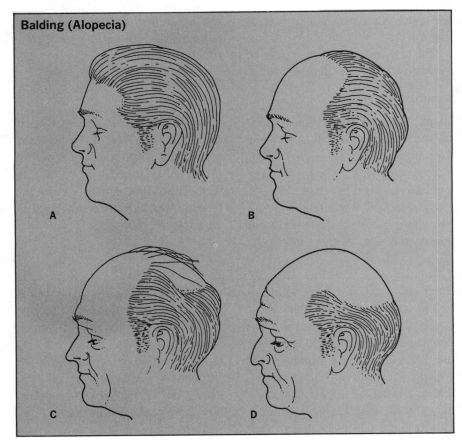

Balding (Alopecia)

A

B

C

D

cia, was approved in 1997. More than 80 percent of men in trials experienced a slowing of hair loss and 60 percent grew new hair. Propeicia is available by prescription only.

Other forms of baldness may be the result of bacterial or fungal infections, allergic reactions to particular medicines, radiation, or continual friction. It has been suggested that stress from hair curlers or tight ponytails can cause loss of hair. These forms of baldness usually disappear when the cause is eliminated.

Although diet has very little to do with baldness, poor nutrition can result in hair that is dry, dull, and brittle enough to break easily. Any serious illness can lead to hair loss as well. It is thought that vitamin A taken in grossly excessive amounts can contribute to hair loss.

Women ordinarily lose some of their hair at the end of pregnancy, after delivery, and during the menopause, but regrowth can be expected in a few months.

A surgical procedure for treating male pattern baldness and baldness in women is called hair transplantation; it is discussed in Ch. 20, *Surgery.*

Hair Removal

Over the centuries and around the world, fashions in whiskers and beards come and go, but the average American male still subjects at least part of his face to daily shaving. Although feminine shaving practices are a more recent phenomenon, most American women now consider it part of good grooming to remove underarm and leg hair with a razor as often as twice a week. Shaving removes not only the dead skin cells that make up the protective layer of the body's surface but also some of the living skin underneath. Instead of being harmful, this appears to stimulate rather than damage new skin growth.

Male Shaving

The average beard grows about two-tenths of an inch a day. However, the density of male face hair varies a great deal depending on skin and hair color. In all races, the concentration is usually greatest on the chin and in the area between the nose and upper lip.

There is no proof that an electric razor is safer or better for all types of skin than a safety razor. Both types result in nicks and cuts of the living skin tissue, depending on the closeness of the shave.

Twice as many men prefer wet shaving to dry because the use of soap and hot water softens the hair stubble and makes it easier to remove. Shaving authorities point out that thorough soaking is one of the essentials of easy and safe shaving. Leaving the shaving lather on the face for at least two minutes will also soften whiskers a good deal.

The razor should be moistened with hot water throughout the proc- ess, and the chin and upper lip left for last so that the heavier hair concentration in these areas has the longest contact with moisture and lather.

Oily Skin

Men with oily skin should use an aerosol shaving preparation or a lather-type applied with a brush. These are really soaps and are more effective in eliminating the oils that coat the face hair, thus making it easier to shave.

Dry Skin

A brushless cream is advisable for dry skin, since it lubricates the skin rather than further deprives it of oil.

Ingrown Hairs

One of the chief problems connected with shaving is that it often causes ingrown hairs, which can lead to pore-clogging and infection. Hair is more likely to turn back into the skin if it is shaved against the grain, or if the cutting edge of the blade is dull and rough rather than smooth. Men with coarse, wiry, curly, rather than fine, hair may find that whisker ends are more likely to become ingrown than men with fine hair. The problem is best handled by shaving with the grain, using a sharp blade, and avoiding too close a shave, particularly in the area around the neck.

Shaving and Skin Problems

For men with acne or a tendency to skin problems, the following advice is offered by Dr. Howard T. Behrman, Director of Dermatological Research, New York Medical College:

- Shave as seldom as possible, perhaps only once or twice a week, and always with the grain.

- If wet shaving is preferred, use a new blade each time, and shave as lightly as possible to avoid nicking pimples.

- Wash face carefully with plenty of hot water to make the beard easy to manage, and after shaving, rinse with hot water followed by cold.

- Use an antiseptic astringent face lotion.

- Instead of plucking out ingrown hairs, loosen them gently so that the ends do not grow back into the skin.

- Although some people with skin problems find an electric shaver less irritating, in most cases, a wet shave seems best.

Female Shaving

Millions of American women regularly shave underarm and leg hair, and most of them do so with a blade razor. In recent years, various types of shavers have been designed with blade exposure more suited to women's needs than the standard type used by men. To make shaving easier and safer, the following procedures are recommended.

- Since wet hair is much easier to cut, the most effective time to shave is during or immediately following a bath or shower.

- Shaving cream or soap lather keeps the water from evaporating, and is preferred to dry shaving.

- Underarm shaving is easier with a contoured razor designed for this purpose. If a deodorant or antiperspirant causes stinging or irritation after shaving, allow a short time to elapse before applying it.

- Light bleeding from nicks or scrapes can be stopped by applying pressure to a sterile pad placed on the injured area.

Unwanted Hair

The technical word for excess or unwanted hair on the face, chest, arms, and legs is *hirsutism*. The condition varies greatly among different ethnic strains, and so does the attitude toward it. Women of southern European ancestry are generally hairier than those with Nordic or Anglo-Saxon ancestors. Caucasoid peoples are hairier than Negroid peoples. The sparsest amount of body hair is found among the Mongolian races and American Indians. Although heredity is the chief factor of hirsutism, hormones also influence hair growth. If there is a sudden appearance of coarse hair on the body of a young boy or girl or a woman with no such former tendency, a glandular disturbance should be suspected and investigated by a physician.

A normal amount of unwanted hair on the legs and under the arms is usually removed by shaving. When the problem involves the arms, face, chest, and abdomen, other methods of removal are available.

Temporary Methods of Hair Removal

Bleaching

Unwanted dark fuzz on the upper lip and arms can be lightened almost to invisibility with a commercially prepared bleach or with a homemade paste consisting of baking soda, hydrogen peroxide (bleaching strength), and a few drops of ammonia. Soap chips can be used instead of baking soda. The paste should be left on the skin for a few minutes and then washed off. It is harmless to the skin, and if applied repeatedly, the hair will tend to break off as a result of constant bleaching.

Chemical Depilatories

These products contain alkaline agents that cause the hair to detach easily at the skin surface. They can be used on and under the arms, and on the legs and chest. However, they should not be used on the face unless the label says it is safe to do so. Timing instructions should be followed carefully. If skin irritation results, this type of depilatory should be discontinued in favor of some other method.

Abrasives

Devices that remove hair from the skin surface by rubbing are cheap but time-consuming. However, if an abrasive such as pumice is used regularly, the offending hairs will be shorter with each application. A cream or lotion should be applied to the skin after using an abrasive.

Waxing

The technique of applying melted wax to the skin for removal of excess facial hair is best handled by an experienced cosmetician. The process involves pouring hot wax onto the skin and allowing it to cool. The hairs become embedded in the wax, and are plucked out from below the skin surface when the wax is stripped off. Because this method is painful and often causes irritation, it is not very popular, although the results are comparatively long-lasting.

Plucking

The use of tweezers for removing scattered hairs from the eyebrows, face, and chest is slightly painful but otherwise harmless. It is not a practical method for getting rid of dense hair growth, however, because it takes too much time.

Permanent Hair Removal by Electrolysis

The only permanent and safe method of removing unwanted hair is by *electrolysis*. This technique destroys each individual hair root by transmitting electric current through fine wire needles into the opening of the hair follicle. The hair thus loosened is then plucked out with a tweezer. The older type of electrolysis machine uses galvanic current. The newer type, sometimes called an *electrocoagulation machine*, uses modified high-frequency current. In either case, the efficiency and safety of the technique depends less on the machine than on the care and skill of the operator.

Because the process of treating each hair root is expensive, time-consuming, and uncomfortable, it is not recommended for areas of dense hair growth, such as the arms or legs. Before undertaking electrolysis either at a beauty salon or at home, it would be wise to consult a dermatologist about individual skin reaction.

Nails

Fingernails and toenails are an extension of the epidermis, or outer layer of the skin. They are made of elastic tissue formed from keratin, the substance that gives hair its strength and flexibility.

Some of the problems associated with fingernails are the result of too much manicuring. White spots, for example, are often caused by too much pressure at the base of the nail when trying to expose the "moon"— the white portion that contains tissue not yet as tough as the rest of the nail.

To ensure the health of toenails, feet should be bathed once a day and the nails cleaned with a brush dipped in soapy water. Shoes should fit properly so that the toenails are not subjected to pressure and distortion. To avoid ingrown toenails, trimming should be done straight across rather than by rounding or tapering the corners.

Splitting

Infection or injury of the tissue at the base of a fingernail may cause its surface to be rigid or split. Inflammation of the finger joints connected with arthritis will also cause nail deformity. For ordinary problems of splitting and

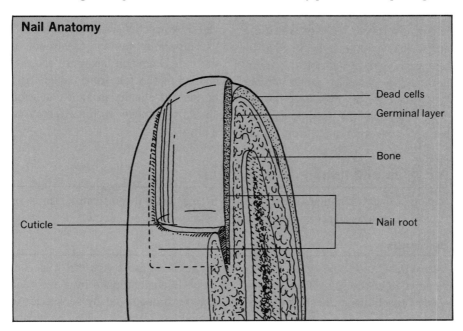

Nail Anatomy

Dead cells

Germinal layer

Bone

Nail root

Cuticle

peeling, the nails should be kept short enough so that they don't catch and tear easily. For practical purposes, the top of the nail should not be visible when the palm is held about six inches from the eye. As the nails grow stronger, they can be grown longer without splitting.

Brittleness

This condition seems to be caused by such external factors as the chemicals in polish removers, soaps, and detergents. It is also a natural consequence of aging. Commercial nail-hardening preparations that contain formaldehyde are not recommended, because they are known to cause discoloration, loosening, or even loss of nails in some cases.

Nail damage can be reduced by wearing rubber gloves while doing household chores. Hand cream massaged into the skin around the nails will counteract dryness and lessen the possibility of hangnails. Although nail polish provides a shield against damage, it should not be worn all the time, particularly if the nail is polished right down to the base; this prevents live tissue from "breathing."

Disorders of the Skin

The skin is subject to a large number of disorders, most of which are not serious even though they may be temporarily uncomfortable. A disorder may be caused by one or another type of allergy; by excessive heat or cold; or by infection from fungi, bacteria, viruses, or parasites. Many skin ailments are caused or aggravated by emotional disturbances.

The symptoms and treatment of the more common disorders are discussed in the following pages. Any persistent change in skin condition should be brought to the attention of a physician.

Allergies and Itching

Itching and inflammation of the skin may be caused by an allergic reaction, by exposure to poisonous plants, or by a generalized infection.

Dermatitis

Dermatitis is the term used for an inflammation of the skin. The term for allergic reactions of the skin resulting from surface contact with outside agents is *contact dermatitis*. This condition is characterized by a rash and may be brought out by sensitivity to cosmetics, plants, cleaning materials, metal, wool, and so on. Other forms of dermatitis can be caused by excesses of heat or cold, by friction, or by sensitivity to various medicines. Dermatitis is usually accompanied by itching at the site of the rash.

Poison Ivy

This common plant, unknown in Europe but widespread everywhere in the United States except in California and Nevada, produces an allergic reaction on the skin accompanied by a painful rash and blisters. Some people are so sensitive to it that they are affected by contact not only with the plant itself but with animal fur or clothing that might have picked up the resin weeks before.

A mild attack of poison ivy produces a rash and small, watery blisters that get progressively larger. The affected area of the skin becomes crusty and dry, and after a few weeks, all symptoms vanish. If the exposed area is thoroughly washed with cold, running water immediately after contact, the poison may not penetrate the skin.

If the symptoms do develop, they can be relieved with applications of over-the-counter medications such as Domeboro or calamine lotion. If the symptoms are severe, and especially if the area around the eyes is involved, a physician should be consulted. He may prescribe an application or an injection of cortisone.

The best way to avoid the unpleasantness of a poison ivy attack is to learn to recognize the plant and stay away from it. Children especially should be warned against putting the leaves and berries in their mouths.

Poison oak and poison sumac produce somewhat the same symptoms and should also be avoided.

Under no circumstances should these plants be burned to eliminate them, because the inhaling of the contaminated smoke even from a distance can cause a serious case of poisoning. The application of special sprays, if the instructions are followed carefully, will get rid of the plants without affecting people or the neighborhood greenery.

Hives

These are large, irregularly shaped swellings on the skin that burn and itch. The cause is unknown, but allergic reactions to certain foods and medicine or to insect bites have been suggested as possible causes. The swellings of hives usually disappear within a day or so, but they can be very uncomfortable while they last. The itching and burning can often be relieved by applying cold water and a calamine solution. However, some people are sensitive to cold and develop wheals when subjected to intense cold. Commercial preparations containing surface anesthetics are seldom effective and may cause allergic reactions.

If the outbreak of hives can be traced to a specific food, such as shellfish or strawberries, the food should be eliminated from the diet. If a medicine such as penicillin or a sulfa drug is the cause, a physician should be told about the reaction.

Eczema

This condition is an allergic reaction that produces itching, swelling, blistering, oozing, and scaling of the skin. It is more common among children than among adults and may sometimes cover the entire body, although the rash is usually limited to the face, neck, and folds of the knees and elbows. Unlike contact dermatitis, it is likely to be caused by an allergy to a food or a pollen or dust. Advertised cures for eczema cannot control the cause and sometimes make the condition worse. A physician should be consulted if the symptoms are severe, particularly if the patient is an infant or very young child.

Itching

The technical name for the localized or general sensation on the skin that can be relieved by scratching is *pruritus*. Itching may be caused by many skin disorders, by infections, by serious diseases such as nephritis or leukemia, by medicines, or by psychological factors such as tension. A physician should always be consulted to find the cause of persistent itching, because it may be the symptom of a basic disorder. Repeated scratching may provide some relief, but it can also lead to infection.

Anal Pruritus

If itching in the anal area is so severe that only painful scratching will relieve it, the condition is probably *anal pruritus*. It is often accompanied by excessive rectal mucus that keeps the skin irritated and moist. This disorder is most commonly associated with hemorrhoids, but many other conditions, such as reactions to drugs, can cause it. Anxiety or tension can also contribute to it. Sitz baths with warm water are usually recommended. Every effort should be made to reduce scratching and to keep the anal skin clean and dry. Cortisone cream may be prescribed in persistent cases.

Skin Irritations and Weather

Extremes of weather produce local inflammations and other skin problems for many people.

Chapping

In cold weather, the sebaceous glands slow down the secretions that lubricate the skin, causing it to become dry. When dry skin is exposed to wintry weather, it becomes irritated and is likely to crack, particularly around the lips. Chapped skin is especially sensitive to harsh soaps. During such periods of exposure, the skin can be protected with a mild cream or lotion. A lubricating ointment should be used on the lips to prevent them from cracking. Children who lick their lips continually no matter what the weather can benefit from this extra protection. Chapped hands caused by daily use of strong soaps and detergents can be helped by the use of a lubricating cream and rubber gloves during housework.

Frostbite

Exposure to extreme cold for a prolonged period may cause freezing of the nose, fingers, toes, or ears, thus cutting off the circulation to the affected areas. Frostbitten areas are of a paler color than normal and are numb. They should not be rubbed with snow or exposed to intense heat. Areas should be thawed gradually, and a physician should be consulted for aftercare in extreme cases.

Chilblain

A localized inflammation of the skin called *chilblain* is common among people who are particularly sensitive to cold because of poor circulation. Chilblain may occur in the ears, hands, feet, and face, causing itching, swelling, and discoloration of the skin. Anyone prone to chilblain should dress protectively during the cold weather and use an electric pad or blanket at night. Affected parts should not be rubbed or massaged, nor should ice or extreme heat be applied directly, since these measures may cause additional damage. Persistent or extreme attacks of chilblain should be discussed with a physician.

Chafing

This condition is an inflammation of two opposing skin surfaces caused by the warmth, moisture, and friction of their rubbing together. Diabetics, overweight people, and those who perspire heavily are particularly prone to chafing. Chafing is accompanied by itching and burning, and sometimes infection can set in if the superficial skin is broken. Parts of the body subject to chafing are the inner surfaces of the thighs, the anal region, the area under the breasts, and the inner surfaces between fingers and toes.

To reduce the possibility of chafing, lightweight clothing should be worn and strenuous exercise avoided during hot weather. Vaseline or a vitamin A and D ointment may be applied to reduce friction. In general, the treatment is the same as that for diaper rash in infants. If the condition becomes acute, a physician can prescribe more effective remedies.

Prickly Heat

This skin rash is usually accompanied by itching and burning. It is caused by an obstruction of the sweat ducts such that perspiration does not reach the surface of the skin but backs up and causes pimples the size of a pinhead. If the obstruction is superficial, the pimples are white; if it is deeper, they are red. The condition can be brought on by other minor skin irritations, by continued exposure to moist heat, such as a compress, or by exercise in humid weather. Infants and people who are overweight are especially prone to prickly heat.

The discomfort can be eased by wearing lightweight, loose-fitting clothing, especially at night, and keeping room temperature low. Alcoholic beverages, which tend to dehydrate the body, should be avoided. Tepid baths and the application of cornstarch to the affected skin areas will usually relieve itching. If the rash remains for several days, a physician should be consulted to make sure it does not arise from some other cause.

Calluses and Corns

As a result of continued friction or pressure in a particular area, the skin forms a tough, hard, self-protecting layer known as a *callus*. Calluses are common on the soles of the feet, the palms of the hands, and, among guitarists and string players, on the tips of the fingers. A heavy callus that presses against a bone in the foot because of poorly fitted shoes can be very painful. The hard surface can be reduced somewhat by the use of pumice, or by gently paring it with a razor blade that has been washed in alcohol.

Corns are a form of callus that appear on or between the toes. They usually have a hard inner core that causes pain when pressed against underlying tissue by badly fitted shoes.

A hard corn that appears on the surface of the little toe can be removed by soaking for about ten minutes and applying a few drops of ten percent salicylic acid in collodion. The surface should be covered with a corn pad to reduce pressure, and the corn lifted off when it is loose enough to be released from the skin. Anyone suffering from a circulatory disease and particularly from diabetes should avoid home treatment of foot disturbances. Those with a tendency to callus and corn formations should be especially careful about the proper fit of shoes and hose. A *chiropodist* or *podiatrist* is a trained specialist in foot care who can be visited on a regular basis to provide greater foot comfort.

Fungus Infections

Fungi are plantlike parasitic growths found in the air, in water, and in the soil. They comprise a large family that includes mushrooms, and are responsible for mildew and mold. Only a small number cause disease.

Ringworm

This condition is caused not by a worm but by a group of fungi that live on the body's dead skin cells in those areas that are warm and damp because of accumulated perspiration. One form of ringworm attacks the scalp, arms, and legs, especially of children, and is often spread by similarly affected pets. It appears as reddish patches that scale and blister and frequently feel sore and itchy. Ringworm is highly contagious and can be passed from person to person by contaminated objects such as combs and towels. It should therefore be treated promptly by a physician. Ringworm can best be prevented by strict attention to personal cleanliness.

Athlete's Foot

Another form of ringworm, *athlete's foot,* usually attacks the skin between the toes and under the toenails. If not treated promptly, it can cause an itching rash on other parts of the body. Athlete's foot causes the skin to itch, blister, and crack, and as a result, leaves it vulnerable to more serious infection from other organisms. The disorder can be treated at home by gently removing the damaged skin, and, after soaking the feet, thoroughly drying and dusting between the toes with a medicated foot powder. Some of the powder should be sprinkled into shoes. If the condition continues, a fungicidal ointment can be applied in the morning and at night. Persistent cases require the attention of a physician.

Scabies

An insectlike parasite causes the skin irritation called *scabies,* otherwise known as "the itch." The female itch mite burrows a hole in the skin, usually in the groin or between the fingers or toes, and stays hidden long enough to build a tunnel in which to deposit her eggs. The newly hatched mites then work their way to the skin surface and begin the cycle all over again. There is little discomfort in the early period of infestation, but in about a week, a rash appears, accompanied by extreme itching, which is usually most severe at night. Constant scratching during sleep can lead to skin lesions that invite bacterial infection.

Scabies is very contagious and can spread rapidly through a family or through a community, such as a summer camp or army barracks. It can also be communicated by sexual contact.

Treatment by a physician involves the identification of the characteristic tunnels from which sample mites can be removed for examination. Hot baths and thorough scrubbing will expose the burrows, and medical applications as directed by the physician usually clear up the condition in about a week.

Bacterial Infections

The skin is susceptible to infection from a variety of bacteria. Poor diet and careless hygiene can lower the body's resistance to these infectious agents.

Boils

These abscesses of the skin are caused by bacterial infection of a hair follicle or a sebaceous gland. The pus that accumulates in a boil is the result of the encounter between the bacteria and the white blood cells that fight them. Sometimes a boil subsides by itself and disappears. Sometimes the pressure of pus against the skin surface may bring the boil to a head; it will then break, drain, and heal if washed with an antiseptic and covered with a sterile pad. Warm-water compresses can be applied for ten minutes every hour to relieve the pain and to encourage the boil to break and drain. A fresh, dry pad should be applied after each period of soaking.

Anyone with a serious or chronic illness who develops a boil should consult a physician. Since the bacteria can enter the bloodstream and cause a general infection with fever, a physician should also be consulted for a boil on the nose, scalp, upper lip, or in the ear, groin, or armpit.

Carbuncles

This infection is a group of connected boils and is likely to be more painful and less responsive to home treatment. Carbuncles may occur as the result of poor skin care. They tend to occur in the back of the neck where the skin is thick, and the abscess tends to burrow into deeper tissues. A physician usually lances and drains a deep-seated carbuncle, or he may prescribe an antibiotic remedy.

Impetigo

This skin infection is caused by staphylococcal or streptococcal bacteria, and is characterized by blisters that break and form yellow crusted areas. It is spread from one person to another and from one part of the body to another by the discharge from the sores. Impetigo occurs most frequently on the scalp, face, and arms and legs. The infection often is picked up in barber shops, swimming pools, or from body contact with infected people or household pets.

Special care must be taken, especially with children, to control the spread of the infection by keeping the fingers away from infected parts. Bed linens should be changed daily, and disposable paper towels, as well as paper plates and cups, should be used during treatment. A physician should be consulted for proper medication and procedures to deal with the infection.

Barber's Itch

Sycosis, commonly called *barber's itch,* is a bacterial infection of the hair follicles of the beard, accompanied by inflammation, itching, and the formation of pus-filled pimples. People with stiff, curly hair are prone to this type of chronic infection, because their hair is more likely to curve back and reenter the skin. The infection should be treated promptly to prevent scarring and the destruction of the hair root.

In some cases, physicians recommend antibiotics. If these are not effective, it may be necessary to drain the abscesses and remove the hairs from the inflamed follicles. During treatment, it is best to avoid shaving, if possible. If one must shave, the sterilization of all shaving equipment and the use of a brushless shaving cream are recommended.

Erysipelas

An acute streptococcal infection of the skin, *erysipelas* can be fatal, particularly to the very young or very old, if not treated promptly. One of its symptoms is the bright redness of the affected areas of the skin. These red patches enlarge and spread, making the skin tender and painful. Blisters may appear nearby. The patient usually has a headache, fever, chills, and nausea. Erysipelas responds well to promptly administered antibiotics, particularly penicillin. The patient is usually advised to drink large amounts of fluid and to eat a nourishing, easily digested diet.

Viral Infections

The most common skin conditions caused by viruses are cold sores, shingles, and warts, discussed below.

Cold Sores

Also called fever blisters, *cold sores* are technically known as *herpes simplex.* They are small blisters that appear most frequently in the corners of the mouth, and sometimes around the eyes and on the genitals. The presumed cause is a virus that lies dormant in the skin until it is activated by infection or by excessive exposure to sun or wind. There is no specific cure for cold sores, but the irritation can be eased by applying drying or cooling agents such as camphor ice or cold-water compresses. Recurrent cold sores, especially in infants, should be called to a physician's attention.

Recent studies have shown that a variety of the herpes simplex virus called HSV-II (for herpes simplex virus-Type II) can be a serious danger to the fetus of a pregnant woman. For a discussion of this condition, see Ch. 25, *Women's Health.* The variety that causes cold sores is called Type I.

Shingles

The virus infection of a sensory nerve, accompanied by small, painful blisters that appear on the skin along the path of the nerve—usually on one side of the chest or abdomen—is called *shingles.* The medical name for the disorder, which is caused by the chicken pox virus, is *herpes zoster,* Latin for "girdle of blisters." When a cranial nerve is involved, the blisters appear on the face near the eye. The preliminary symptom is neuritis with severe pain and, sometimes, fever. The blisters may take from two to four weeks to dry up and disappear. Valtrex, which inhibits the activity of the herpes virus, has recently been approved for the treatment of shingles. Aspirin may also be used to alleviate pain.

Warts

These growths are caused by a virus infection of the epidermis. They never become cancerous, but can be painful when found on the soles of the feet. In this location, they are known as *plantar warts,* and they cause discomfort because constant pressure makes them grow inward. Plantar warts are most likely to be picked up by children because they are barefooted so much of the time, and by adults when their feet are moist and they are walking around in showers, near swimming pools, and in locker rooms. Warts can be spread by scratching, by shaving, and by brushing the hair. They are often transmitted from one member of the family to another. Because warts can spread to painful areas, such as the area around or under the fingernails, and because they may become disfiguring, it is best to consult a physician whenever they appear.

In many ways, warts behave rather mysteriously. About half of them go away without any treatment at all. Sometimes, when warts on one part of the body are being treated, those in another area will disappear. The folklore about "witching" and "charming" warts away has its foundation in fact, because apparently having faith in the cure, no matter how ridiculous it sounds, sometimes brings success. This form of suggestion therapy is especially successful with children.

There are several more conventional ways of treating warts. Depending on their size and the area involved, electric current, dry ice, or various chemicals may be employed. A physician should be consulted promptly when warts develop in the area of the beard or on the scalp, because they spread quickly in these parts of the body and thus become more difficult to eliminate.

Sebaceous Cysts

When a sebaceous gland duct is blocked, the oil that the gland secretes cannot get to the surface of the skin. Instead, it accumulates into a hard, round, movable mass contained in a sac. This mass is known as a *sebaceous cyst.* Such cysts may appear on the face, back, ears, or in the genital area. A sebaceous cyst that forms on the scalp is called a *wen,* and may become as large as a billiard ball. The skin in this area will become bald, because the cyst interferes with the blood supply to the hair roots.

Some sebaceous cysts just disappear without treatment. However, those that do not are a likely focus for secondary infection by bacteria, and they may become abscessed and inflamed. It is therefore advisable to have cysts examined by a physician for possible removal. If such a cyst is superficial, it can be punctured and drained. One that is deeper is usually removed by simple surgical procedure in the physician's office.

Acne

About 80 percent of all teenagers suffer from the skin disturbance called *acne.* It is also fairly common among women in their twenties. Acne is a condition in which the skin of the face, and often of the neck, shoulders, chest, and back, is covered to a greater or lesser extent with pimples, blackheads, whiteheads, and boils.

The typical onset of acne in adolescence is related to the increased activity of the glands, including the sebaceous glands. Most of the oil that they secrete gets to the surface of the skin through ducts that lead into the pores. When the surface pores are clogged with sebaceous gland secretions and keratin, or when so much extra oil is being secreted that it backs up into the ducts, the result is the formation of the skin blemishes characteristic of acne. Dirt or makeup does not cause acne.

The blackheads are dark not because they are dirty but because the fatty material in the clogged pore is oxidized and discolored by the air that reaches it. When this substance is infected by bacteria, it turns into a pimple. Under no circumstances should such pimples be picked at or squeezed, because the pressure can rupture the surrounding membrane and spread the infection further.

Although a mild case of acne usually clears up by itself, it is often helpful to get the advice of a physician so that it does not get any worse.

Cleanliness

Although surface dirt does not cause acne, it can contribute to its spread. Therefore, the affected areas should be cleansed with a medicated soap and hot water twice a day. Hair should be shampooed frequently and brushed away from the face. Boys who are shaving should soften the beard with soap and hot water. The blade should be sharp and should skim the skin as lightly as possible to avoid nicking pimples.

Creams and Cosmetics

Nonprescription medicated creams and lotions may be effective in reducing some blemishes, but if used too often, they make the skin dry. They should be applied according to the manufacturer's instructions and should be discontinued if they cause additional irritation. If makeup is used, it should have a nonoily base and be completely removed before going to bed.

Forbidden Foods

Although acne is not caused by any particular food, it can be made worse by a diet overloaded with candy, rich pastries, and fats. Chocolate and cola drinks must be eliminated entirely in some cases.

Professional Treatment

A serious case of acne, or even a mild one that is causing serious emotional problems, should receive the attention of a physician. He or she may prescribe antibiotics, usually considered the most effective treatment, or recommend sunlamp treatments. A physician can also be helpful in dealing with the psychological aspects of acne that are so disturbing to teenagers.

Psoriasis

Psoriasis is a noncontagious chronic condition in which the skin on various parts of the body is marked by bright red patches covered with silvery scales. The areas most often affected are the knees, elbows, scalp, and trunk, and less frequently, the areas under the arms and around the genitals.

The specific cause of psoriasis has not yet been discovered, but it is thought to be an inherited abnormality in which the formation of new skin cells is too rapid and disorderly. In its mild form, psoriasis responds well to a variety of long-term treatments. When it is acute, the entire skin surface may be painfully red, and large sections of it may scale off. In such cases, prompt hospitalization and intensive care are recommended.

Conditions That Can Bring On an Outbreak

The onset or aggravation of psoriasis can be triggered by some of the following factors:

- bruises, burns, scratches, and overexposure to the sun

- sudden drops in temperature—a mild, stable climate is most beneficial
- sudden illness from another source, or unusual physical or emotional stress

- infections of the upper respiratory tract, especially bacterial throat infections and the medicines used to cure them

Treatment

Although there is no specific cure for psoriasis, these are some of the recommended treatments:

- controlled exposure to sunlight or an ultraviolet lamp

- creams or lotions of crude coal tar or tar distillates, used alone or in combination with ultraviolet light

- psoralen and ultraviolet light (PUVA), a combined systemic-external therapy in which a psoralen drug is taken orally before exposure to ultraviolet light

- systemic drugs, such as methotrexate, which can be taken orally

- steroid hormone medications applied to the skin surface under dressings

Pigment Disorders and Birthmarks

The mechanism that controls skin coloration is described above under "Skin Color." Abnormalities in the creation and distribution of melanin result in the following disorders, some of which are negligible.

Freckles

These are small spots of brown pigment that frequently occur when fair-skinned people are exposed to the sun or to ultraviolet light. For those whose skin gets red rather than tan during such exposure, freckles are a protective device. In most cases, they recede in cold weather. A heavy freckle formation that is permanent can be covered somewhat by cosmetic preparations. No attempt should be made to remove freckles with commercial creams or solutions unless supervised by a physician.

Liver Spots

Flat, smooth, irregularly placed markings on the skin, called *liver spots,* often appear among older people, and result from an increase in pigmentation. They have nothing to do with the liver and are completely harmless. Brownish markings of similar appearance sometimes show up during pregnancy or as a result of irritation or infection. They usually disappear when the underlying cause is eliminated.

Liver spots are permanent, and the principal cause is not aging but the accumulated years of exposure to sun and wind. They can be disguised and treated in the same way as freckles. A liver spot that becomes hard and thick should be called to a physician's attention.

Moles

Clusters of melanin cells, called *moles,* may appear singly or in groups at any place on the body. They range in color from light tan to dark brown; they may be raised and hairy or flat and smooth. Many moles are present at birth, and most make their appearance before the age of 20. They rarely turn into malignancies, and require medical attention only if they become painful, if they itch, or if they suddenly change in size, shape, or color.

There are several ways of removing moles if they are annoying or particularly unattractive. They can be destroyed by the application of an electric needle, by cauterizing, and by surgery. A mole that has been removed is not likely to reappear. The hairs sometimes found in moles can be clipped close to the surface of the skin, or they can be permanently removed. Hair removal often causes the mole to get smaller.

Vitiligo

Vitiligo is an autoimmune disease in which the body's white cells attack its pigment cells, causing a loss of pigment in the skin. About 1 percent of the U.S. population suffers from this condition, which can appear any time up to middle age and is believed to be inherited. Vitiligo can occur anywhere on the body, from small spots to large patches, but the nose, hands, feet, and genital area are the most common areas affected.

There is no cure for vitiligo, but it can be treated with drugs and exposure to ultraviolet A radiation. The condition itself is not physically painful, but many vitiligo sufferers, particularly dark-skinned persons, experience emotional pain and embarrassment.

Birthmarks

About one-third of all infants are born with the type of birthmark called *a hemangioma,* also known as a vascular birthmark. These are caused by a clustering of small blood vessels near the surface of the skin. The mark, which is flat, irregularly shaped, and either pink, red, or purplish, is usually referred to as "port wine stain." There is no known way to remove it, but with cosmetic covering creams, it can usually be successfully masked.

The type of hemangioma that is raised and bright red—called a strawberry mark—spontaneously disappears with no treatment in most cases during early childhood. If a strawberry mark begins to grow rather than fade, or if it begins to ulcerate, a physician should be promptly consulted.

See Ch. 18, *Cancer,* for a discussion of skin cancer; see Ch. 3, *The Teens,* for a discussion of adolescent skin problems; see Ch. 23, *Aches, Pains, Nuisances, Worries,* for further discussion of minor skin problems.

22

The Teeth and Gums

Although a human baby is born without teeth, a complete set of 20 *deciduous,* or baby, teeth (also called *primary teeth*) already has formed within the gums of the offspring while it still is within the mother's womb. The buds of the permanent or secondary teeth are developing even before the first baby tooth appears at around the age of six months. The baby teeth obviously are formed from foods eaten by the mother. Generally, if the mother follows a good diet during pregnancy, no special food items are required to ensure an adequate set of deciduous teeth in the baby.

It takes about two years for the full set of deciduous teeth to appear in the baby's mouth. The first, usually a central incisor at the front of the lower jaw, may erupt any time between the ages of three and nine months. The last probably will be a second molar at the back of the upper jaw. As with walking, talking, and other characteristics of infants, there is no set timetable for the eruption of baby teeth. One child may get his first tooth at three months while another must wait until nine months, but both would be considered within a normal range of tooth development.

The permanent teeth are never far behind the deciduous set. The first permanent tooth usually appears around the age of six years, about four years after the last of the baby teeth has erupted. As the baby teeth gradually fall out, they are replaced by permanent teeth. The chart below shows the usual ages for the appearance and shedding of baby teeth.

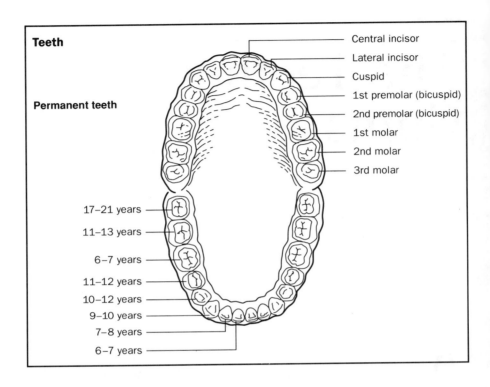

UPPER JAW			LOWER JAW		
central incisor	8-12 mos	6-7 yrs	central incisor	6-10 mos	6-7 yrs
lateral incisor	9-13 mos	7-8 yrs	lateral incisor	10-16 mos	7-8 yrs
canine (cuspid)	16-22 mos	10-12 yrs	canine (cuspid)	17-23 mos	9-12 yrs
first molar	13-19 mos	9-11 yrs	first molar	14-18 mos	9-11 yrs
second molar	25-33 mos	10-12 yrs	second molar	23-31 mos	10-12 yrs

Types of Teeth

The permanent teeth number 32. In advancing from deciduous to permanent teeth, the human gains six teeth in the lower jaw, or *mandible,* and six in the upper jaw, or *maxilla,* of the mouth. In general, each kind of tooth appears first in the lower jaw. The usual ages for the appearance of the permanent teeth are as follows:

	LOWER	UPPER
incisors	6-8 yrs	7-9 yrs
cuspids	9-10 yrs	11-12 yrs
bicuspids	10-12 yrs	10-12 yrs
first molars	6-7 yrs	6-7 yrs
second molars	11-13 yrs	12-13 yrs
wisdom teeth	17-21 yrs	17-21 yrs

An *incisor* is designed to cut off particles of food, which is then pushed by muscles of the tongue and cheeks to teeth farther back in the mouth for grinding. The front teeth, one on each side, upper and lower, are central incisors. Next to each central incisor is a lateral incisor.

A *cuspid* is so named because it has a spear-shaped crown, or *cusp*. It is designed for tearing as well as cutting. Cuspids sometimes are called *canine teeth* or *eyeteeth;* canine teeth owe their name to the use of these teeth by carnivorous animals, such as dogs, for tearing pieces of meat. There are four cuspids in the mouth, one on the outer side of each lateral incisor in the upper and lower jaws.

Bicuspids sometimes are identified as *premolars*. The term "bicuspid" suggests two cusps, but a bicuspid may in fact have three cusps. The function of the bicuspids is to crush food passed back from the incisors and cuspids. The permanent set of teeth includes a total of eight bicuspids.

The *molars,* which also number eight and are the last teeth at the back of the mouth, are the largest and strongest teeth, with the job of grinding food. The third molars, or wisdom teeth, are smaller, weaker, and less functional than the first and second molars.

Structure of the Tooth

The variety of shapes of teeth make them specialized for the various functions in preparing food for digestion—biting, chewing, and grinding. All varieties, however, have the same basic structure. Each tooth has a crown (the part of the tooth visible above the gum line) and a root, which is embedded in a socket in the jaw.

Enamel

The outer covering of the crown is *enamel,* the hardest substance in the human body. Enamel is about 97 percent mineral and is as tough as some gemstones. It varies in thickness, with the greatest thickness on the surfaces that are likely to get the most wear and tear.

Enamel begins to form on the first tooth buds of an embryo at the age of about 15 weeks, depending upon substances in the food eaten by the mother for proper development. Once the tooth has formed and erupted through the gum line, there is nothing further that can be done by natural means to improve the condition of the enamel. The enamel has no blood supply, and any changes in the tooth surface will be the result of wearing, decay, or injury.

While the health and diet of the mother can affect the development of tooth enamel in the deciduous teeth, certain health factors in the early life of a child can result in defective enamel formation of teeth that have not yet erupted. Some infectious or metabolic disorders, for example, may result in enamel pitting.

Dentin

Beneath the enamel surface of a tooth is a layer of hard material—though not as hard as enamel—called *dentin,* which forms the bulk of a tooth. The dentin forms at the same time that enamel is laid down on the surface of a developing tooth, and the portion beneath the crown of the tooth probably is completed at the same time as the enamel. However, the dentin, which is composed of calcified material, is not as dense as the enamel; it is formed as myriad tubules that extend downward into the pulp at the center of the tooth. There is some evidence that dentin formation may continue slowly during the life of the tooth.

Cementum

The *cementum* is a bonelike substance that covers the root of the tooth. Though harder than regular bone, it is softer than dentin. It contains attachments for fibers of a periodontal ligament that holds the tooth in its socket. The periodontal ligament serves as a kind of hammock of fibers that surround and support the tooth at the cementum surface, radiating outward to the jawbone. This arrangement allows the tooth to move a little while still attached to the jaw. For example, when the teeth of the upper and lower jaws are brought together in chewing, the periodontal ligament allows the teeth to sink into their sockets. When the teeth of the two jaws are separated, the hammocklike ligament permits the teeth to float outward again.

Pulp

The cavity within the dentin contains the *pulp*. There is a wide pulp chamber under the crown of the tooth and a pulp canal that extends from the

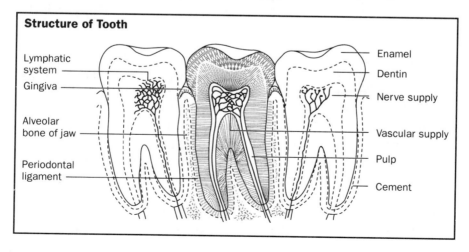

Structure of Tooth

Lymphatic system
Gingiva
Alveolar bone of jaw
Periodontal ligament

Enamel
Dentin
Nerve supply
Vascular supply
Pulp
Cement

chamber down through the root or roots. Some teeth, such as the molars, may contain as many as three roots, and each of the roots contains a pulp canal.

The pulp of a tooth contains the nerve fibers, lymphatic vessels, blood vessels, and connective tissue. Although the blood supply arrangement is not the same for every tooth, a typical pattern includes a dental artery entering through each passageway, or *foramen*, leading into the root of a tooth. The artery branches into numerous capillaries within the root canal. A similar system of veins drains the blood from the tooth through each foramen. A lymphatic network and nerve system also enter the tooth through a foramen and spread through the pulp, as branches from a central distribution link within the jawbone. The nerve fibers have free endings in the tooth, making them sensitive to pain stimuli.

Supporting Structures

The soft, pink gum tissue that surrounds the tooth is called the *gingiva,* and the bone of the jaw that forms the tooth socket is known as *alveolar bone.* The gingiva, alveolar bone, and periodontal ligaments sometimes are grouped into a structural category identified as the *periodontium.* Thus, when a dentist speaks of periodontal disease, he is referring to a disorder of these supporting tissues of the teeth. The ailment known as *gingivitis* is an inflammation of the gingiva, or gum tissue around the teeth.

Care of the Teeth and Gums

Years ago, loss of teeth really was unavoidable. Today, thanks to modern practices of preventive dentistry, it is possible for nearly everyone to enjoy the benefits of natural teeth for a lifetime. But natural teeth can be preserved only by daily oral-hygiene habits and regular dental checkups.

The Dental Examination

Dental checkups should begin in early childhood and continue throughout adult life. A child should see a dentist at the age of two or two-and-a half, once all the primary teeth have emerged. Children who require special attention in treating dental problems can benefit from seeing a pedodontist, a dentist who specializes in the care of children. After the permanent teeth have become established, the dentist should be visited every six months, or at whatever intervals the dentist recommends for an individual patient who may need more or less care than the typical patient.

The dentist, like the family physician, usually maintains a general health history of each patient, in addition to a dental health history. He examines each tooth, the gums and other oral tissues, and the *occlusion,* or bite. A complete set of X-ray pictures may be taken on the first visit and again at intervals of perhaps five to seven years. During routine visits, the dentist may take only a couple of X-ray pictures of teeth on either side of the mouth; a complete set of X rays may result in a file of 18 or 20 pictures covering every tooth in the mouth.

X rays constitute a vital part of the dental examination. Without them the dentist cannot examine the surfaces between the teeth or the portion of the tooth beneath the gum, a part that represents about 60 percent of the total length of the tooth. The X rays will reveal the condition of the enamel, dentin, and pulp; any impacted wisdom teeth; and the alveolar bone, or tooth sockets. Caps, fillings, abscessed roots, and bone loss resulting from gum disease also are clearly visible on a set of X rays.

Other diagnostic tests may be made, such as a test of nerve response. Sometimes the dentist will make an impression of the teeth, an accurate and detailed reverse reproduction, in plaster of paris, plastic impression compound, or other material. Models made from these impressions are used to study the way the teeth meet. Such knowledge is often crucial in deciding the selection of treatment and materials.

After the examination, the dentist will present and explain any proposed treatment. After oral restoration is completed, the dentist will ask the patient to return at regular intervals for a checkup and *prophylaxis,* which includes cleaning and polishing the teeth. Regular checkups and prophylaxis help prevent periodontal diseases affecting the gum tissue and underlying bone. Professional cleaning removes hard deposits that trap bacteria, especially at the gum line, and polishing removes stains and soft deposits.

Dental Care in Middle Age

Although periodontal disease and cavities—called *dental caries* by dentists—continue to threaten oral health, two other problems may assume prominence for people of middle age: replacing worn-out restorations, or fillings, and replacing missing teeth. No filling material will last forever. The whitish restorations in front teeth eventually wear away. Silver restorations tend to crack and chip with age because they contract and expand slightly when cold or hot food and drinks come in contact with them. Even gold restorations, the most permanent kind, are subject to decay around the edges, and the decay may spread underneath.

If a needed restoration is not made or a worn-out restoration is not replaced, a deep cavity may result. When the decay reaches the inner layer of the tooth—the dentin—temporary warning twinges of pain may occur. If the tooth still is not restored, the decay will spread into the pulp that fills the inner chamber of the tooth. A toothache can result from inflammation of the pulp, and although the pain may eventually subside, the pulp tissue dies and an abscess can form at the root of the tooth.

Dental Care During Pregnancy

It may be advisable for a pregnant woman to arrange for extra dental checkups. Many changes take place during pregnancy, among them increased hormone production. Some pregnant women develop gingivitis (inflammation of the gums) as an indirect consequence of hormonal changes. A checkup by the dentist during the first three months of pregnancy is needed to assess the oral effects of such changes, and to make sure all dental problems are examined and corrected. Pregnant women should take special care to brush and floss their teeth to minimize these problems.

Infection

To avoid the problem of toxic substances or poisons circulating in the mother's bloodstream, all sources of infection must be removed. Some of these sources can be in the mouth. An abscessed tooth, for example, may not be severe enough to signal its presence with pain, but because it is directly connected to the bloodstream it can send toxic substances and bacteria through the mother's body, with possible harmful effects to the embryo.

It is during pregnancy that tooth buds for both the deciduous and permanent teeth begin to form in the unborn child. If the mother neglects her diet or general health care during this period, the effects may be seen in the teeth of her child.

Maintaining Good Oral Hygiene

Fluoridation

Among general rules to follow between dental checkups are using fluorides, maintaining a proper diet, and removing debris from the teeth by brushing and by the use of dental floss. Fluorides are particularly important for strengthening the enamel of teeth in persons under the age of 15. Many communities add fluorides to the water supply, but if the substance is not available in the drinking water, the dentist can advise the patient about prescription fluoride rinses and treatments. Studies show that fluoride keeps teeth and gums healthy for older adults as well as for children and teenagers.

Dental sealants are also used in the prevention of tooth decay. The dentist brushes a plastic protective coating on the chewing surfaces of the back teeth, creating a barrier against food particles and bacteria. Since sealants can prevent up to 80 percent of all cavities, the American Dental Association recommends this treatment for all children.

Diet

Although a good diet for total health should provide all of the elements needed for dental health, several precautions on sugars and starches should be added. Hard or sticky sweets should be avoided. Such highly refined sweets as soft drinks, candies, cakes, cookies, pies, syrups, jams, jellies, and pastries should be limited, especially between meals. One's intake of starchy foods, such as bread, potatoes, and pastas, should also be controlled. Natural sugars contained in fresh fruits can provide sweet flavors with less risk of contributing to decay if the teeth are brushed regularly after eating such foods. Regular chewing gum may help remove food particles after eating, but it deposits sugar; if you chew gum, use sugarless gum.

Because decay is promoted each time sugars and other refined carbohydrates are eaten, between-meals snacks of sweets should be curtailed to lessen the chances of new or additional caries. Snack foods can be raw vegetables, such as carrots or celery, apples, cheese, peanuts, or other items that are not likely to introduce refined carbohydrates into the mouth between meals.

Brushing

Brushing the teeth is an essential of personal oral hygiene. Such brushing rids the mouth of most of the food debris that encourages bacterial growth. Brush with a fluoride toothpaste at least twice a day, more often if your dentist recommends it. A complete cleaning of brushing and flossing should take three to five minutes.

There is no one kind of toothbrush that is best for every person. Most dentists, however, recommend a brush with soft end-rounded or polished bristles. The size and shape of the brush should allow you to reach every tooth. Replace your toothbrush every three or four months, sooner if the bristles become worn, frayed or splayed. A hard, brittle brush can injure the gums. An interdental brush, a small brush tip at the end of a handle, is useful for cleaning between widely spaced teeth, between a tooth and an artificial crown or a bridge, or any tooth surface that is hard to reach.

Although several different methods may be used effectively, the following is the technique most often recommended. Brush the outside, inside, and chewing surfaces of the teeth with short, gentle strokes. Hold the brush with the bristle tips angled against the gum line at 45 degrees. Use a slight side-to-side motion. Brush the outside surface of each tooth before proceeding to the next tooth. Use the same technique on the inside surface of each tooth as well. For the hard-to-brush inside surfaces of the front teeth hold the handle of the brush in front of the mouth and apply the tip in an up-and-down motion. Next, carefully brush the chewing surfaces, or tops, of the back upper and lower teeth. Then brush the tongue to remove food particles and bacteria.

Some people prefer electric toothbrushes, which require less effort to use than ordinary toothbrushes. These are available with two basic motions—up and down and back and forth. Your dentist may advise which kind best serves an individual's needs and proper use of equipment. Some dentists point out that back-and-forth brushing applied with too much pressure can have an abrasive effect on tooth enamel because it works against the grain of the mineral deposits. The American Dental Association also evaluates electric toothbrushes and issues reports on the safety and effectiveness of various types.

Removing Debris with Dental Floss

Brushing often does not clean debris from between the teeth. But plaque and food particles that stick between the teeth usually can be removed with dental floss. A generous length of floss, about 18 inches, is needed to do an effective job. The ends can be wrapped several times around the first joint of the middle finger of each hand. Using the thumbs or index fingers, the floss is inserted between the teeth with a gentle, sawing, back-and-forth motion. Then it is slid gently around part of a tooth in the space at the gum line and gently pulled out; snapping the floss in and out may irritate the gums. After brushing and flossing, the mouth should be rinsed with water. A mouthwash is unnecessary, but it may be used for the good taste it leaves in the mouth.

The dentist may recommend the use of an oral irrigating device as part of dental home care. These units pro-

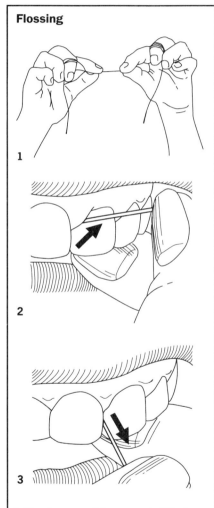

Flossing

1. Wrap floss several times around middle fingers and pull center section taut between thumbs or index fingers.
2. Insert floss between teeth and gently slide back and forth against every tooth. Work floss into the space between tooth and gumline.
3. To remove, pull floss gently downward along the angle of the tooth. Snapping it in and out may cause gum irritation.

duce a pulsating stream of water that flushes food debris from between teeth. They are particularly useful for patients wearing orthodontic braces or for those who have had recession of the gums, creating larger spaces between the teeth.

People who want to see the areas of plaque on their teeth can chew a *disclosing tablet,* available at most pharmacies, which leaves a harmless temporary stain on plaque surfaces. Some dentists recommend the use of disclosing tablets about once a week so that patients can check on the effectiveness of their tooth-cleaning techniques.

Dental Care in Emergencies

If a tooth is knocked out, you should immediately rinse the tooth gently in water to remove dirt or debris. Then place the tooth back in its socket. If reinsertion isn't possible, place the tooth in a cup of milk or water since it is important not to let the tooth dry

out. Then see a dentist or go to a hospital emergency room immediately. Studies show that if a tooth is placed back into its socket within 30 minutes of being knocked out, there is a 50 percent chance of saving the tooth.

If a tooth is pushed out of place (inward or outward) but not knocked out of its socket, gently clean any dirt or debris from the injured area with warm water. Push (but do not force) the tooth back into place and hold it in the socket with a moist tissue or gauze. Go to a dentist or emergency room immediately.

When you have a toothache, rinse your mouth thoroughly with warm water to clean out food particles. Use dental floss to remove any food that might be wedged between the teeth. Take an aspirin or other pain reliever to help dull the ache. An over-the-counter medication containing benzocaine can be applied to the tooth. See your dentist as soon as possible.

Tooth Decay

In addition to wear, tear, and injury, the major threat to the health of a tooth is tooth decay, or *caries.* Tooth decay and gum diseases are the leading causes of tooth loss. Tooth decay is caused by the bacteria that are normally present in the mouth and in the foods we eat. The bacteria digest the sugars and starches in the particles of food that remain in the mouth and begin to produce harmful acids within 20 minutes after eating. Although saliva and the actions of the tongue generally wash away some of the harmful material, decay will occur in places where bacteria and food particles accumulate and remain undisturbed.

The bacteria and acids build up in the mouth and become part of *plaque*, a sticky, transparent substance that forms a film over the surface of the teeth. Plaque forms on a continuous basis, which is the reason teeth must be flossed and brushed daily. Plaque can grow between the teeth and gums and irritate the soft tissues that support the teeth. The acids in plaque can eat through tooth enamel, creating a cavity. Plaque that is not removed combines with minerals in the saliva and hardens into a rough-textured substance called *tartar*, or *dental calculus*. Tartar can only be removed with a professional cleaning.

Other Causes of Decay

Bacterial acid is not the only way in which the tooth enamel may be damaged to permit the entry of decay bacteria. Certain high-acid foods and improper dental care can erode the molecules of enamel. Temperature extremes also can produce cracks and other damage to the enamel; some dental scientists have suggested that repeated exposure to rapid temperature fluctuations of 50° F, as in eating alternately hot and cold foods or beverages, can cause the enamel to develop cracks.

Complications of Tooth Decay

Tooth decay occurs gradually. It begins on the tooth's outer enamel surface where plaque has formed. The initial stage of tooth decay is usually painless and often goes unnoticed. Once decay activity breaks through the hard enamel surface, the bacteria can attack the dentin. Because the dentin is about 30 percent organic material, compared to 5 percent in the enamel layer, the decay process can advance more rapidly there. If the tooth decay is not stopped at the dentin layer, the disease organisms can enter the pulp chamber, which contains sensitive nerve endings. The decay can produce an acute inflammation, or abscess, which, if unchecked, can spread to adjoining teeth or other parts of the body. Osteomyelitis, an infection of the bone and bone marrow, and endocarditis, an inflammation of the lining of the heart, are among diseases in other parts of the body that can begin with untreated tooth decay.

Periodontal disease, described below, is another possible complication of tooth decay.

Treatment of Tooth Decay

The portion of a tooth invaded by decay is called a *cavity;* it may be compared to an ulcer that develops because of disease in soft tissues. In treating the decay process, the dentist tries to prevent further destruction of the tooth tissue. The dentist also tries to restore as much as possible the original shape and function of the diseased tooth. The procedure used depends on many factors, including the surfaces affected (enamel, dentin, etc.) and the tooth face and angle involved, as well as whether the cavity is on a smooth area or in a pit or fissure of the tooth surface.

The decayed portions of the tooth are removed with various kinds of carbide burrs and other drill tips, as well as with hand instruments. The dentist may also use a caries removal system that reduces or eliminates drilling. In this system two solutions are combined in one liquid and squirted in a pulsating stream onto the decayed area. The stream does not harm gums or healthy teeth; rather, it softens the caries so that it can easily be scraped away. Used, generally, in conjunction with rotary or hand instruments, the "squirt" system may make anesthesia unnecessary.

In other cases an anesthetic may be injected for the comfort of the patient. The dentist usually asks whether the patient prefers to have an anesthetic before work commences. In the cleaning process, an effort is made to remove all traces of diseased enamel or dentin, but no more of the tooth material than is necessary.

The cleaned cavity is generally filled in a layering procedure. The layers of liners and bases used before insertion of the filling are determined by the depth of the cavity and other factors. If pulp is exposed, special materials may be applied to help the pulp recover from the irritation of the procedure and to form a firm base for the amalgam, inlay, plastic resin, or other restorative substance that becomes the filling.

Tooth Extraction

When it becomes necessary to remove a diseased, damaged, or malpositioned tooth, the procedure is handled as a form of minor surgery, usually with administration of a local anesthetic to the nerves supplying the tooth area. However, there is no standard routine for extraction of a tooth, because of the numerous individual variations associated with each case. The dentist usually has a medical history of the patient available, showing such information as allergies to drugs, and medications used by the patient that might react with those employed in oral surgery. Because the mouth contains many millions of bacteria, all possible precautions are taken to prevent entry of the germs into the tooth socket.

The condition of the patient is checked during and immediately after tooth extraction, in the event that some complication develops. The patient is provided with analgesic (pain killing) and other needed medications, along with instructions regarding control of any postoperative pain or bleeding. The dentist also may offer special diet information with suggested meals for the recovery period, which usually is quite brief.

Root Canal Therapy

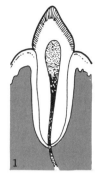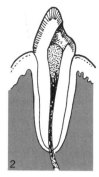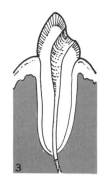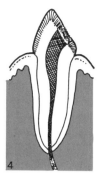

(1) The first step of root canal, or removal of the nerve of a tooth, begins with examining the infected pulp to determine its vitality. (2) The depth of the root is measured by X ray and, after administering local anesthetic, the dentist extracts the pulp with drill or hand instrument marked to indicate when the end of the root has been reached. (3) When the entire pulp and nerve have been removed the canal is sterilized to prevent infection. (4) After filling the tooth with silver or a tough plastic substance known as *gutta-percha*, or sometimes a combination of both, the dentist then caps the tooth.

Dry Socket

Severe pain may develop several days after a tooth has been extracted if a blood clot that forms in the socket becomes dislodged. The condition, commonly called *dry socket*, can involve infection of the alveolar bone that normally surrounds the roots of the tooth; loss of the clot can expose the bone tissue to the environment and organisms that produce *osteitis,* or inflammation of the bone tissue. Dry socket may be treated by irrigating the socket with warm salt water and packing it with strips of medicated gauze. The patient also is given analgesics, sedatives, and other medications as needed to control the pain and infection.

General anesthetics are sometimes necessary for complicated oral surgery. In such cases, there are available dental offices or clinics that are as well equipped and staffed as hospital operating rooms.

Endodontic Therapy

Tooth extraction because of caries is less common today than in previous years, although an estimated 25 million Americans have had all of their teeth removed. Modern preventive dentistry techniques of *endodontics* now make it possible to save many teeth that would have been extracted in past decades after the spread of decay into the pulp canal. The procedures include *root canal therapy, pulp capping,* and *pulpotomy.*

Root Canal Therapy

Once the tooth has fully developed in the jaw, the nerve is not needed, so if the pulp is infected, the nerve as well as the pulp can be removed. Only minor effects are noticeable in the tooth structure after the pulp is removed, and the dentist compensates for these in filling the tooth after root canal therapy.

Briefly, the procedure of root canal work begins by examination and testing of the pulp viability. The pulp may be tested by heat, cold, or an electrical device called a *vitalometer,* which measures the degree of sensation the patient feels in a tooth. If the pulp is dead, the patient will feel no sensation, even at the highest output of current.

After the degree of vitality in the pulp has been determined, a local anesthetic is injected and the dentist begins removing the pulp, using rotary drills and hand instruments. By means of X-ray pictures, the dentist measures the length of the root, which may be about one and a half times the length of the crown. Stops or other markers are placed on the root excavation tools to show the dentist when the instrument has reached the end of the root. The canal is then sterilized and filled with gutta-percha—a tough plastic substance—silver, or a combination of the two, and a cap is added.

Pulp Capping

Pulp capping consists of building a protective cover, or cap, over the exposed pulp with layers of calcium hydroxide paste, which is covered by zinc oxide and topped with a firm cement.

Pulpotomy

A pulpotomy procedure involves removal of the pulp in the pulp chamber within the crown of the tooth, while leaving the root canal pulp in place. The amputated pulp ends are treated and a pulp-capping procedure is used to restore the crown of the tooth.

Periodontal Disease

It is important in the middle years of life and later to continue good oral-hygiene habits and the practice of having regular dental checkups. Studies have found that after the age of 50 more than half the people in America have periodontal disease. At the age of 65, nearly everybody has this disease.

The Course of the Disease

Periodontal disease is an infection of the tissues surrounding and supporting the teeth. This includes the gums (gingiva), connective tissue (period-

Periodontal Disease

(1) If allowed to build up at the gumline, deposits of plaque and calculus result in damage to the gum tissues (periodontal disease). (2) As gums become increasingly irritated and inflamed, they may bleed easily and begin to recede from the tooth itself. (3) Untreated, the inflammation spreads to the roots of the teeth. Bacteria and particles of food lodge in the pockets between tooth and gums, aggravating the condition. (4) A tooth held by the diseased gum loses most of its bony support structure, causing it to loosen and move out of position. Eventually, such teeth may need to be extracted.

ontal ligament), and tooth sockets (alveolar bone). It is caused by plaque, a sticky, colorless film of bacteria that constantly forms on the teeth. If plaque isn't removed each day by brushing and flossing, it hardens and turns into tartar, or calculus. The toxins (poisons) produced by the bacteria in plaque and tartar irritate the gums.

Gingivitis, an inflammation of the gums, is the mildest form of periodontal disease. At first there is a slight redness and swelling of the gum tissue around one or more teeth. Later the redness and swelling become more pronounced and the gums tend to bleed easily. Bleeding that occurs during flossing or toothbrushing is one of the earliest signs of periodontal disease. Gingivitis is reversible with professional treatment and with good home oral care.

Periodontitis, also called *pyorrhea*, is an advanced stage of gum disease.

Symptoms include persistent bad breath; receding and shrinking gums; loose or separating teeth; a hypersensitivity to hot, cold, or sweet foods or beverages; and a change in the way your teeth fit together when you bite.

Periodontitis occurs when plaque and tartar extend below the gum line. The gums separate from the teeth, forming pockets that fill up with more plaque and bacteria. As the disease progresses, the bacteria weakens the bone supporting the teeth and the affected teeth begin to loosen and drift from their normal position. Finally, if the disease is left untreated, the teeth may be lost.

Another form of periodontal disease is an acute infection called *trench mouth*. It is also known as *necrotizing gingivitis* or *Vincent's infection*. The condition is very painful and is characterized by profuse bleeding at the slightest pressure or irritation. The affected areas become inflamed and develop blisters. A grayish-yellow membrane covers the infected areas and unpleasant breath odor is usually present. Other parts of the mouth, such as the insides of the cheeks and the tonsils, sometimes become infected. The disease was given the name trench mouth during World War I, when soldiers living in trenches contracted the disease. The infection is associated with poor oral hygiene and poor nutrition.

Causes

The accumulation of bacterial plaque and tartar between the gums and teeth is the chief cause of most periodontal diseases. If plaque is not removed daily by brushing and flossing, bacteria produce infections that destroy the supporting tissues around the teeth, including the bone.

Other factors can contribute to the development of gum disease. The hormonal changes that occur during puberty and pregnancy can make the gums more susceptible to bacterial infection. Poor nutrition and a diet rich in sugar-containing foods and beverages can increase the risk of gum disease. People who use tobacco products are more likely to get periodontal diseases and suffer from the more severe forms. Diseases such as leukemia or AIDS lower resistance to infection and can make gum disease more severe or harder to control.

Bruxism

Bruxism—the nervous habit, often unconsciously done, of clenching and grinding the teeth—can contribute to the development of periodontal disease. Bruxism frequently occurs during sleep.

Malocclusion

Another contributing cause to periodontal disease is repeated shock or undue pressure on a tooth because of *malocclusion,* or an improper bite. This effect accelerates damage to the tooth and gum structure during such simple activities as biting and chewing.

Treatment

Periodontal treatment may include a variety of techniques ranging from plaque removal to oral surgery. Early periodontal disease, when the beginnings of gum recession are seen, is treated by nonsurgical deep cleaning around the teeth below the gums. This procedure, called *scaling and root planing*, removes tartar and bacteria from tooth surfaces. As a result, the surfaces of the teeth become smoother both above and below the gum line, making it difficult for bacteria to attach themselves to the tooth.

In advanced periodontal disease dentists need to perform a surgical procedure, such as flap surgery or a gum tissue graft. Flap surgery involves pulling back gum tissue and cleaning both the infected side of the root and the bottom of the periodontal pocket. Then the flap is sutured back in place. Gum tissue grafts involve surgically removing a small piece of healthy gum tissue from the mouth, transferring it to receded gum tissue, and suturing it in place.

Guided tissue regeneration is another surgical treatment. It is a technique for regenerating periodontal ligament and bone. A mesh-like barrier is placed around the tooth root. The barrier keeps the gum tissue away from underlying ligaments and bone and leaves space for the ligaments and bones to grow.

After periodontal treatment, the patient should visit the dentist for a professional teeth cleaning every three or four months to maintain good oral health.

Dental Implants & Dentures

If it becomes necessary to have some teeth removed, they should be replaced as soon as possible with dental implants, a bridge, or partial or full dentures.

Why Missing Teeth Must Be Replaced

Most patients show some concern over the replacement of natural teeth with dentures, associating the loss of teeth with old age in the same way that others resist wearing eyeglasses or using a hearing aid. Millions of persons of all ages have improved their eating, speaking, and physical appearance by obtaining attractive and well-fitted dental implants or dentures.

Also, each tooth functions to hold the teeth opposite and on either side in place. Missing teeth would mean shifting teeth and a host of other problems. For example, food particles could lodge in the spaces created by the shifting teeth, followed by the formation of plaque and the development of periodontal disease, resulting in the loss of additional teeth.

Dental Implants

Dental implants, or *osseointegration,* are an effective alternative to ordinary dentures because they serve as substitutes for natural tooth roots that rely on the jawbone for support. Implants are capable of supporting dentures or replacing individual teeth or bridges.

Although physicians have been experimenting with dental implants for centuries, researchers only recently developed the most advanced version of the implant using titanium, whose primary advantage is that bone tissue actually fuses to it.

An implant consists of a small post

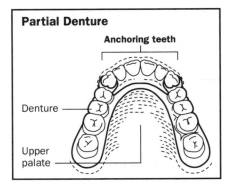

Partial Denture

Anchoring teeth

Denture

Upper palate

that protrudes from the gum tissue and is anchored either in the jaw bone (endosseous) or fitted directly over the jaw bone (subperiosteal). Prosthetic teeth are attached to the posts. These prosthetic teeth can be permanent or removable; cleaning and care depends upon the type.

Because it is a surgical procedure that can take up to three visits over a period of three to six months, most implant surgery occurs in two stages. First, the general dentist or oral surgeon implants the metal "roots" and then, in a second surgery, attaches the metal posts with the prosthetic teeth.

Not everyone is a candidate for implants. You must have healthy gums and an adequate amount of jawbone to secure the implant. You must be in general good health and not have a disease or condition, such as diabetes, that would interfere with the healing process after surgery. Meticulous oral hygiene is essential once you have an implant. Failing to brush, floss, and care properly for implants can lead to gum inflammation and bone loss. Consult with your dentist to determine if this procedure is compatible with your dental problems.

Fitting of Dentures

Modern techniques and materials of construction and the skill of modern dentists should assure well-fitting, natural-looking dentures. The dentist selects the tooth shade and shape that are best for an individual's face size, contours, and coloring. No one, however, has perfectly arranged, perfectly white natural teeth. Tooth coloring depends upon genetic factors and changes as one grows older.

Bridges and Partial Dentures

Several different types of dental appliances may be constructed to fill empty spaces. Some, such as dental bridges, may be cemented to the remaining natural teeth. Others, such as complete sets of dentures, are removable.

A bridge may be made entirely of gold, a combination of gold and porcelain, or combinations of gold and porcelain and other materials. If there is a sound natural tooth on either side of the space, an artificial tooth (or *pontic*) may be fused to the metal bridge. The crown retainer on either side of the pontic may then be cemented to crowns of the neighboring natural teeth.

If there are no natural teeth near the space created by an extracted tooth, a partial denture may be constructed to replace the missing teeth.

This appliance usually fastens by a clasp onto the last tooth on each side of the space. A bar on the inside of the front teeth provides stability for the partial denture. A "Maryland bridge," a fixed partial denture, eliminates the need for crowns to anchor false teeth.

A removable partial denture should be taken out and cleaned with special brushes whenever the natural teeth are brushed. Your dentist should check bridges and partial dentures periodically to make sure they have not become loosened. A loose clasp of a partial denture can rock the teeth to which the device is attached, causing damage and possible loss.

New materials have brought bonding into more common use as an alternative to crowning and for cosmetically restoring chipped, malformed, stained, or widely spaced teeth. In the bonding process the dentist applies first liquid plastic and then thin layers of tooth-colored materials known as composite resins and laminate veneers. The layers are sculpted and polished.

Complete Dentures

Before a full set of removable dentures is constructed, the dentist determines whether there are any abnormalities in the gum ridges, such as cysts or tooth root tips that may have to be removed. If the gums are in poor condition, treatments may be needed to improve the surfaces of the ridges on which the dentures will be fitted. The dentist may also have to reconstruct the bone underlying the gums—the alveolar ridge. Human bone "harvested" from another part of the patient's body was used in such reconstruction for decades but has been replaced by ceramic materials such as arehydroxylapatite and beta tricalcium phosphate.

The dentist now makes an impression of the patient's mouth. Tooth and shade choices are discussed. Several other appointments may be arranged before the new dentures are delivered to the patient, either for "try-ins" of dentures as they are being constructed or for adjustments after completion of the set.

Although dentures do not change with age, the mouth does. Therefore, it is necessary for the denture-wearer to have occasional check-ups during which the dentist examines oral tissues for irritation and determines how the dentures fit with respect to possible changing conditions of the mouth, and if a replacement should be recommended. The dentist also seeks to correct any irritations of the oral tissues of the mouth and polishes the dentures, making them smooth and easier to clean between check-ups.

Care of Dentures

Dentures should be cleaned daily with a denture brush and toothpaste; each night at bedtime dentures should be removed and soaked for seven or eight hours in a denture cleaner or in water. To avoid breaking them during the brushing process, fill a wash basin with water and place it under the dentures while they are being cleaned; if they are dropped, the dentures will be cushioned by the water. A harsh abrasive that could scratch the denture surface should not be used. Scratches allow stains to penetrate the surface of the dentures, creating permanent discoloration.

The use of adhesives and powders is only a temporary solution to ill-fitting dentures. In time, the dentist may rebuild the gum side of the denture to conform with the shape of the patient's gum ridge. The patient should never try to make his own changes in the fit of dentures. Rebuilding the gum side of the dentures, or relining, as it is called, usually begins with a soft temporary material if the patient's gums are in poor condition, and requires several appointments over a period of two or three weeks while the gum tissues are being restored to good health.

Orthodontics

Orthodontics is a term derived from the Greek words for straight, or normal, teeth. Straight teeth are easier to keep clean and they make chewing food more efficient. There also is a cosmetic benefit in being able to display a smile with a set of straight teeth, although many dentists consider the cosmetic aspect of orthodontics as secondary to achieving proper occlusion, or bite.

Causes of Improper Bite

Orthodontic problems can be caused by hereditary factors, by an infectious or other kind of disease, by the premature loss of primary teeth, by the medications used in treatment, or by individual factors such as injury or loss of permanent teeth. A person may have congenitally missing teeth resulting in spaces that permit drifting of neighboring teeth or collapse of the dental arch. Or he may develop extra (supernumerary) teeth resulting from an inherited factor. The supernumerary teeth may develop during the early years of life while the deciduous teeth are in use. A supernumerary tooth may force permanent teeth into unnatural positions.

Nutritional disorders can also affect the development of jaws and teeth, while certain medications can cause abnormal growth of gingival, or gum, tissues, resulting in increased spaces between the teeth.

Teeth that erupt too early or too late, primary teeth that are too late in falling out when permanent teeth have developed, and habits such as grinding of the teeth, thumb-sucking, or pushing the tongue against the teeth are among other factors that can result in *malocclusion,* or improper bite, and the need for orthodontic treatment.

Diagnosis of Orthodontic Problems

Each child should visit a dentist before the eruption of the permanent teeth for an examination that may determine the need for orthodontic treatment. Because there are many genetic and other influences that help shape the facial contours and occlusion of each individual, there are no standard orthodontic procedures that apply to all children. The dentist may recommend what treatment, if any, would be needed to produce normal occlusion and when it should begin; some dentists advise only that necessary procedures for correcting malocclusion be started before the permanent set of teeth (excluding wisdom teeth) has become established, or around the age of 12 or 13. However, there are few age limits for orthodontic care, and increasing numbers of adults are receiving treatment today for malocclusion problems that were neglected during childhood.

In the normal or ideal occlusion positions of the teeth, the first and second permanent upper molars fit just slightly behind the same molars of the lower jaw; all of the teeth of the upper jaw are in contact with their counterparts of the lower jaw. In this pattern of occlusion, all of the biting surfaces are aligned for optimum use of their intended functions of cutting, tearing, or grinding.

There are numerous variations of malocclusion, but generally, in simple deformities, the teeth of the upper jaw are in contact with lower jaw teeth once removed from normal positions. Other variations include an *open bite,* in which the upper and lower incisors do not contact each other, or *closed bite,* in which there is an abnormal degree of overlapping (*overbite*) of the front teeth.

Diagnosis is made with the help of X-ray pictures, photographs of the face and mouth, medical histories, and plaster models of the patient's teeth and jaws. The plaster models are particularly important because the dentist can use them to make experimental reconstructions without touching an actual tooth of a patient. For example, the dentist can remove one or more teeth from the plaster model and reorganize neighboring teeth in the jawbones to get an accurate representation of the effects of extracting teeth or forcing teeth into different developmental situations.

Orthodontic Appliances

Once a plan of orthodontic treatment has been determined by the dentist, he may choose from a dozen or more types of bands, braces, or other orthodontic appliances, some removable and some nonremovable, for shaping the teeth and jaws of the patient. A typical orthodontic appliance may include small curved strips or loops of metal, ceramic, or plastic cemented to the surfaces of the teeth as anchors for arch wires that pass around the dental arch. Springs and specially designed rubber bands, called elastics, are sometimes used to bring about alignment of the two jaws, or to align teeth within a dental arch.

In addition to the appliances that are attached to and between the upper and lower dental arches, the dentist may prescribe the use of an elastic tape device with a strap that fits around the back of the patient's neck and is attached also to the arch wire inside the mouth, thus providing a force from outside the mouth to bring teeth into alignment.

Orthodontic appliances are custom-designed and built for the individual patient. This requires several rather long sessions or one all-day session in the dental chair while the appliance is being organized and properly anchored. Thereafter, the patient must return at regular intervals spaced a few weeks to a month apart so the dentist can make adjustments in the appliance, determine if any of the bands have pulled away from tooth surfaces, and prevent plaque from

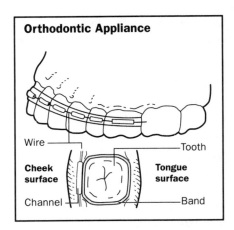

building up in places that the braces may make impervious to brushing.

The patient, meanwhile, must follow a diet that prohibits sticky foods or items that may damage the appliance or any of its parts. A conscientious program of oral hygiene, including regular cleaning by the dentist or hygienist, also is necessary because, as indicated above, it is more difficult to do a thorough job of cleaning the teeth when orthodontic appliances are in the mouth.

Orthodontics for Adults

Although orthodontic treatment originally was applied only to children, adults are undergoing treatment with increasing frequency to correct a variety of facial and dental disorders. Receding chins, buck teeth, sunken cheeks, sunken mouths, and other abnormalities have been treated successfully in adults beyond the age of 40. Orthodontists have observed that adult patients usually are more patient and cooperative during the long periods of treatment than youngsters.

The upper age limit for orthodontic work has not really been established, but doctors at the National Institute of Dental Research believe it is possible to treat adult patients with protrusion of the upper jaw and related disfigurements until the age of 70. This is possible because the upper jaw does not completely unite with the frontal bone of the skull, according to the experts, until after the

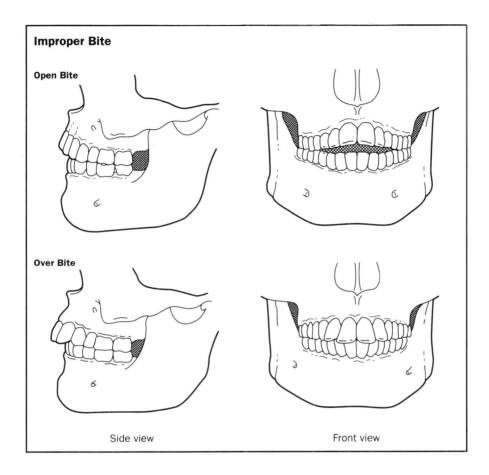

Improper Bite

Open Bite

Over Bite

Side view   Front view

age of 70 in most people.

Orthodontic treatments can be relatively expensive and involve many visits to a dentist's office over a long period of time. Any parent of a prospective patient or a responsible older patient seeking orthodontic work for himself should have a frank discussion with the dentist regarding the time and money to be invested in the corrective procedures before making an agreement to begin the work. In nearly every case some arrangement can be made for covering the costs of dental work that is vital to the health and welfare of a patient.

TMD: Temporomandibular Disorder

T he temporomandibular joints connect both sides of the lower jaw (mandible) to the temporal bone of the skull. Ligaments, tendons, and muscles attached to and surrounding the joints control the up-and-down and side-to-side movement of the jaw. Temporomandibular (jaw) disorders, formerly called temporomandibular joint (TMJ) syndrome, include problems with the jaw joints and the muscles that control chewing and talking.

TMD symptoms include pain or tenderness in the jaw muscles; pain that radiates to the face, neck, or shoulders; clicking, popping, or grating noises in a jaw joint when opening or closing the mouth; locking or limited movement of the jaw. There is typically no single cause of temporomandibular disorders. A severe injury to the jaw or dislocation of the jaw joint can cause TMD. Some experts believe that anxiety and stress can lead to *bruxism* (the clenching and grinding of teeth at night), which can cause muscle spasms and pain. Malocclusion (an improper bite) and arthritis in a jaw joint may contribute to TMD.

TMD symptoms should be evaluated by a dentist or physician. In most cases the problems causing TMD pain are temporary and simple treatment is all that is needed to relieve discomfort. Simple remedies a dentist may suggest include eating soft, nonchewy foods; avoiding extreme jaw movements, such as wide yawning and gum chewing; applying hot or cold compresses to the chewing muscles along the sides of the face; and taking aspirin or other anti-inflammatory medication.

The dentist may prescribe a mouth guard that is worn over the teeth while sleeping. The guard can reduce bruxism and ease muscle tension and joint stress. Other conservative treatments include biofeedback and relaxation therapies, muscle-relaxant medications, and physical therapy. Surgery and other permanent changes to the mouth or jaw are usually not necessary and may make TMD discomfort worse.

23

Aches, Pains, Nuisances, Worries

And Other Things You Can Live With But Could Get Along Very Well Without

None of the variety of discomforts discussed in this chapter is a laughing matter. The best thing about most of them is that they will pass, given your commonsense attention, or will disappear if you follow your physician's advice. This includes taking the medications prescribed by your physician exactly as directed. In a few cases, such as allergies or gout, long-term drug therapy may be necessary on a self-supervised basis, once treatment has been established by a physician. Of course, when symptoms of any kind persist or get worse, you should waste no time in seeking a professional diagnosis.

There may be somebody, somewhere, who has never felt rotten a day in his life. But most of us are not so fortunate. Among the most common nuisance ailments are:

- upper respiratory infections
- allergies
- occasional headaches
- backaches
- weight problems
- weather discomforts
- disturbances of normal sleep patterns
- aching feet
- indigestion

The unpleasant feeling associated with any of these common disorders can almost always be banished with a modicum of care and thought. For example, allergic reactions to particular foods can be curtailed by identifying the offending food and avoiding it.

Self-diagnosis and self-discipline can often enable one to cope with weight problems. A backache may be cured by attention to posture, or adjusting your office chair. A sensible approach to clothing and exposure can often do away with weather discomforts.

For many minor disorders and discomforts, particularly those caused by stress, massage may be the answer. Massage is a process that is at least 3,000 years old and has been used to help relieve tension, increase muscle tone, improve blood and oxygen circulation, and aid major body functions. Massage has also helped alleviate aches and pains resulting from exercise, improve posture, and increase joint flexibility. Among the disorders for which massage should not be used are osteoporosis, varicose veins, inflamed joints, herniated discs, tumors, and some cardiovascular problems.

Massage invariably involves kneading, manipulation, and methodical pressure on various body parts. The process should never be painful. The three kinds of massage in most common use are Swedish, a pleasant, muscle-kneading procedure; Shiatsu, or "acupressure," which depends on finger and hand pressure on so-called energy meridians in the body; and reflexology, a system that calls for pressure on various points of the foot.

When symptoms do not respond to self-help—as when sporadic difficulty in sleeping burgeons into a string of near-sleepless nights, or when abdominal pain you interpret as indigestion is intense or frequent in spite of avoiding rich or heavy foods, it's time to see a physician.

The Common Cold and Upper Respiratory Infections

Common cold is the label attached to a group of symptoms that can be caused by one or more of some 20 different viruses. Colds are considered highly contagious, but some physicians think that people don't entirely catch others' colds—in a sense they catch their own. While the viruses that carry the infection are airborne and practically omnipresent, somebody in good health is usually less susceptible to a cold than someone who is run down. Both environmental factors (such as air pollution) and emotional ones (such as anxiety or depression) seem to increase susceptibility.

Symptoms

Symptoms differ from person to person and from cold to cold with the same person. Generally, a cold starts with sneezes, a running nose, teary eyes, and a stuffed head. Sometimes the nasal membranes become so swollen that a person can breathe only through the mouth; sometimes the senses of smell and taste simply disappear. The throat may be sore; a postnasal drip may cause a constant cough when the person is lying down at night.

When these symptoms are acute and are accompanied by fever and aching joints, the illness is usually referred to as influenza or "the flu." There are many different viruses that cause influenza, and new ones are always turning up. Unfortunately, there is as yet no medicine that can cure either a cold or a flu attack, although many people do get relief from symptoms by taking various cold remedies. Antibiotics are sometimes prescribed by doctors to prevent more serious bacterial diseases, such as pneumonia, from developing, but antibiotics are not effective against the cold viruses.

Treatment

Some people can get away with treating a cold with contempt and an occasional aspirin, and go about their business. Others are laid low for a few days. If you are the type who is really hit hard by a cold, it isn't coddling yourself to stay home for a couple of days. In any event, a simple cold usually runs its course, lasting anywhere from a few days to two weeks.

Discomfort can be minimized and recovery speeded by a few simple steps: extra rest and sleep, drinking more liquids than usual, and taking aspirin as needed. Sucking on zinc gluconate lozenges within 24 hours of the first sign of a cold may help lessen the duration of a cold, although this has not been proven definitively. Antihistamine preparations or nose drops should be avoided unless specifically prescribed by a physician.

A painful sore throat accompanied by fever, earache, a dry, hacking cough, or pains in the chest are symptoms that should be brought to the attention of a physician.

Prevention

A person typically becomes infected with a cold by touching his or her eyes or nose after touching a surface—or another person's hand—that is contaminated with the cold virus. Since cold viruses can live for hours on hands and surfaces, one of the most effective defenses against catching a cold is to avoid touching your face and to wash your hands frequently, particularly after being in public places, before and after using the bathroom, and after blowing your nose. Taking large doses of vitamin C, a practice favored by some people, is of little help in preventing or curing colds.

Inoculation against particular types of viruses is recommended by many physicians in special cases: for pregnant women, for the elderly, and for those people who have certain chronic heart and lung diseases. Flu shots are effective against a particular virus or viruses for a limited period.

Allergies

Discomforts of various kinds are considered allergies when they are brought on by substances or conditions that ordinarily are harmless. Not too long ago, perturbed allergy sufferers would say things like:

"I can't use that soap because it gives me hives."

"Smelling roses makes me sneeze."

Nowadays, such complaints are commonly recognized as indications of allergies.

Symptoms

Allergic symptoms can range from itching eyes, running nose, coughing, difficulty in breathing, welts on the skin, nausea, cramps, and even going into a state of shock, depending upon the severity of the allergic individual's response. Almost any part or system of the body may be affected, and almost anything can pose an allergic threat to somebody.

Allergens

Substances that trigger an allergic reaction are called *allergens.* The system of an allergic individual reacts to such substances as if they were germs, producing *antibodies* whose job it is to neutralize the allergens. But the body's defense mechanism overreacts: in the process of fighting off the effects of the allergens, various chemicals, particularly *histamines,* are dumped indiscriminately into the bloodstream. It is the over-abundance of these "good" chemicals that causes the discomforts associated with allergies.

Allergens are usually placed in the following categories:

- Those that affect the respiratory tract, or *inhalants,* such as pollens, dust, smoke, perfumes, and various airborne, malodorous chemicals. These bring on sneezing, coughing, and breathing impairment.

- Food substances that affect the digestive system, typically eggs, seafood, nuts, berries, chocolate, and pork. These may cause not only nausea and diarrhea but also hives and other skin rashes.

- Medicines and drugs, such as penicillin, or a particular serum used in inoculations.

- Agents that act on the skin and mucous membranes, such as insecticides, poison oak, and poison ivy, particular chemical dyes, cosmetics, soaps, metals, leathers, and furs.

- Environmental agents, such as sunlight or excessive cold.

- Microbes, such as particular bacteria, viruses, and parasites.

Treatment

In general, approaches to treatment for allergies fall into three categories:

removing or avoiding as many allergens from the environment as possible; using creams, inhalers, pills, and other medications to control the symptoms; and undergoing immunotherapy (allergy shots) to reduce the allergic response. The type of treatment selected often depends on test findings that indicate what is causing the allergic reaction; the tests may produce such identification quickly or they may have to be continued for weeks or months before the allergen is finally tracked down.

As soon as the source of the allergen is identified, the obvious course is to avoid it, if possible. Avoidance may not, however, be possible. Few persons can avoid breathing pollen in the spring and fall. Giving up a house pet may be almost as difficult, but may be necessary as a health or comfort measure.

New medications that control the symptoms of allergies have been marketed in recent years. Newer antihistamines, for example, relieve allergic reactions but do not cause the drowsiness associated with earlier medications. Other medicines that have been used to treat allergies include adrenaline, ephedrine, and cortisone. Aerosol drugs may be used to attack specific symptoms. Some, for example, may be inhaled to treat the linings of the nose and throat.

In addition to histamines, other body chemicals are released during an allergy "attack." Researchers have found that these chemicals include leukotrienes. Consequently, antileukotrienes have tested as medications.

Direct or specific immunotherapy constitutes the third approach to treatment of allergy. The shots are effective in reducing allergic responses. A person with a substance allergy receives increasing amounts of the substance over a period of years. For example, a person who is allergic to insect stings receives injections of the particular insect's venom.

A life-threatening allergic reaction calls for emergency treatment, usually with adrenalin. Physicians suggest that persons with very intense food allergies or who are allergic to insect stings should carry special kits that include an adrenalin-filled syringe. The allergy victims administer the medication to themselves in case of *anaphylaxis* — an acute, life-threatening response (see "Allergic Shock" in Ch. 31, *Medical Emergencies*).

Persons subject to severe, disabling allergy attacks by a known allergen should also carry a card describing both the allergen and the allergic reactions. Detailed information on the latest developments in allergy treatment is available from the Asthma and Allergy Foundation of America, 1125 15th St. NW, Suite 502, Washington, DC 20005. See also Ch. 24, *Allergies and Hypersensitivities*.

Headaches

The common headache is probably as ancient as primitive man. The headache, a pain or ache across the forehead or within the head, may be severe or mild in character, and can last anywhere from under half an hour to three or four days. It may be accompanied by dizziness, nausea, nasal stuffiness, or difficulty in seeing or hearing. It is not a disease or illness but a symptom.

Causes

Headaches in today's modern world can arise from any of a number of underlying causes. These include excessive drinking or smoking, lack of sleep, hunger, drug abuse, and eyestrain. Eyestrain commonly results from overuse of the eyes, particularly under glaring light, or from failure to correct defective vision.

Treatments for headaches are as varied as the causes of headaches. Diagnosis may take some time, but if you suffer from severe or chronic headaches, it is important to consult your doctor. Headaches may point to an underlying problem, such as high blood pressure.

Headaches that are non-debilitating may be treated with analgesics such as aspirin or ibuprofen. Debilitating headaches such as tension, migraine, or cluster headaches can be treated with prescription drugs if your doctor advises it.

Chronic headaches should be diagnosed so the sufferer does not have to always depend on medication to treat the problem. Long-term solutions may include meditation, relaxation exercises, and exercise to reduce tension and stress. Dietary changes such as eliminating chocolate, caffeine, cheese, alcohol, sugar, or other products may also help.

Migraine

Migraine, also called *sick headache,* is a particularly severe, intense kind of headache. An attack may last several days and necessitate bed rest. Dizziness, sensitivity to light, and chills may accompany a migraine headache.

The exact cause of migraine is unknown, but researchers suspect a hereditary link, since the majority of migraine patients have one or more close relatives with migraine.

Migraine headaches can occur from changes in body hormone balances, sudden body temperature changes, bright light or noise, shifts in barometric pressure, and alcohol and drug use. It may also be caused by a combination of these triggers.

For chronic migraine sufferers, keeping a daily journal of food consumed, activities done, emotional status, and (for women) menstrual cycles, may help provide an indication of why migraines occur.

Migraines can be avoided by eliminating any apparent triggers. The fluctuation in estrogen is believed to be a major cause of migraines. Some foods only bring on headaches during certain times of the menstrual cycle. Hormone replacement therapy, some types of birth control pills, and menopause may increase incidence of migraines, although menopause may also end migraines

in women who had them for years.

Tension Headaches

Tension headaches are characterized by a painful pressure in the head. Such headaches can be caused by stress, depression, or poor posture and should be treated with analgesics such as aspirin and ibuprofen, a mas- sage or a cold shower. Tension head- aches can occur at any time; you can even wake up with one. The best long-term treatment is learning to re- duce or manage the stress in your life.

Cluster Headaches

Cluster headaches cause pain around a specific area of the head, and eye tearing, nasal stuffiness, and a burn- ing sensation on the side of the head affected. The headaches usually last only a few hours but are usually de- scribed as excruciating. These head- aches usually occur after a person has fallen asleep and typically affect men and heavy smokers. Since the pain is resistant to over-the-counter medi- cine, cluster headaches can be treat- ed with corticosteroids, such as predni- sone, or inhaling 100 percent oxygen.

Backaches

"Oh, my aching back" is probably the most common complaint among peo- ple past the age of 40. Most of the time, the discomfort—wherever it occurs, up or down the backbone— can be traced to some simple cause. However, there are continuous back- aches that have their origin in some internal disorder that needs the atten- tion of a physician. Among the more serious causes are kidney or pancreas disease, spinal arthritis, and peptic ul- cer.

Some Common Causes

Generally a backache is the result of strain on the muscles, nerves, or lig- aments of the spine. It can occur be- cause of poor posture, carelessness in lifting or carrying heavy packages, sitting in one position for a long time in the wrong kind of chair, or sleeping on a mattress that is too soft. Back- ache often accompanies menstrua- tion, and is common in the later stages of pregnancy. Emotional ten- sion can also bring on back pain.

Prevention

In general, maintaining good posture during the waking hours and sleeping on a hard mattress at night—if neces- sary, inserting a bed board between the mattress and bedsprings—are the first line of defense against back- aches. Anyone habitually carrying heavy loads of books or groceries, or even an overloaded attaché case, should make a habit of shifting the weight from arm to arm so that the spine doesn't always get pulled in one direction. Workers who are sedentary for most of the day at a desk or factory table should be sure that the chair they sit in provides firm support for back muscles and is the right height for the working surface.

Treatment

Most cases of simple backache respond to rest, aspirin, and the application of heat, applied by a hot water bottle or heating pad. In cases where the pain persists or becomes more acute, a physician should be consulted. He may find that the trouble is caused by the malfunctioning of an internal organ, or by pressure on the sciatic nerve (*sciatica*). With X rays he may also locate a slipped disk or other abnormality in the alignment of the vertebrae of the spine. See "Back Pain and Its Causes" in Ch. 7, *Diseases of the Skeletal System.*

Weight Problems

A few people can maintain the weight that is right for their body build without ever having to think about it. However, most experts believe that just about half the people in the United States may be risking shorter lives because they are too heavy. By one estimate, approximately one out of five American men and one out of four American women are 10 percent or more overweight, a group that may be called the borderline obese.

There is no longer any reasonable doubt that, if you are overweight, you have statistically a greater chance of high blood pressure, diabetes, and *atherosclerosis* (lumpy deposits in the arteries). And because atherosclerotic heart disease alone accounts for 20 percent of deaths among adults in the United States, it is understandable why physicians consider weight truly a national problem.

Causes

In practically all cases, weighing too much is the result of eating too much and exercising too little. In many cases, the food eaten is of the wrong kind and leisure time is used for riding around in a car rather than walking, or for watching television rather than playing tennis.

Many people like to think that they weigh too much only because they happen to like good food; but the real explanations may be considerably more complicated. In some cases, overeating has been found to have emotional sources: feelings of inadequacy; the need to compensate for a lack of affection or approval, or an unconscious desire to ward off the attention of the opposite sex. Psychological weight problems of this kind can be helped by consulting a psychiatrist or psychologist.

Treatment

There are many overweight people who merely need the support and encouragement that come from participating in a group effort, and for them, joining one of the various weight-control organizations can be extremely beneficial in taking off extra pounds and keeping them off.

Permanent results are rarely achieved by crash diets, faddish food combinations, or reducing pills. Not only are such solutions usually temporary; they may actually be harmful. See "Weight" in Ch. 27, *Nutrition and Weight Control,* for further information about weight problems.

Weather Discomforts

Using good sense about clothing, exercise, and proper diet is probably our best protection against the discomforts caused by extremes of temperature. Sometimes circumstances make this exercise of good sense impossible, with unpleasant but rarely serious results, if treatment is promptly administered. Following are some of the more common disorders resulting from prolonged exposure to excessive heat or cold, and what you can do to alleviate them.

Heat Cramps

In a very hot environment, a person may drink great quantities of water while "sweating buckets" of salty perspiration. Thus, the body's water is replaced, but its salt is not. This salt–water imbalance results in a feeling of faintness and dizziness accompanied by acute stomach cramps and muscle pains in the legs. When the symptoms are comparatively mild, they can be relieved by taking coated salt tablets in five-to-ten-grain doses with a full glass of tepid or cool—not iced—water. Salt tablets along with plenty of fluids should be taken regularly as a preventive measure by people who sweat a great deal during hot weather.

Sunburn

If you have not yet been exposed to much sun, as at the beginning of summer, limit your exposure at first to a period of 15 to 20 minutes, and avoid the sun at the hours around midday even if the sky is overcast. Remember, too, that the reflection of the sun's rays from water and beach sand intensifies their effect. Some suntan lotions give effective protection against burning, and some creams even prevent tanning; but remember to cover all areas of exposed skin and to reapply the lotion when it's been washed away after a swim.

Treatment

A sunburn is treated like any other burn, depending upon its severity. See "Burns" in Ch. 31, *Medical Emergencies*. If there is blistering, take care to avoid infection. Extensive blistering requires a physician's attention.

Heat Exhaustion

This condition is different from heatstroke or sunstroke, discussed below. Heat exhaustion sets in when large quantities of blood accumulate in the skin as the body's way of increasing its cooling mechanism during exposure to high temperatures. This in turn lowers the amount of blood circulating through the heart and decreases the blood supply to the brain. If severe enough, fainting may result. Other symptoms of heat exhaustion include unusual pallor and profuse cold perspiration. The pulse may be weak, and breathing shallow.

Treatment

A person suspected of having heat exhaustion should be placed in a reclining position, his clothing loosened or removed, and his body cooled with moist cloths applied to his forehead and wrists. If he doesn't recover promptly from a fainting spell, smelling salts can be held under his nose to revive him. As soon as he is conscious, he can be given salt tablets and a cool sugary drink—either tea or coffee—to act as a stimulant. Don't give the patient any alcoholic beverages.

Sunstroke or Heatstroke

Sunstroke is much more of an emergency than heat exhaustion and requires immediate attention. The characteristic symptom is extremely high body temperature brought on by cessation of perspiration. If hot, dry, flushed skin turns ashen gray, a physician must be called immediately. Too much physical activity during periods of high temperature and high humidity is a direct contributing cause.

Treatment

See "Heatstroke" in Ch. 31, *Medical Emergencies,* for a description of the emergency treatment recommended for this condition.

Chapped Skin

One of the most widespread discomforts of cold weather is *chapped skin.* In low temperatures, the skin's sebaceous glands produce fewer oils that lubricate and protect the skin, causing it to become dry. Continued exposure results in reddening and cracking. In this condition, the skin is especially sensitive to strong soaps.

Treatment

During cold, dry weather, less soap should be used when washing, a bath oil should be used when bathing, and a mild lotion or creme should be applied to protect the skin from the damaging effects of wind and cold. A night cream or lotion containing lanolin is also helpful, and the use of cleansing cream or oil instead of soap can reduce additional discomfort when cleansing chapped areas. The use of a colorless lip pomade is especially recommended for children when they play out of doors in cold, dry weather for any length of time.

Chilblain

A *chilblain* is a local inflammation of the skin brought on by exposure to cold. The condition commonly affects people overly sensitive to cold because of poor circulation. When the hands, feet, face, and ears are affected, the skin in these areas itches and burns, and may swell and turn reddish blue.

Treatment

The best way to avoid chilblains is to wear appropriate clothing during cold weather, especially warm socks, gloves, and ear coverings. The use of bed socks and a heating pad at night is also advisable. Once indoors, cold, wet feet should be dried promptly, gently, and thoroughly. Rubbing or massaging should be avoided, because these can cause further irritation. People who suffer from repeated attacks of chilblains should consult a physician for diagnosis of circulatory problems.

Frostbite

Frostbite is a considerably more serious condition than chilblains, because it means that a part or parts of the body have actually been frozen. The fingers or toes, the nose, and the ears are most vulnerable. If frostbitten, these areas turn numb and pale and feel cold when touched. The dangerous thing about frostbite is that pain may not be a warning. If the condition is not treated promptly, the temperature inside the tissues keeps going down and eventually cuts off blood circulation to the overexposed parts of the body. In such extreme cases, there is a possible danger of gangrene.

Treatment

In mild cases, prompt treatment can slowly restore blood circulation. The frozen parts should be rewarmed *slowly* by covering them with warm clothing or by soaking them in lukewarm water. Nothing hot should be applied—neither hot water nor a heating pad. Nor should the patient be placed too close to a fireplace or radiator. Because the affected tissues can be easily bruised, they should not be massaged or rubbed. If you are in doubt about restoring circulation, a physician should be called promptly or the patient taken to a hospital for emergency treatment.

Sleep and the Lack of It

Until rather recently, it was assumed that sleep was the time when the body rested and recovered from the activities of wakefulness. Although there is still a great deal to learn about why we sleep and what happens when we are sleeping, medical researchers have now identified several different phases of sleep, all of them necessary over the long run, but some more crucial than others.

How much sleep a person needs varies a great deal from individual to individual; and the same individual may need more or less at different times. Children need long periods of unbroken sleep; the elderly seem to get along on very little. No matter what a person's age, too little sleep over too long a time leads to irritability, exhaustion, and giddiness.

Insomnia

Almost everybody has gone through periods when it is difficult or impossible to fall asleep. Excitement before bedtime, temporary worries about a pressing problem, spending a night in an unfamiliar place, changing to a different bed, illness, physical discomfort because of extremes of temperature—any of these circumstances can interfere with normal sleep patterns.

But this is quite different from *chronic insomnia,* when a person consistently has trouble falling asleep for no apparent reason. If despite all your commonsense approaches insomnia persists, a physician should be consulted about the advisability of taking a tranquilizer or a sleeping pill. Barbiturates should not be taken unless prescribed by a physician.

The Vulnerable Extremities

Aches and pains in the legs and feet occur for a wide variety of reasons, some trivial and easily corrected, others serious enough to require medical attention. Those that originate in such conditions as arthritis and rheumatism can often be alleviated by aspirin or some of the newer prescription medications.

Gout

Gout, which is usually a metabolic disorder, is a condition that especially affects the joint of the big toe, and sometimes the ankle joint, causing the area to become swollen, hot, and acutely painful. Although the specific cause of gout is not yet clearly understood, the symptoms can be alleviated by special medication prescribed by a physician. An attack of gout can be triggered by a wide variety of causes: wearing the wrong shoes, eating a diet too rich in fats, getting a bad chill, surgery in some other part of the body, or chronic emotional anxiety, as well as the use of certain medicines, such as diuretics ("waterpills"). See also "Gout" in Ch. 7, *Diseases of the Skeletal System.*

Fallen Arches

Fallen arches can cause considerable discomfort because the body's weight is carried on the ligaments of the inside of the foot rather than on the sole. When the abnormality is corrected by orthopedic shoes with built-in arches for proper support, the pressure on the ligaments is relieved. A physician rather than a shoe salesman should be consulted for a reliable diagnosis. In some cases, the physician may also recommend special exercises to strengthen the arch.

Flat Feet

Flat feet can usually be revealed by a simple test—making a footprint on level earth or hard-packed sand. If the print is solid rather than indented by a curve along the big-toe side of the foot, the foot is flat. Aching ligaments in the area of the instep are often a result, but can be relieved by proper arch supports inside the shoes. Corrective arch supports are particularly important for young children, for anyone who is overweight, and for anyone who has to stand a great deal of the time.

Blisters

Although blisters are sometimes a sign of allergy, fungus infection, or sunburn, they most commonly appear on the feet because of the friction of a shoe or of hosiery that does not fit properly. A *water blister* is a collection of lymph that forms inside the upper level of the skin; a *blood blister* goes down deeper and contains some blood released from broken capillaries. A normal amount of walking in shoes and hosiery that fit comfortably—neither too loose nor too tight—rarely results in blisters. When blisters do appear, it is best to protect them from further friction by the use of a sterile bandage strip.

Treatment

A blister that causes acute pain when one is walking can be treated as follows: after cleaning the area with soap and water, pat it dry and swab it with rubbing alcohol. Sterilize the tip of a needle in a flame, let it cool a little, and then puncture the edge of the blister, absorbing the liquid with a sterile gauze. The loose skin can be removed with manicure scissors that have been sterilized by boiling for ten minutes. The surface of raw skin should then be covered with an adhesive bandage. This procedure is best done before bedtime so that healing can begin before shoes are worn again.

If redness appears around the area of any blister and inflammation appears to be spreading, a physician should be consulted promptly.

Bunions

A *bunion* is a deformation in the part of the foot that is joined by the big toe. The swelling and pain at the joint is caused by inflammation of the *bursa* (a fluid-filled sac) that lubricates the joint. Although bunions often develop because of wearing shoes that don't fit correctly, they most frequently accompany flat feet. Pain that is not too severe can be relieved by the application of heat; the condition may eventually be cured by doing foot exercises recommended by a physician, who will also help in the choice of correct footwear. A bunion that causes acute pain and difficulty in walking can be treated by a simple surgical procedure.

Calluses

A *callus* is an area of the skin that has become hard and thick as a result of constant friction or pressure against it. Pain results when the callus is pressed against a nerve by poorly fitting shoes. A painful callus can be partially removed by rubbing it—very cautiously—with a sandpaper file or a pumice stone sold for that purpose. The offending shoes should then be discarded for correctly fitted ones. Foot care by a podiatrist is recommended for anyone with recurring calluses and corns (see below), and especially for those people who have diabetes or any disorder of the arteries.

Corns

A *corn* is a form of callus that occurs on or between the toes. When the thickening occurs on the outside of the toe, it is called a *hard corn;* when it is located between the toes, it is called a *soft corn.* The pain in the affected area is caused by pressure of the hard inside core of the corn against the tissue beneath it. The most effective treatment for corns is to wear shoes that are the right size and fit. Corns can be removed by a podiatrist, but unless footwear fits properly, they are likely to return.

Treatment

To remove a corn at home, the toes should be soaked in warm water for about ten minutes and dried. The corn can be rubbed away with an emery file, or it can be treated with a few drops of 10 percent salicylic acid in collodion, available from any druggist. Care should be exercised in applying the solution so that it doesn't reach surrounding tissue; it is highly irritating to normal skin. The area can then be covered with a corn pad to relieve pressure. This treatment may have to be repeated several times before the corn becomes soft enough to lift out. Diabetics or those suffering from any circulatory disorder should never treat their own corns.

Bursitis

Bursitis is a pain and swelling in a joint caused when the bursa, a sac-like cushion between the bones and tendons, becomes worn or torn from constant use.

Forms of bursitis include: housemaid's knee, characterized by a swollen kneecap that has become inflamed by injury or constant pressure; bunions, where the joint of the big toe is swollen and inflamed by poorly fitting shoes; and weaver's bottom, where the bursa around the pelvic girdle become damaged from long periods of sitting on hard surfaces.

Bursitis can be treated by resting the inflamed joint, applying heat, taking an anti-inflammatory drug, such as aspirin or ibuprofen, or getting a corticosteroid injection or antibiotic therapy. For chronic bursitis, surgery may be required, and physical therapy to repair the joint may follow treatment.

Tendinitis

Tendinitis is inflammation of a tendon, and tenosynovitis is inflammation of the tendon sheath from injury. These problems tend to occur together. The tendon becomes injured by excessive or unusual use, such as a weekend athlete might experience, or from extreme strain on the tendon by overexertion in lifting, carrying, or moving something heavy. The tendon may also be injured by repetitive movement. The areas most susceptible to tendon injuries are the shoulder, hips, hamstrings, ankles, and heels.

Tendinitis can be treated with aspirin or ibuprofen, corticosteroid injections, elevating the injured limb and applying ice, and using a sling. Tendinitis can be avoided by doing warm-up exercises before engaging in an athletic activity, and by not overexerting.

If the pain is persistent, you should seek professional medical advice. Because rest and then gradually increased exercise of the injured area is required, your doctor will have to help you develop a plan for recovery.

Carpal tunnel syndrome

Carpal tunnel syndrome is caused when a median nerve, which provides feeling in the wrist, thumb and fingers, is compressed and becomes swollen and inflamed. The result is a painful stiffness of the hand, wrist, or fingers. The pain also can reach an arm or shoulder.

The debilitating condition is caused by repetitive motion caused by overusing the wrist. It typically affects people who type, such as secretaries and reporters, and is common among carpenters, meat cutters, gymnasts, and supermarket checkers. Water retention and weight gain in pregnant women often causes them to develop carpal tunnel syndrome which disappears after the baby is born.

Treatments include halting the activity that caused the syndrome, performing the activity differently, and using a splint to keep the wrist from bending while it heals. Anti-inflammatory drugs are also used. In severe cases, a carpal tunnel sufferer may be injected with corticosteroid drugs or undergo surgery to cut the bandlike ligament that is pressing on the median nerve.

Unnecessary delays in treating carpal tunnel may cause loss of function, although the condition need not reach such a stage.

The Exposed Integument

Common skin and scalp annoyances such as rashes, itches, dandruff, excessive perspiration, and infections of various kinds (such as athlete's foot and ringworm), as well as acne, wrinkles, and baldness, are discussed in Ch. 21, *Skin and Hair.*

Splinters

If lodged superficially in the hand, a splinter will usually work its own way out, but a splinter of no matter what size in the sole of the foot must be removed promptly to avoid its becoming further embedded by pressure and causing infection. The simplest method of removal is to pass a needle through a flame; let the needle cool; then, after the skin surface has been washed with soap and water or swabbed with alcohol, press the point of the needle against the skin, scraping slightly until the tail of the splinter is visible and loosened. It can then be pulled out with tweezers that have been sterilized in boiling water or alcohol.

Hangnails

Hangnails are pieces of partly living skin torn from the base or side of the fingernail, thus opening a portion of the underskin to infection. A hangnail can cause considerable discomfort. It should not be pulled or bitten off; but the major part of it can be cut away with manicuring scissors. The painful and exposed area should then be washed with soap and water and covered with a sterile adhesive bandage. Hangnails are likely to occur when the skin is dry. They can therefore be prevented by the regular use of a hand cream or lotion containing lanolin.

"Normal" Disorders of the Blood and Circulation

Almost everybody is bothered occasionally by minor disturbances of the circulatory system. Most of the time these disturbances are temporary, and in many cases where they are chronic they may be so mild as not to interfere with good health. Among the more common disturbances of this type are the following.

Anemia

Anemia is a condition in which there is a decrease in the number of red blood cells or in the hemoglobin content of the red blood cells. *Hemoglobin* is the compound that carries oxygen to the body tissues from the lungs. Anemia in itself is not a disease but rather a symptom of some other disorder, such as a deficiency of iron in the diet; excessive loss of blood resulting from an injury or heavy menstrual flow; infection by industrial poisons; or kidney or bone marrow disease. A person may also develop anemia as a result of hypersensitivity (allergy) to various medicines.

In the simple form of anemia, caused by a deficiency of iron in the diet, the symptoms are rarely severe. There may be feelings of fatigue, a loss of energy, and a general lack of vitality. Deficiency anemia is especially common among children and pregnant women, and can be corrected by adding foods high in iron to the diet, such as liver, lean meat, leafy green vegetables, whole wheat bread, and dried peas and beans.

If the symptoms persist, a physician should be consulted for diagnosis and treatment. For more information on anemia, see "Diseases of the Blood" in Ch. 9, *Diseases of the Circulatory System.*

Varicose Veins

Varicose veins are veins that have become ropy and swollen, and are therefore visible in the leg, sometimes bulging on the surface of the skin. They are the result of a sluggish blood flow (poor circulation), often combined with weakened walls of the veins themselves. The condition is common in pregnancy and occurs frequently among people who find it necessary to sit or stand in the same position for extended periods of time. A tendency to develop varicose veins may be inherited.

Even before the veins begin to be visible, there may be such warning symptoms as leg cramps, feelings of fatigue, or a general achiness. Unless the symptoms are treated promptly, the condition may worsen, and if the blood flow becomes increasingly impeded, ulcers may develop on the lower area of the leg.

Treatment

Mild cases of varicose veins can be kept under control, or even corrected, by giving some help to circulation, as follows:

- Several times during the day, lie flat on your back for a few minutes, with the legs slightly raised.

- Soak the legs in warm water.

- Exercise regularly.

- Wear lightly reinforced stockings or elastic stockings to support veins in the legs.

If varicose veins have become severe, a physician should be consulted. He or she may advise injection treatment or surgery. See also "The Inflammatory Disorders" in Ch. 9, *Diseases of the Circulatory System.*

Chronic Hypertension

Hypertension, commonly known as *high blood pressure,* is a condition that may be a warning of some other disease. In many cases, it is not in itself a serious problem and has no one underlying specific cause: this is called *functional, essential,* or *chronic hypertension.* The symptoms of breathing difficulty, headache, weakness, or dizziness that accompany high blood pressure can often be controlled by medicines that bring the pressure down, by sedatives or tranquilizers, and in cases where overweight is a contributing factor, by a change in diet, or by a combination of these.

More serious types of high blood pressure can be the result of kidney disease, glandular disturbances, or diseases of the circulatory system. Acute symptoms include chronic dizziness or blurred vision. Any symptoms of high blood pressure call for professional advice and treatment. See "Hypertensive Heart Disease" in Ch. 10, *Heart Disease.*

Tachycardia

Tachycardia is the medical name for a condition that most of us have felt at one time or another—abnormally rapid heartbeat, or a feeling that the heart is fluttering, or pounding too quickly. The condition can be brought on by strong feelings of fear, excitement, or anxiety, or by overtaxing the heart with sudden exertion or too much exercise. It may also be a sign of heart disease, but in such cases, it is usually accompanied by other symptoms.

The most typical form of occasional rapid heartbeat is called *paroxysmal tachycardia,* during which the beat suddenly becomes twice or three times as fast as it is normally, and then just as suddenly returns to its usual tempo. When the paroxysms are frequent enough to be disturbing and can be traced to no specific source, they can be prevented by medicines prescribed by a physician.

Nosebleed

Nosebleeds are usually the result of a ruptured blood vessel. They are especially common among children, and among adults with high blood pressure. If the nosebleed doesn't taper off by itself, the following measures should be taken: the patient should be seated—but not lying down—clothing loosened, and a cold compress placed on the back of the neck and the nose. The soft portion of the nostril may be pressed gently against the bony cartilage of the nose for at least six minutes, or rolled wads of absorbent cotton may be placed inside each nostril, with part of the cotton sticking out to make its removal easier. The inserted cotton should be left in place for several hours and then gently withdrawn.

Fainting

Fainting is a sudden loss of consciousness, usually caused by an insufficient supply of blood and oxygen to the brain. Among the most common causes of fainting are fear, acute hunger, the sight of blood, and prolonged standing in a room with too little fresh air. Fainting should not be confused with a loss of consciousness resulting from excessive alcohol intake or insulin shock. A person about to faint usually feels dizzy, turns pale, and feels weak in the knees.

Treatment

If possible, the person should be made to lie down, or to sit with his head between his knees for several minutes. Should he lose consciousness, place him so that his legs are slightly higher than his head, loosen his clothing, and see that he gets plenty of fresh air. If smelling salts or aromatic spirits of ammonia are available, they can be held under his nose. With these procedures, he should revive in a few minutes. If he doesn't, a physician should be called.

Troubles Along the Digestive Tract

From childhood on, most people are occasionally bothered by minor and temporary disturbances connected with digestion. Most of the disturbances listed below can be treated successfully with common sense and, if need be, a change in habits.

The Mouth

The digestive processes begin in the mouth, where the saliva begins chemically to break down some foods into simpler components, and the teeth and the tongue start the mechanical breakdown. Disorders of the teeth such as a malocclusion or poorly fitted dentures that interfere with proper chewing, should promptly be brought to the attention of a dentist.

Inflammation of the Gums

Also known as *gingivitis,* inflammation of the gums is caused by the bacteria that breed in food trapped in the spaces between the gums and the teeth. The gums become increasingly swollen, may bleed easily, and be sore enough to interfere with proper chewing. The condition can be prevented by cleaning the teeth thoroughly and frequently, which includes the use of dental floss or the rubber tip on the toothbrush to remove any food particles lodged in the teeth after eating. Because gingivitis can develop into the more serious condition of *pyorrhea,* persistent gum bleeding or soreness should receive prompt professional treatment. See Ch. 22, *The Teeth and Gums.*

Canker Sores

Canker sores are small ulcers inside the lips, mouth, and cheeks. Their specific cause is unknown, but they seem to accompany or follow a virus infection, vitamin deficiency, or emotional stress. They may be additionally irritated by citrus fruit, chocolate, or nuts. A canker sore usually clears up in about a week without special treatment. A bland mouth rinse will relieve pain and, in some cases, speed the healing process.

Coated Tongue

Although a coated tongue is commonly supposed to be a sure sign of illness, this is not the case. The condition may occur because of a temporary lack of saliva.

Glossitis

Glossitis, an inflammation of the tongue causing the tongue's surface to become bright red or, in some cases, glazed in appearance, may be a symptom of an infection elsewhere in the body. It may also be a symptom of anemia or a nutritional deficiency, or it may be an adverse reaction to certain forms of medication. If the inflammation persists and is accompanied by acute soreness, it should be called to a physician's attention.

Halitosis or Bad Breath

Contrary to the millions of commercial messages on television and in print, bad breath cannot be cured by any mouthwash, lozenge, spray, or antiseptic gargle now on the market. These products can do no more than mask the odor until the basic cause is diagnosed and cured. Among the many conditions that may result in bad breath (leaving out such fleeting causes as garlic and onions) are the following: an infection of the throat, nose, or mouth; a stomach or kidney disorder; pyorrhea; respiratory infection; tooth decay; improper mouth hygiene; and excessive drinking and smoking. Anyone who has been made self-conscious about the problem of bad breath should ask his physician or dentist whether his breath is truly offensive and if it is, what to do about it.

Gastritis

Gastritis, one of the most common disorders of the digestive system, is an inflammation of the lining of the stomach that may occur in acute, chronic, or toxic form. Among the causes of *acute gastritis* are various bacterial or viral infections; overeating, especially heavy or rich foods; excessive drinking of alcoholic beverages; or food poisoning. An attack of acute gastritis may be severely painful, but the discomfort usually subsides with proper treatment. The first symptom is typically sharp stomach cramps, followed by a bloated feeling, loss of appetite, headache, and nausea. When vomiting occurs, it rids the stomach of the substance causing the attack but usually leaves the patient temporarily weak. If painful cramps persist and are accompanied by fever, a physician should be consulted about the possibility of medication for bacterial infection. For a few days after an attack of acute gastritis, the patient should stay on a bland diet of easily digested foods, taken in small quantities.

Toxic Gastritis

Toxic gastritis is usually the result of swallowing a poisonous substance, causing vomiting and possible collapse. It is an emergency condition requiring prompt first aid treatment and the attention of a physician. See "Poisoning" in Ch. 31, *Medical Emergencies.*

Chronic Gastritis

Chronic gastritis is a recurrent or persisting inflammation of the stomach lining over a lengthy period. The condition has the symptoms associated with indigestion, especially pain after eating. It can be caused by excessive drinking of alcoholic beverages, constant tension or anxiety, or deficiencies in the diet. The most effective treatment for chronic gastritis is a bland diet from which caffeine and alcohol have been eliminated. Heavy meals should be avoided in favor of eating small amounts at frequent intervals. A tranquilizer or a mild sedative prescribed by a physician may reduce the tensions that contribute to the condition. If the discomfort continues, a physician should be consulted about the possibility of ulcers. See Ch. 11, *Diseases of the Digestive System.*

Gastroenteritis

Gastroenteritis is an inflammation of the lining of both the stomach and the intestines. Like gastritis, it can occur in acute or toxic forms as a result of food poisoning, excessive alcohol intake, viral or bacterial infections, or food allergies. Vomiting, diarrhea, and fever may be more pronounced and of longer duration. As long as nausea and vomiting persist, no food or fluid should be taken; when these symptoms cease, a bland, mainly fluid diet consisting of strained broth, thin cereals, boiled eggs, and tea is best. If fever continues and diarrhea doesn't taper off, a physician should be called.

Diarrhea

Diarrhea is a condition in which bowel movements are abnormally frequent and liquid. It may be accompanied by cramps, vomiting, thirst, and a feeling of tenderness in the abdominal region. Diarrhea is always a symptom of some irritant in the intestinal tract; among possible causes are allergy, infection by virus or bacteria, accidentally swallowed poisonous substances, or excessive alcohol. Brief attacks are sometimes caused by emotions, such as overexcitement or anxiety.

Diarrhea that lasts for more than two days should be diagnosed by a physician to rule out a more serious infection, a glandular disturbance, or a tumor. Mild attacks can be treated at home by giving the patient a light, bland diet, plenty of fluids, and the prescribed dosage of a kaolin-pectin compound available at any drugstore.

Constipation

Many people have the mistaken notion that if they don't have a bowel movement every day, they must be constipated. This is not necessarily so. From a physician's viewpoint, constipation is determined not by an arbitrary schedule of when the bowel should be evacuated but by the individual's discomfort and other unpleasant symptoms. In too many instances, overconcern and anxiety about bowel movements may be the chief cause of constipation.

The watery waste that results from the digestion of food in the stomach and small intestine passes into the large intestine, or colon, where water is absorbed from the waste. If the waste stays in the large intestine for too long a time, so much water is removed that it becomes too solid and compressed to evacuate easily. The efficient removal of waste material from the large intestine depends on wavelike muscular contractions. When these waves are too weak to do their job properly, as often happens in the elderly or the excessively sedentary, a physician may recommend a mild laxative or mineral oil.

Treatment

Constipation is rarely the result of an organic disorder. In most cases, it is caused by poor health habits; when these are corrected, the disorder corrects itself. Often, faulty diet is a major factor. Make sure that meals contain plenty of roughage in the form of whole-grain cereals, fruit, and leafy green vegetables. Figs, prunes, and dates should be included from time to time. Plenty of liquid intake is important, whether in the form of juices, soups, or large quantities of water. Scheduling a certain amount of exercise each day strengthens the abdominal muscles and stimulates muscle activity in the large intestine. Confronting the sources of worries and anxieties, if necessary with a trained therapist, may also be helpful.

An enema or a laxative should be considered only once in a while rather than as regular treatment. The colon should be given a chance to function properly without relying on artificial stimulation. If constipation resists these commonsense approaches, the problem should be talked over with a physician.

Hemorrhoids

Hemorrhoids, commonly called *piles,* are swollen veins in the mucous membrane inside or just outside the rectum. When the enlargement is slight, the only discomfort may be an itching sensation in the area. Acute cases are accompanied by pain and bleeding. Hemorrhoids are a very common complaint and occur in people of all ages. They are usually the result of straining to eliminate hard, dry stools. The extra pressure causes a fold of the membranous rectal lining to slip down, thus pinching the veins and irritating them.

Because hemorrhoids may be a symptom of a disorder other than constipation, they should be treated by a physician. If neglected, they may bleed frequently and profusely enough to cause anemia. Should a blood clot develop in an irritated vein, surgery may be necessary.

Treatment

Advertised cures should be avoided because they are not only ineffective but can cause additional irritation. Laxatives and cathartics, which may temporarily solve the problem of constipation, are likely to aggravate hemorrhoids.

If pain or bleeding becomes acute, a physician should be consulted promptly. Treatment can be begun at home. Sitting for several minutes in a hot bath in the morning and again in the evening (more frequently if necessary) will provide temporary relief.

Preventing constipation is of the utmost importance.

Anal Fissure

This is a condition in which a crack or split or ulcerated place develops in the area of the two anal sphincters, or muscle rings, that control the release of feces. Such breaks in the skin are generally caused by something sharp in the stool, or by the passage of an unusually hard and large stool. Although discomfort often accompanies a bowel movement when there is a fissure, the acute pain typically comes afterward. Healing is difficult because the injured tissue is constantly open to irritation. If the condition persists, it usually has to be treated by a minor surgical procedure. Intense itching in this area is called *anal pruritis*.

Minor Ailments in the Air Pipes

In addition to all the respiratory discomforts that go along with the common cold, there are various other ailments that affect breathing and normal voice production.

Bronchitis

Usually referred to as a chest cold, *bronchitis* is an inflammation of the bronchial tubes that connect the windpipe and the lungs. If bronchitis progresses down into the lungs, it can develop into pneumonia. Old people and children are especially susceptible to acute bronchitis. The symptoms include pain in the chest, a feeling of fatigue, and a nagging cough. If the infection is bacterial, it will respond to antibiotics. If it is viral, there are no specific medicines. The attack usually lasts for about ten days, although recovery may be speeded up with bed rest and large fluid intake.

Chronic Bronchitis

Chronic bronchitis is a condition that may recur each winter, or may be present throughout the year in the form of a constant cough. The condition is aggravated by smoking and by irritants such as airborne dust and smog. The swollen tissues and abnormally heavy discharge of mucus interfere with the flow of air from the lungs and cause shortness of breath. Medicines are available that lessen the bronchial phlegm and make breathing easier. People with chronic bronchitis often sleep better if they use more than one pillow and have a vaporizer going at night.

Coughing

Coughing is usually a reflex reaction to an obstruction or irritation in the trachea (windpipe), pharynx (back of mouth and throat), or bronchial tubes. It can also be the symptom of a disease or a nervous habit. For a simple cough brought on by smoking too much or breathing bad air, medicines can be taken that act as sedatives to inhibit the reflex reaction. Inhaling steam can loosen the congestion (a combination of swollen membranes and thickened mucus) that causes some types of coughs, and hot drinks such as tea or lemonade help to soothe and relax the irritated area. Constant coughing, especially when accompanied by chest pains, should be brought to a physician's attention. For a discussion of whooping cough and croup, see the respective articles under the "Alphabetic Guide to Child Care" in Ch. 2, *The First Dozen Years.*

Laryngitis

Laryngitis is an inflammation of the mucous membrane of the larynx (voice box) that interferes with breathing and causes the voice to become hoarse or disappear altogether. This condition may accompany a sore throat, measles, or whooping cough, or it may result from an allergy. Prolonged overuse of the voice, a common occupational hazard of singers and teachers, is also a cause. The best treatment for laryngitis is to go to bed, keep the room cool, and put moisture into the air from a vaporizer, humidifier, or boiling kettle. Don't attempt to talk, even in a whisper. Keep a writing pad within arm's reach and use it to spare your voice. Drinking warm liquids may help to relieve some of the discomfort. If you must go out, keep the throat warmly protected.

Chronic laryngitis may result from too many acute laryngitis attacks, which can cause the mucous membrane to become so thick and tough that the voice remains permanently hoarse. The sudden onset of hoarseness that lasts for more than two weeks calls for a physician's diagnosis.

Hiccups

Hiccups (also spelled *hiccoughs*) are contractions of the diaphragm, the great muscle responsible for forcing air in and out of our lungs. They may be brought on by an irritation of the diaphragm itself, of the respiratory or digestive system, or by eating or drinking too rapidly. Common remedies for hiccups include sipping water slowly, holding the breath, and putting something cold on the back of the neck. Breathing into a paper bag is usually effective because after a few breaths, the high carbon dioxide content in the bag will serve to make the diaphragm contractions more regular, rather than spasmodic. If none of these measures helps, it may be necessary to have a physician prescribe a sedative or tranquilizer.

The Sensitive Eyes and Ears

Air pollution affects not only the lungs but the eyes as well. In addition to all the other hazards to which the eyes are exposed, airborne smoke, chemicals, and dust cause the eyes to burn, itch, and shed tears. Other common eye troubles are discussed below.

Sty

This pimplelike inflammation of the eyelid is caused by infection, which may be linked to the blocking of an eyelash root or an oil gland, or to general poor health. A sty can be treated at home by applying clean compresses of hot water to the area for about 15 minutes at a time every two hours. This procedure should cause the sty to open, drain, and heal. If sties are recurrent, a health checkup may be indicated.

Pinkeye

Pinkeye, an acute form of *conjunctivitis,* is an inflammation of the membrane that lines the eyelid and covers the eyeball, causing the eyes to become red and the lids to swell and stick together while one is sleeping. The condition may result from bacterial or viral infection—in which case it is extremely contagious—or from allergy or chemical irritation. A physician should be consulted.

Conjunctivitis can be treated by washing the eyes with warm water, drying them with a disposable tissue to prevent the spread of infection, and applying a medicated yellow oxide of mercury ophthalmic ointment (as recommended by your physician) on the inner edges of the lids. This should be done upon rising in the morning and upon retiring at night. The eyes should then be closed until the ointment has spread. Apply compresses of hot water three or four times a day for five-minute periods.

Eyestrain

Eyestrain—with symptoms of fatigue, tearing, redness, and a scratchy feeling in the eyelids—can be caused by a need for corrective glasses, by a disorder of the eye, or by overuse of the eyes. One of the most common causes of eyestrain, however, is improper lighting. Anyone engaged in close work, such as sewing or miniature model building, and at all times when reading, should have light come from behind and from the side so that no shadow falls on the book or object being scrutinized. The light should be strong enough for comfort—not dazzling. Efforts should be made to avoid a shiny or highly polished work surface that produces a glare. To avoid eyestrain when watching television, be sure the picture is in sharp focus; the viewer should sit at least six feet from the screen; and see that the room is not in total darkness.

Ear Infections

Ear infections related to colds, sore throats, or tonsillitis can now be kept from spreading and entering the mastoid bone by the use of sulfa drugs and other antibiotics. Any acute earache should therefore be called to a physician's attention promptly. Aspirin, in adults, can be taken for temporary relief from pain; holding a heating pad or a hotwater bottle to the affected side of the face may also be helpful until proper medication can be prescribed.

Earwax

An excessive accumulation of earwax can cause pain and interfere with hearing. A small wad of cotton should be used to gently clean the ear canal, and sharp objects such as hairpins and matchsticks should never be used.

Hardened earwax can be softened by a few drops of hydrogen peroxide. Sometimes a doctor may have to flush out earwax that is deeply imbedded.

Ear Blockage

A stopped-up feeling in the ear can be caused by a cold, and also by the change in air pressure experienced when a plane makes a rapid descent. The obstruction of the eustachian tube can usually be opened by swallowing hard or yawning.

Ringing in the Ear

The general word for a large variety of noises in the ear is *tinnitus*. Tinnitus can be ringing, buzzing, or other low level continual sounds. Everyone experiences some form of ear ringing on occasion, such as after listening to loud music or noise. However, chronic noise is symptomatic of other problems. Tinnitus can be caused by tension in the jaw muscle from stress, grinding of the teeth, or structural problems with the jaw. It can also be caused by high blood pressure, infections, or as a reaction to chemicals, such as nicotine. If you experience continual or chronic ringing, you should discuss it with your physician.

Tinnitus is treated by avoiding excessive noise, masking irritating ear noises with music or amplified sounds from a hearing aid or cleaning ear wax out of ears. A doctor's opinion should also be sought to determine if the ringing is caused by an inner ear infection. Avoiding caffeine, nicotine and alcohol also helps.

The Path from the Kidneys

Cystitis

Cystitis is the general term for inflammation of the bladder caused by various types of infection. It is more common in women than in men. Infecting microbes may come from outside the body by way of the urethra, or from some other infected organ, such as the kidney. When the bladder becomes inflamed, frequent and painful urination results.

Cystitis may also occur as a consequence of other disorders, such as enlargement of the prostate gland, a structural defect of the male urethra, or stones or a tumor in the bladder. Although there is no completely reliable way to prevent cystitis, some types of infection can be prevented by cleansing the genital region regularly so that the entrance of the urethra is protected against bacterial invasion. Cystitis is usually cured by medicines prescribed by a physician. For a detailed discussion of cystitis and related conditions affecting women, see "Disorders of the Urinary System" in Ch. 25, *Women's Health.*

Prostatitis

Prostatitis is an inflammation of the prostate gland (present in males only), caused by an infection of the urinary tract or some other part of the body. It may occur as a result of venereal infection. The symptoms of painful and excessive urination generally respond favorably to antibiotics. *Acute prostatitis* is less common: the patient is likely to have a high fever, as well as a discharge of pus from the penis. These symptoms should be brought to a physician's attention without delay.

Excessive Urination

A need to empty the bladder with excessive frequency can be merely a nuisance caused by overexcitement or tension, or it can be the sign of a disorder of the urinogenital system. A physician should be consulted if the problem persists.

The All-Important Feet

The *podiatrist* is the specialist who treats foot problems. Causes of foot ailments range from lack of cleanliness to ill-fitting shoes and overindulgence in athletic activities (see "Care of the Feet" in Ch. 5, *The Middle Years,* "The Vulnerable Extremities" in Ch. 23, *Aches, Pains, Nuisances, Worries*).

An ache, pain, or other disorder of the foot can be particularly annoying because it usually hampers mobility. A severe problem can keep a person bedridden, sometimes in the hospital, for substantial periods of time. As humans, we move about on our feet. They deserve the best of care from us, as their owners, and from the podiatrist in case a serious problem arises.

Podiatry, the science of foot care, has become more and more important as Americans have taken to athletics and exercises of various kinds. Most of these activities require the use of the feet. Increasing numbers of persons in the adult years are also taking up walking, jogging, or running as diversions or exercises.

Podiatrists believe that some persons "walk old"—they give the appearance, by the way they walk, of greater age than their chronological years. Others "walk young," or walk normally. Those who walk old may be inviting foot problems, and a fact of podiatric science is that every foot problem has its reflection in another part, or other parts, of the body.

By contrast, good foot and body posture often suggests that the owner of the feet enjoys good health in other parts of the body. Foot care may in effect help other body parts to function better. Because many problems with parts of the body remote from the feet make good foot posture and normal walking difficult or impossible, individuals with diverse problems, such as back pains, sometimes go to a podiatrist for treatment. The back pain may disappear when the feet have been brought into good working order.

Diabetes and the Feet

"Care" for the feet of diabetics means prevention. The diabetic tries to keep his feet so healthy that he avoids major problems. He knows that diabetes affects blood circulation, and that the leg and foot are extremely vulnerable to circulatory problems. Where blood cannot reach a limb or member, gangrene becomes a possibility.

Foot Care

What kind of care serves the diabetic best? Effective care means that the diabetic takes steps quickly to treat such problems as abrasions or ulcers that refuse to heal. Other conditions that warn of possible future problems are dry skin, numbness, and dry or brittle nails. Ulcers that appear in the skin of the foot and that appear to have roots in deeper layers of tissue serve as danger signals. Such ulcers may appear on the site of an injury, cut, or scratch. A physician will usually prescribe medication, dietary adjustments, or other measures.

Ulcers may result from neglect of a corn or callus. But such neglect itself indicates the risks that diabetics incur: they may neglect to have a foot problem such as a corn treated because their disease has, over time, reduced the sensitivity of their feet. They may lose much of their ability to feel pain, heat or cold, or stress in the foot. Because of such problems, diabetics generally follow certain rules of foot care, including the following:

• Give the feet a daily examination for cuts, bruises, or other abnormalities

• Use only prescribed medications in caring for the feet—and avoid over-the-counter preparations

- Visit a podiatrist regularly, as often as once a month, and avoid medical "treatment" of one's own feet or even cutting one's own toenails

- Wash the feet daily in warm, not hot, water and dry them carefully, including the area between the toes

- Use a gentle lubricant on the feet after washing and drying—and never go barefoot

- Avoid the use of items of clothing that may interfere with circulation, including wraparound garters and support hosiery

- Avoid "holey" socks, darned socks, or anything else that may irritate the soles of the feet and

- Avoid constrictive boots or shoes

Jogging and Running

The podiatrist usually tries to learn about a patient's work, his hobbies and sports, and other facts before undertaking treatment. In particular, the podiatrist asks whether the patient runs or jogs or takes part in other strenuous exercises. With such background information, he or she can suggest appropriate treatment.

A podiatrist will advise runners or joggers on the kind of footwear that would be best—especially if problems have been encountered or may be expected. Shoe inserts may be custom-designed if needed. The podiatrist may also advise runners and joggers to run on softer surfaces rather than cement. Jogging or running "in place," without forward movement, is to be avoided if possible; even when jogging inside the home or apartment, the jogger should move from room to room.

Podiatrists point out that even the more serious knee and ankle problems incurred in running and jogging can be treated. "Jogger's ankle," pain resulting from too much jogging and the attendant strain, can be controlled if the jogger will use moderation. Beginning joggers in particular should start slowly and gradually increase their level of participation. Runners' knee problems may be cured in many cases by treatment that enables the feet to carry the weight of the body properly. In part, the treatment requires practice in throwing the body weight onto the balls of the feet, not on the inner sides of the feet. The remainder of the body, including the knees, can be kept in proper alignment with the feet if the weight falls where it should.

Podiatrists also advise runners, joggers, and others taking part in sports to make certain *all* their clothing and equipment are appropriate. That applies especially in skiing, ice-skating, and other sports requiring extensive foot use.

With proper equipment, including good shoes, and a moderate approach, runners and joggers can avoid physical difficulties that could require podiatric care. These others include fallen arches; corns, calluses, and bunions.

24

Allergies and Hypersensitivities

*A*llergy is a broad term used to describe an unusual reaction of the body's tissues to a substance that has no noticeable effect on other persons. About 17 out of every 100 persons in America are allergic, or hypersensitive, to one or more substances that are known to precipitate an unusual reaction. Such substances, known as *allergens,* include a variety of irritants, among them mold spores, pollens, animal dander, insect venoms, and house dust. Some individuals are allergic to substances in soap, which produce a skin irritation. Others react to the smell of a rose by sneezing. Still others react with an outbreak of hives, diarrhea, or other symptoms to allergens in foods.

How Allergens Affect the Body

Allergic symptoms can range from itching eyes, running nose, coughing, difficulty in breathing, and welts on the skin to nausea, cramps, and even going into a state of shock, depending upon the severity of the particular individual's sensitivity and response. Almost any part or system of the body can be affected, and almost anything can pose an allergic threat to somebody.

The Role of Antibodies

The system of an allergic individual reacts to such substances in the way it would react to an invading disease organism: by producing *antibodies* whose job it is to neutralize the allergen. In the process of fighting off the effects of the allergen, the body's defense mechanism may overreact by dumping a chemical mediator, *histamine,* indiscriminately into the individual's bloodstream. It is the overabundance of this protective chemical that causes the discomforts associated with allergies.

At the same time, the antibodies can sensitize the individual to the allergen. Then, with each new exposure to the allergen, more antibodies are produced. Eventually the symptoms of allergy are produced whenever the allergen is encountered. Most allergic reactions, including hay fever, asthma, gastrointestinal upsets, and skin rashes, are of the type just described; their effect is more or less immediate. A second type, known as the delayed type, seems to function without the production of antibodies; contact dermatitis is an example of the delayed type.

Eosinophils

Some individuals seem to be sensitive to only one known allergen, but others are sensitive to a variety of substances. Persons who suffer acute allergic reactions have abnormally high levels of a type of white blood cell called *eosinophil.* The eosinophil contains an enzyme that may have some control over the allergic reaction, and varying degrees of the enzyme's efficiency appear to account for individual differences in the severity of allergic reactions.

Allergic Symptoms in Children

Many of the common allergies appear during the early years of life. It has been estimated that nearly 80 percent of the major allergic problems begin to appear between the ages of 4 and 9. Allergic youngsters may have nasal speech habits, breathe through the mouth, have coughing and wheezing spells, or rub their eyes, nose, and ears because of itching. A not uncommon sign of allergic reaction in a child may be dark circles under the eyes caused by swelling of the mucous membranes to such an extent that blood does not drain properly from the veins under the lower eyelids. Nose twitching and mouth wrinkling also are signs that a youngster has allergic symptoms.

Common Allergens

The allergens responsible for so many unpleasant and uncomfortable symptoms take a variety of forms too numerous and sometimes too obscure for any book to enumerate. Discussed below are some of the more common types of allergens.

Foods

Foods are among the most common causes of allergic reactions. While nearly any food substance is a potential allergen to certain sensitive individuals, those most frequently implicated are cow's milk, orange juice, and eggs, all considered essential in a child's diet. However, substitute foods are almost always available. Many natural foods contain vitamin C, or ascorbic acid, found in orange juice. Ascorbic acid also is available in vitamin tablets. All of the essential amino acids and other nutrients in cow's milk and eggs also can be obtained from other food sources, although perhaps not as conveniently packaged for immediate use. Other common food offenders are chocolate, pork, seafoods, nuts, and berries. An individual may be allergic to the gluten in wheat, rye, and oats, and products made from those grains.

Inhaled Allergens

Allergens also may affect the respiratory tract, bringing on sneezing, coughing, and breathing impairment. The substances involved can be pollens, dust, smoke, perfumes, and various airborne chemicals.

Mold Spores

A person also can become allergic to a certain mold by inhaling the spores, or reproductive particles, of fungus. In the nose, the mold spores trigger a reaction in cells of the tissues beneath the mucous membranes that line the nasal passages. This in turn leads to the symptoms of allergy. Because they are small, mold spores can evade the natural protective mechanisms of the nose and upper respiratory tract to reach the lungs and bring on an allergic reaction in that site. Usually, this leads to the buildup of mucus, wheezing, and difficulty in breathing associated with asthma.

Less frequently, inhaling mold spores can result in skin lesions similar to those of eczema or chronic hives. In all but the very warmest areas of the United States, molds are seasonal allergens, occurring from spring into late fall. But unlike pollens, molds do not disappear with the killing frosts of autumn. Actually, frost may help increase the activity of molds, which thrive on dying vegetation produced by cold temperatures.

Dust and Animal Hair

House dust and animal hair (especially cat and dog hair) are also responsible for respiratory allergies in many people. Asthma attacks are often triggered by contact with these substances. Symptoms of dust allergy are usually most severe in the spring and fall, and tend to subside in the summer.

Man-Made Allergens

An example of respiratory allergy caused by man-made allergens is the complaint known as "meat wrappers' asthma," which results from fumes of the price-label adhesive on the polyvinyl chloride film used to package foods. The fumes are produced when the price label is cut on a hot wire. When the fumes are inhaled, the result is burning eyes, sore throat, wheezing and shortness of breath, upset stomach, and other complaints. Studies show that exposure to the fumes from the heat-activated label adhesive for as little as five minutes could produce airway obstruction in food packagers.

Another source of respiratory allergy is the photochemical smog produced by motor vehicle exhaust in large city areas. The smog is composed of hydrocarbons, oxides of nitrogen, and other chemicals activated by the energy of sunlight. When inhaled in the amounts present along the nation's expressways, the smog has been found to impair the normal function of membranes in the lungs.

Drugs

Medicines and drugs, such as penicillin, or serums used in inoculations, can cause allergic reactions. Estimates of the incidence of allergy among those receiving penicillin range from one to ten percent. The National Institutes of Health has calculated that just three common drugs—penicillin, sulfonamides, and aspirin—account for as much as 90 percent of all allergic drug reactions. The allergic reactions include asthmatic symptoms, skin rash, shock, and other symptoms similar to tissue reactions to other allergens. Medical scientists theorize that chemicals in certain drugs probably combine with protein molecules in the patient's body to form a new substance that is the true allergen. However, it also has been noted that some persons show allergic reactions to placebo drugs, which may contain sugar or inert substances rather than real drugs.

Insect Venom

Insect stings cause serious allergic reactions in about four of every 1,000 persons stung by bees, fire ants, yellow jackets, wasps, or hornets. A single sting to a sensitive person may lead to a serious drop in blood pressure, shock, and possibly death. There are more than 50 reported fatalities a year, and experts suspect that other deaths occur as a result of insect stings but are listed as heart attacks, stroke, or convulsions.

Sensitivity tests of persons who might be acutely allergic to insect stings have been difficult to develop, because allergic individuals reacted in the same way as nonallergic persons to skin tests performed with extracts from insect bodies. More recently, physicians have found that using pure insect venom produces a reaction that determines whether a person is allergic to the sting. Medical scientists also have isolated the major allergen in an insect venom for use in diagnosing and treating patients who are particularly sensitive to stings.

Skin Allergies

Allergies affecting the skin take many forms, the most common being eczema, urticaria (hives), angioedema (swelling of the subcutaneous tissues), and contact dermatitis. Among the most common causes are foods, cosmetics, fabrics, rubber, metals, plants and flowers, plastics, insecticides, furs and leather, jewelry, and many industrial chemicals. Studies of patients who seem to be especially sensitive to skin allergies show that they have higher than average amounts of a body protein called *immunoglobulin E* in their systems.

Contact dermatitis usually is distinguished by skin swelling, hives, or blisters. The area affected is usually the skin that comes in direct contact with the allergen, so a watch band allergy response will appear as a band around the wrist where the watchband touches the skin. Long-term exposure will cause dry, cracked, darkened patches on the skin.

Poisonous Plants

Poison ivy, poison oak, and poison sumac contain an extremely irritating oily resin that sensitizes the body; repeated contact seems to increase the severity of the allergic reactions. About 50 percent of the population who come in contact with the resin will experience a severe form of dermatitis, and up to 10 percent will be temporarily disabled by the effects. Exposure to the resin may come from direct contact with the plant, from contact with other objects or animals that have touched the plant, or from inhaling smoke from the burning plant.

Cosmetics and Jewelry

A wide variety of cosmetics and jewelry can cause allergic reactions through skin contact. Even jewelry that is presumably pure gold can contain a certain amount of nickel that will produce a mild reaction that causes a skin discoloration, sometimes aided by chemical activity resulting from perspiration in the area of jewelry contact. Among cosmetics that may be involved in allergic reactions are certain permanent-wave lotions, eyelash dyes, face powders, permanent hair dyes, hair-spray lacquers, and skin-tanning agents. Of course, not all persons are equally sensitive to the ingredients known to be allergens, and in most cases a similar product with different ingredients can be substituted for the cosmetic causing allergic reactions. For more information on skin allergies, see "Disorders of the Skin" in Ch. 21, *Skin and Hair.*

Environmental Allergies

Environmental agents such as sunlight, excessive cold, and pressure are known to produce allergic reactions in certain individuals. Cold allergy, for example, can result in hives and may even lead to a drop in blood pressure, fainting, severe shock, and sometimes death. Research into the causes of cold allergy has shown that cold urticaria, or hives, results from a histamine released from body tissues as they begin to warm up after a cold stimulus. Extremely high histamine levels coincide with episodes of very low blood pressure, the cause of fainting.

Although reaction of the body tissues to the invasion of microbes, such as bacteria, viruses, and other microorganisms, generally is not thought of as an allergic situation, the manner in which the body musters its defenses against the foreign materials is essentially the same as the way the antibodies are mobilized to neutralize other allergens. Thus, there is a similarity between infectious diseases and allergies.

Temporary Allergies

Occasionally, a change in the body's hormonal balance may trigger a hypersensitivity to a substance that previously had no effect on the individual. Pregnant women are especially susceptible to these temporary allergies, which almost always disappear after childbirth. Some women during pregnancy, on the other hand, experience complete relief from allergies that have plagued them since childhood.

People who suffer from seasonal allergies, such as hay fever, often have heightened allergic reactions to dust, animal dander, and even certain foods, such as chocolate and pineapple, during the season when ragweed pollen or other airborne allergens are plentiful.

Diagnosis of Allergies

Some allergic reactions are outgrown; some don't develop until adulthood; some become increasingly severe over the years because each repeated exposure makes the body more sensitive to the allergen. In many instances, the irritating substance is easily identified, after which it can be avoided. In other cases, it may take a long series of tests before the offending allergen is tracked down.

Medical History

If a person suspects he may have an allergy, the first thing he should do is consult a physician to see if the help of an allergy specialist should be sought. The physician or allergist will first take a complete medical history and check the patient's general health. Not infrequently the source of an allergy can be found by general questioning about the patient's life style. For example, the reaction may occur only on or immediately after the patient eats seafood. Or a patient may have an apparently chronic allergy but be unaware that it may be related to daily meals that include milk and eggs. A patient who keeps several cats or sleeps every night with a dog in the bedroom may not realize that an asthmatic condition actually is an allergic reaction to dander from the fur of a pet animal.

The history taken by the physician will include questions about other known allergies, allergies suffered by other members of the family, variations in symptoms according to the weather, time of day, and season of the year. The symptoms may be related to a change in working conditions or the fact that the symptoms, if perhaps a result of house dust, diminish during periods of outdoor exercise. A person sensitive to cold may unwittingly exacerbate the symptoms with cold drinks, while another person who is sensitive to heat may not realize that symptoms can be triggered by hot drinks but relieved by cold drinks, and so on.

Skin Testing

If the patient is referred to an allergy specialist, the allergist will continue the detective story by conducting skin tests.

Scratch Test

Based on information in the medical history of the patient and the allergist's knowledge of molds, pollens, and other airborne allergens in the geographical area, "the allergist" will conduct what is called a *scratch test.*

A diluted amount of a suspected allergen is applied to a small scratch on the patient's arm or back. If the results of the scratch test are inconclusive, a more sensitive test may be tried.

Intracutaneous Test

In the *intracutaneous* test, a solution of the suspected allergen is injected into the underlayer of skin called the *dermis.* The intracutaneous test also may be used to verify the results of a positive scratch test. With either test, a positive reaction usually consists of a raised reddish welt, or *wheal.* The welt should develop within 15 or 20 minutes if that particular allergen is the cause of the symptoms.

Culture Plates

If the allergen has been identified, or if the allergist still suspects a substance in the environment of the patient despite negative or inconclusive tests, the patient may be given a set of culture plates to place around his home and office or work area. If the allergen has been identified, the culture plates can help the physician and patient learn where his exposure to the substance takes place. If the allergen is not known, the cultures may pick up samples of less common allergens that the specialist can test.

Mucosal Test

Another kind of approach sometimes is used by allergists when skin tests fail to show positive results despite good evidence that a particular allergen is the cause of symptoms. It is called the *mucosal test.* The allergist using the mucosal test applies a diluted solution of the suspected allergen directly to the mucous membranes of the patient, usually on the inner surface of a nostril or by aerosol spray into the bronchial passages. In some cases, the allergic reaction occurs immediately and medication is administered quickly to counter the effects. Because of the possibility of a severe reaction in a hypersensitive patient, the mucosal test is not employed if other techniques seem to be effective.

Relief from Allergies

Other Tests

Allergists have other ways to test for allergies. They can, for example, use the *prick test,* a kind of skin test in which a physician or nurse pricks the skin as many as 30 or 40 times. On each pricked spot a drop of a watery solution is dropped; the solution contains a small amount of one allergen. A red welt appears on the spot within 15 to 30 minutes if the patient is allergic. Using another approach, an *elimination diet,* an allergist may specify a diet that omits certain foods for stated periods. Improvement in the patient's condition while avoiding certain foods usually indicates that the individual has an allergy to that food.

A variation of the prick test involves injection of small amounts of food in solution under the skin or application of the solution under the tongue. If the injection or drops provoke reactions, an allergy is indicated.

Avoidance

For a patient sensitive to a particular type of allergen, such as molds, complete avoidance of the substance can be difficult, but some steps can be taken to avoid undue exposure. For example, the mold allergy sufferer should avoid areas of his home, business, or recreational areas that are likely spots for mold spores to be produced. These would include areas of deep shade or heavy vegetation, basements, refrigerator drip trays, garbage pails, air conditioners, bathrooms, humidifiers, dead leaves or wood logs, barns or silos, breweries, dairies, any place where food is stored, and old foam, rubber pillows and mattresses.

Medication

To supplement avoidance measures, the allergist may prescribe medications that will significantly reduce or relieve the irritating symptoms of the allergic reaction. Antihistamines, corticosteroids, and a drug called cromolyn sodium are among medications that may be prescribed, depending upon the nature and severity of the patient's reactions to the allergen.

Immunotherapy

If avoidance measures and medications do not control the symptoms effectively, the allergist may suggest *immunotherapy*. Immunotherapy consists of injections of a diluted amount of the allergen, a technique similar to that used in the skin tests. A small amount of a very weak extract is injected once or twice a week at first. The strength of the extract is gradually increased, and the injections are given less frequently as relief from the symptoms is realized. The injections are continued until the patient has experienced complete relief of the symptoms for a period of two or three years. However, some people may have to continue the injections for longer time spans. Even though the treatments may relieve the symptoms, they may not cure the allergy.

Identification Cards

Any person subject to severe disabling allergy attacks by a known allergen should carry a card describing both the allergic reaction and the allergen. Detailed information can be obtained from the Asthma and Allergy Foundation of America, 1302 18th St., NW, Washington, DC 20036. See also "Allergic Respiratory Diseases" in Ch. 12, *Diseases of the Respiratory System,* and "Asthma Attack" in Ch. 31, *Medical Emergencies.*

25

Women's Health

The special health matters that are related to a woman's reproductive system belong to the branch of medicine known as *gynecology*. *Obstetrics* is a closely related specialty associated with pregnancy and childbirth. The distinction is something of a technicality for most patients, since obstetricians usually are quite capable of handling gynecological cases and vice versa. The practice of obstetrics and gynecology is commonly combined in a medical service identified by the contraction *Ob-Gyn*. However, there are medical matters that are specifically concerned with female reproductive organs and related tissues but have little to do with obstetrics. For a discussion of obstetrics, see "Infertility, Pregnancy, and Childbirth" in Ch. 4, *The Beginning of a Family.*

The Gynecological Examination

What should a woman expect on her first visit to a gynecologist? First, the gynecologist will interview her, asking about her family, her medical history, and any fears or apprehensions she may have about her personal health. The woman's answers and comments are written into her medical records for future reference. The information can contain important clues that may help in diagnosing any present or future disorders.

A sample of urine and a sample of blood are usually obtained for laboratory tests. During the ensuing physical examination, the woman lies on a special examination table with her feet in metal stirrups and her knees apart. A nurse will be present to assist the doctor. While she is in the *lithotomy position,* the woman's abdomen will be palpated for lumps or other abnormalities. The breasts also will be palpated for possible lumps. Then an external inspection of the vulva and surrounding areas is made by the physician, followed by internal inspection, in which a speculum is used to spread apart the sides of the vagina so that the cervix is exposed. A digital examination (using the fingers) is made of the walls of the vagina and rectum and the neighboring tissue areas, in a search for possible growths or other abnormal conditions. And a sample of cells and secretions from the cervix is taken for a Pap-smear test.

In addition to the examination of the breasts and reproductive system, the gynecologist usually conducts a general physical examination, recording information about height, weight, blood pressure, heart and lung condition, and so on. The routine physical examination, like the medical history,

provides additional clues that, when added to the results of the examination of the breasts and reproductive system, will give a complete picture of the patient's gynecological health.

Following the examination, the gynecologist discusses his appraisal of the woman's condition and answers questions. He will discuss whatever treatment she needs. Medications can be explained at this time, including reasons why certain drugs can or should not be taken. If any surgery or further testing is recommended, those aspects of the health picture also should be discussed in some detail. Any important information that might be misunderstood or forgotten should be jotted down for future reference.

Results of some laboratory tests and the Pap smear are not usually available for several days. But the physician or nurse will contact the patient when the results are available and advise if she should return in the near future for follow-up testing. The American Cancer Society and the American College of Obstetricians and

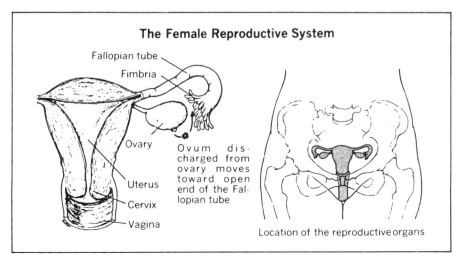

The Female Reproductive System

Fallopian tube

Fimbria

Ovary

Ovum discharged from ovary moves toward open end of the Fallopian tube

Uterus

Cervix

Vagina

Location of the reproductive organs

Gynecologists agree (1) that all women should have their first Pap smear when they become sexually active or at age 18, whichever occurs first; (2) that every woman should have a yearly Pap smear for the following two years; and (3) that later tests should be administered at the physician's discretion if the first three Pap smears are negative. The woman also should discuss arrangements for future checkups or Pap smear tests rather than wait until signs or symptoms of a serious disorder warrant an immediate visit.

Menstrual Disorders

Among the health concerns of women that specifically belong to gynecology are menstrual disorders. Normally, the first menstrual period (menarche) occurs about age 12 or 13, or sometimes earlier or later. Periods are generally irregular for the first year or two, and then they tend to recur at intervals of 24 to 32 days. Each period begins about two weeks after ovulation, or the release of an egg cell (ovum) from the ovary—unless, of course, the ovum happens to be fertilized in the interval and pregnancy interrupts the whole process.

The menstrual flow, which lasts from three to seven days, is composed mainly of serum, mucus, and dead cells shed from the lining (endometrium) of the uterus. The loss of blood is minimal, usually from two to four ounces. The volume of flow, as well as the time schedule, tends to be fairly regular for most women. When one's menstrual pattern varies noticeably from the expected pattern, and in the absence of pregnancy, it may be a sign of a physical or emotional disorder.

Amenorrhea

Failure to menstruate is called *amenorrhea*. Amenorrhea is a natural effect of pregnancy and of nursing a baby. In an older woman, it may be a sign of menopause. But if a nonpregnant or nonnursing woman after menarche and before menopause (say between the ages of 17 or 18 and 52) fails to menstruate for two or more periods, she should bring it to the attention of a doctor—unless, of course, she has undergone a hysterectomy or other surgical or medical treatment that eliminates menstruation.

Primary Amenorrhea

When menarche has not occurred by the age of 16 or 17, the absence of menstruation is called *primary amenorrhea*. In such a case, a physical examination may show that an imperforate hymen or a closed cervix is obstructing the flow of menses, or a congenital defect may be interfering with menstruation. In almost all cases, menarche can be started with a bit of minor surgery, by treatment of any existing systemic disease, or by the injection of sex hormones; or it will start spontaneously later.

Secondary Amenorrhea

When menstrual periods cease after menarche, the condition is known as *secondary,* or *acquired, amenorrhea.* Secondary amenorrhea may involve missing a single menstrual period or many periods in consecutive months. Among possible causes of interrupted menstruation are certain medications, drugs of abuse, emotional stress, normal fluctuations in ovarian activity in the first few years after menarche, and a number of organic diseases. Medicines that can disrupt normal menstrual activity include tranquilizers and other psychotropic (mind-affecting) drugs that apparently influence hormonal activity in the brain centers, amphetamines, and oral contraceptives. When a particular medication is found to be the cause of amenorrhea, the medical treatment may be judged to be more important than maintaining normal menstrual cycles. When the use of oral contraceptives is followed by amenorrhea for six or more months, normal menstrual activity may resume eventually, but it can often be started sooner by a prescribed medication. Among drugs of abuse known to cause amenorrhea are alcohol and opium-based drugs.

Just as the mind-altering effects of psychotropic drugs involve the hypothalamus and pituitary glands in the brain, which control the hormones that regulate menstrual functions, emotional stress seems to have a parallel influence on the incidence of amenorrhea. *Anorexia nervosa,* a disorder associated with emaciation resulting from an emotional disturbance, also can result in an interruption of menstruation.

Other factors contributing to secondary amenorrhea are measles, mumps, and other infections; cysts and tumors of the ovaries; changes in the tissues lining the vagina or uterus; premature aging of the ovaries; diabetes; obesity; anemia; leukemia; and Hodgkin's disease. In many cases, normal or near-normal menstrual function can be restored by medical treatment, such as administration of hormones, or by surgery, or both. In one type of amenorrhea, marked by adhesion of the walls of the uterus, curettage (scraping of the uterus) is followed by insertion of an intrauterine contraceptive device (IUD) to help hold the uterine walls apart.

Menorrhagia

Almost the opposite of amenorrhea is *menorrhagia,* an excessive menstrual flow. The causes of menorrhagia are as varied as those associated with amenorrhea. They include influenza and other infectious diseases, emotional stress, polyps of the cervical or uterine tissues, hypertension, congestive heart failure, leukemia, and blood coagulation disorders. Menorrhagia may occur during the early stages of a young woman's re-productive life soon after reaching puberty, and medical treatment may be necessary to control the excessive loss of blood. In some cases, dilation and curettage is recommended in addition to the administration of hormones and other medications, such as iron tablets to correct anemia resulting from the loss of red blood cells.

Dilation and Curettage

Dilation and curettage, generally referred to as *D and C,* is a procedure in which the cervix is dilated and the cavity of the uterus is cleaned out by a scooplike instrument, a curette. The same procedure is sometimes used to abort an embryo or to remove a tumor or a polyp.

Although it takes only a few minutes to perform a D and C, the procedure is done in a hospital while the patient is anesthetized. There is no afterpain, only a dull discomfort in the lower pelvic region similar to menstrual awareness.

A physical examination is usually made to determine if there are tumors anywhere in the reproductive organs. Except where tumors are found to be a causative factor, most women will resume normal menstrual cycles after treatment of menorrhagia with medications and D and C. For women beyond the age of 40, the physician may recommend a hysterectomy to prevent recurrence of excessive menstrual blood loss.

Polymenorrhea and Metrorrhagia

These medical terms refer to two other ways in which menstrual periods may depart from typical patterns. *Polymenorrhea* is abnormally frequent menstruation, so that menstrual periods occur at intervals of less than 21 days. This short interval may be the natural established pattern for some women. If it is not, the cause may be physical or emotional stress. *Metrorrhagia* is marked by menstrual bleeding that occurs erratically at unpredictable times. It may be the result of a cyst in the lining of the uterus, a tumor in the reproductive tract, polyps, or some hormonal imbalance, including a disorder of the thyroid gland.

Dysmenorrhea

Abdominal or pelvic pain occurring just before or along with the onset of menstruation is known as *dysmenorrhea.* The symptoms include severe colicky abdominal cramps, backache, headache, and, in some cases, nausea and vomiting. As with amenorrhea, there are two general types of dysmenorrhea, primary and secondary.

Primary Dysmenorrhea

This type includes all cases in which no organic disorder is associated with the symptoms, which are presumed to be a result of uterine contractions and emotional factors. More than 75 percent of all cases are of this type. Primary dysmenorrhea generally begins before age 25, but it may appear at any time from menarche to menopause. It frequently ends with the birth of the first child.

Since primary dysmenorrhea by definition occurs in the absence of organic disease, the diagnosis can be made only after a careful medical history is compiled and a special study of the reproductive organs is made to ensure that no disorder has been overlooked. In some cases, oral contraceptives may be prescribed because of the effect such drugs have in suppressing ovulation; the contraceptives prevent the natural production of the hormone progesterone, which is responsible for certain tissue changes associated with the discomfort of dysmenorrhea. Analgesic drugs to relieve pain and medications that help to relax muscles may be prescribed. Medication is often less beneficial, however, than emotional support—including the easing of any stress at home, school, or work, and reassurance about the worries sometimes associated with menstruation.

Secondary Dysmenorrhea

This condition comprises all menstrual pain that is a result of or associated with an organic disease of the reproductive organs, such as endometriosis, to cite just one example. Secondary dysmenorrhea can occur at any age.

Premenstrual Syndrome

Premenstrual syndrome (PMS) has emerged in recent years as a major challenge to the medical profession. PMS clinics have begun to offer specialized counseling, physical examinations, and treatment for women unable to cope with the disorder. Treatment regimens or therapies range from aspirin to large doses of sex hormones, diet programs, and exercise.

A group of related symptoms, PMS involves both psychological and physical changes. Among the psychological are lethargy, tension, irritability, depression, and feelings of aggression. The physical signs may include headache, bloating, asthma, and more exotic problems, such as recurrent herpes or hives. In all, more

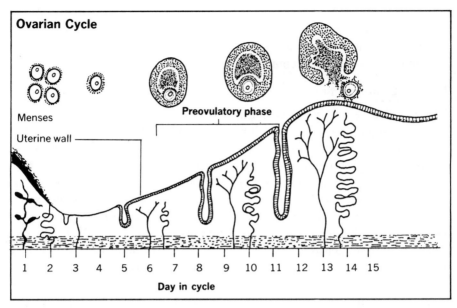

Ovarian Cycle

Menses

Preovulatory phase

Uterine wall

1 2 3 4 5 6 7 8 9 10 11 12 13 14 15

Day in cycle

than 300 different symptoms have been attributed to PMS.

The symptoms, gynecologists warn, should become "disturbing" before they are labeled PMS. Restlessness, minor cramps, and other premenstrual problems may indicate that menstruation is about to start but do not necessarily point to PMS. Such minor problems are called *menstrual molimina*. Cramping and other painful conditions occurring during menstruation are referred to as *dysmenorrhea* (see above).

Of the many treatments for PMS, none has proved uniformly effective. This is because the cause or causes of PMS are not totally understood. Most commonly, physicians believe the disorder represents some basic imbalance in the major female hormones, estrogen and progesterone. Thus one treatment calls for administration of "natural" progesterone to correct the supposed imbalance.

Another common treatment suggested for PMS is vitamin B_6, although the treatment remains partly experimental. Some researchers and physicians, however, have reported disturbing neurological side-effects.

Other theories and treatments exist. Some physicians who have studied PMS and its symptoms believe *prolactin*, a pituitary hormone that stimulates milk secretion, and PMS are associated. A diet and nutrition theory has evolved out of findings that some women report improvement after going on a hypoglycemic diet.

Treated over a substantial period, PMS victims often find that diagnostic tests combined with diet and exercise regimens and vitamin therapy bring good results. If such initial attempts fail, the physician may prescribe medications. In all cases of PMS, according to researchers, psychological support for the sufferer may be important to treatment effectiveness.

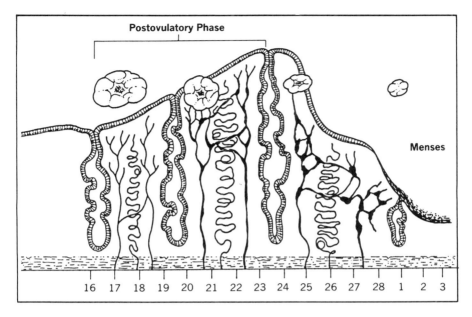

Postovulatory Phase

Menses

16 17 18 19 20 21 22 23 24 25 26 27 28 1 2 3

Minor Menstrual Problems

Blood Clots

There is not usually any cause for alarm if blood clots are expelled during menstruation. Ordinarily, the menstrual flow is completely liquefied, but a few clots tend to appear when the flow is profuse. However, if many clots appear and the flow seems excessive, medical advice is recommended, since these conditions may be a sign of fibroid tumors in the uterus.

Oral Contraceptives

Women on combination birth-control pills can expect to see a changed menstrual pattern. The flow becomes slighter than before and very regular. For a discussion of oral contraceptives, see "Birth Control" in Ch. 4, *The Beginning of a Family.*

Odor

The menstrual flow of a healthy woman generally has a mild odor that develops when it is exposed to the air or to the vulva. Some women are concerned about this odor, although it usually is not offensive. When it is, it tends to be associated with inade-quate bathing. Detergents are added to some commercial tampons and pad products, and special deodorants have been developed to mask the odor. However, such materials produce allergic reactions in some women, and they can have the unfortunate effect of masking an odor that may be the sign of an abnormal con-dition.

Onset of Menopause

Menstrual irregularities almost always precede the natural cessation of menstrual function. For a full discussion of menopause, see Ch. 5, *The Middle Years.*

Postmenopausal Bleeding

Bleeding that occurs after the final cessation of menstrual activity should be seen as an urgent signal to seek medical advice. The bleeding may be painless or painful and may range from occasional spotting that is brownish or bright red to rather profuse bleeding that continues for several days or more. The various signs and symptoms should be noted carefully because they can help suggest to a physician the possible cause of bleeding. Bleeding after the menopause is often a sign of cancer of the cervix or the lining of the uterus, but there is a wide variety of other possible causes, including polyps, ulcers, hypertensive heart disease, an ovarian tumor, or infection. In many cases, the problem can be treated by dilation and curettage or withdrawal of any hormone medications, such as estrogens prescribed for menopausal symptoms, or both. In these cases, if D and C and treatment and discontinuance of hormone therapy fail, the physician may advise a hysterectomy.

Infections of the Reproductive Tract

Vaginal and other reproductive tract infections are among the most common gynecological problems, and among the most stubborn to treat successfully.

Leukorrhea

A whitish, somewhat viscid discharge from the vagina, which is known medically as *leukorrhea,* may be quite normal, especially if it is not continual but occurs only intermittently—prior to menstruation, for example, or associated with sexual excitation. It may also be increased when oral contraceptives are used.

Constant leukorrhea, on the other hand, often is a symptom of an abnormality. Leukorrhea resulting from disease can occur at any age. It is generally associated with an infection of the lower reproductive tract. The discharge may occur without any discomfort, but in some cases there is itching, irritation, and *dyspareunia*—or painful intercourse.

Laboratory tests of vaginal secretions may be needed to help identify the precise cause of the discharge. Leukorrhea can result from vaginal ul-cers; a tumor of the vagina, uterus, or fallopian tubes; gonorrhea; or infection by any of various disease organisms of the vulva, vagina, cervix, uterus, or tubes. It may also result from an abnormality of menstrual function, or even emotional stress.

Treatment, of course, depends on the cause. If the discharge is because of an infection, care must be taken to avoid being reinfected or transmitting the disease organism through sexual contact or possibly contaminated underclothing, etc.

Moniliasis

Moniliasis, also known as *candidiasis,* is an infection by a yeastlike fungus that invades mucous membrane and sometimes skin in various parts of the body. Inside the mouth, the organism causes thrush, most commonly in babies. When the organism invades the vaginal area, it causes a scant white discharge of a thick consistency resembling that of cottage cheese. There is itching, burning, and swelling of the labial and vulvar areas. The symptoms tend to worsen just before the menstrual period. The occurrence of the disease is thought by some researchers to be fostered by oral contraceptives. Antibiotic therapy may increase the moniliasis organism because it destroys many of the benign organisms that regularly share the same environment.

Moniliasis is treated with suppositories, creams, and other medications. The woman's partner should be treated at the same time to prevent a cycle of reinfection because the fungus will otherwise spread to the genital tissues of the man.

Trichomoniasis

A type of leukorrhea that consists of a copious yellow to green frothy and fetid discharge is caused by infection by the *Trichomonas* organism. The organism causes an irritating itching condition that tends to set in or worsen just after a menstrual period. The condition is diagnosed by a test similar to a Pap smear, made with a specimen taken from the vagina. Trichomonas organisms, if present, are easy to identify under a microscope;

they are pear-shaped protozoa with three to five whiplike tails.

The organism favors warm, moist areas, such as genital tissues, but it can also survive in damp towels and washcloths, around toilet seats, and on beaches and the perimeters of swimming pools. Thus it can spread from one member of a family to other members and from one woman to other women. *Trichomoniasis* is not technically a venereal disease, but it can be transmitted by sexual contact. When one partner is infected with trichomoniasis, both must be treated at the same time and a condom must be worn during intercourse.

Several drugs are available for treating trichomoniasis, including tablets taken orally and suppositories inserted in the vagina. The tablets are taken for ten days, then an examination is made to determine if any *Trichomonas* organisms are still present. Medication may be continued for several months if the infection resists the drug—studies show that the organism appears to survive in about 10 percent of treated cases.

Herpes Simplex Virus Type 2

Herpes is acquired by contact with the mucous membranes of an infected person. The mucous membrane of the mouth and lips, the genitals, or the rectum may be affected. The causative agent is known as *herpes simplex virus Type II*, or *HSV-II*. It is similar to but not the same as the virus that causes fever blisters, or cold sores, which is Type *I* (HSV-I). The virus is associated with some sponta- neous abortions. If the mother has blisters at the time of delivery, the virus can be transmitted to the baby as he or she passes through the vagina. The central nervous system, including the brain, may be damaged by the virus if the baby becomes infected. To avoid exposure to the virus, a caesarian delivery is recommended.

Symptoms

Patients with their first HSV-II infection usually complain of intense itching, painful blisterlike eruptions, and ulcerated patches with a discharge. Other symptoms may include genital pain and vaginal bleeding. Fever, swelling, difficult urination, and a gen- eral feeling of ill health and lack of appetite may accompany the infection.

Symptoms may subside after a few weeks, but recurrences are common, though they are less painful and of shorter duration. There is no known cure for the viral infection.

Treatment

No drug has been found to attack the viruses while they are "hibernating" in cells at the base of the spine. But one antiviral drug, *acyclovir*, has been found to reduce recurrent outbreaks and to block flareups for up to several months. Taken orally in pill form, acyclovir is ingested daily. Some patients can stop taking acyclovir and still have no further flare-ups. Researchers have discovered that the capsules kill or neutralize the herpes viruses only when they are active. Because of evidence that the virus may be related to the subsequent development of cervical cancer, women sufferers should have Pap-smear tests at intervals of six months instead of the usual twelve.

Pelvic Inflammatory Disease

Pelvic inflammatory disease, or PID, is on the increase in the female population. Commonly caused by bacteria from other diseases such as chlamydia or gonorrhea, PID may go for years without detection. Frequently symptomless, PID infects and destroys the interior of the reproductive system. It attacks the fallopian tubes and uterine lining, leaving permanent scarring. The increase in the number of ectopic pregnancies (fallopian tube pregnancies) is believed to stem from the increase in women who have scarring from PID. The increase in sterility in the population is also linked directly to PID scarring.

One is seven women in the United States has been infected with PID. Treatment for both partners involves antibiotics to kill the bacteria, and treatment of any original disease that may have caused it. Douching should be avoided if PID is suspected. Symptoms include abdominal tenderness or pain, vaginal discharge, or dull ache or twitching in the uterine cavity.

Blood tests and cultures for chlamydia or other diseases should be done. Two-thirds of PID cases are from sexual transmission. If left untreated, PID can cause sterility, miscarriage, ectopic pregnancy, blood infection, and eventually death.

Disorders of the Urinary System

Both men and women are subject to disorders of the urinary system. There are, however, a few disorders that affect women chiefly or women only, for reasons related to anatomical structure. See also Ch. 17, *Diseases of the Urinogenital System.*

Inflammation of the Bladder

Any inflammation of the bladder is known medically as *cystitis*. Factors such as urinary tract stones, injury, and obstructions to the normal flow of urine can aggravate or cause cystitis in either sex. Cystitis resulting from infectious organisms, however, is much more common in women than in men. This is understandable in view of the relative shortness of the female urethra—the tube through which urine is discharged from the bladder and through which infectious organisms can reach the bladder from the outside. In addition, the anus and the vagina, both of which may frequently be sources of infection, are situated relatively close to the external opening of the female urethra.

In women generally, the symptoms of cystitis may include a burning sensation around the edges of the vulva. There is usually a frequent urge to urinate and difficulty or pain (*dysuria*) associated with urination. Urinary retention and dehydration, which are generally under the control of the individual, can contribute to the spread of infection once it begins. The lining of the urinary bladder is relatively resistant to infection by most microorganisms as long as the normal flow of liquids through the urinary tract is maintained. In cases that do not yield quickly to copious fluid intake, there are medications that may be prescribed to cure the infection. Where urinary frequency or difficulty is accompanied by the appearance of blood in the urine, a physician should be consulted immediately.

Honeymoon Cystitis

One type of cystitis tends to occur mostly in young women during the first few weeks of frequent sexual activity, to which it is attributed. Sexual activity may result in swelling of the urethra and the neck of the bladder, making urination difficult. The inflammation of these tissues can in turn make them more susceptible to infection. A treatment recommended specifically for honeymoon cystitis is to drink large quantities of water or other fluids and to empty the bladder before and after engaging in sexual intercourse. Adequate lubrication, such as K-Y Jelly℠ or a water-soluble product, is also important. Medical care should be sought if the condition persists.

Urethral Disorders

The urethra is perforce involved in the inflammation of cystitis because it is the route by which infectious organisms reach the bladder. In addition, there are disorders that are essentially confined to the urethra.

Urethral Caruncle

Urethral caruncle is a rather uncommon urinary tract disorder that tends to be confined to women after the menopause. A *caruncle* (not to be confused with *carbuncle*) is a small, red, fleshy outgrowth. It may be visible near the opening of the urethra. A caruncle growing from the cells of the urethra may be a sign of a bacterial infection, a tumor, or any of several other possible conditions. Symptoms may include vaginal bleeding, pain, tenderness, painful sexual intercourse (dyspareunia), a whitish, viscid discharge, and difficulty in urinating. A physician should be consulted when such symptoms are present. A tissue biopsy and Pap smear may be taken to diagnose the condition. Caruncles are easily treated and of no long-term consequence.

Urethral Diverticulum

Another disorder of the urethra is a *urethral diverticulum,* or outpocketing of the urethra. The problem can be caused by a developmental malformation, an injury, inflammation, a cyst, a urinary stone, or a venereal disease. Stones are a common cause, and in some patients there may be more than one diverticulum. The symptoms may include discomfort and urinary difficulty, as well as dyspareunia. The disorder can be diagnosed with the help of X-ray photographs of the region of the urethra and bladder after they have been filled with a radiopaque substance that flows into any diverticula that may be present.

Treatment of a urethral diverticulum includes antibiotics to stop infection, medications to relieve pain and discomfort, and douches. In some cases, surgery is needed to eliminate the diverticula.

Structural Anomalies

Various kinds of injury may be sustained by the female reproductive system and other abdominal organs, chiefly as a result of childbearing. The structural damage can generally be repaired by surgical measures.

Fistula

An abnormal opening between two organs or from an organ to the outside of the body is known as a *fistula*. Fistulas may involve the urinary and reproductive systems of a woman. Damage to the organs during pregnancy or surgery, for example, can result in a fistula between the urethra and the vagina, causing urinary incontinence. A similar kind of fistula can develop between the rectum and the vagina as a result of injury, complications of pregnancy, or surgery. Disorders of this sort must be repaired surgically.

Prolapsed Uterus

The uterus normally rests on the floor of the pelvis, held in position by numerous ligaments. Damage to the ligaments and other supporting tissues causes the uterus to descend, or *prolapse,* into the vagina. There are various degrees of prolapse, ranging from a slight intrusion of the uterus into the vagina to a severe condition in which the cervix of the uterus protrudes out of the vaginal orifice. Prolapse of the uterus resembles a hernia but is not a true hernia, because the opening through which the uterus protrudes is a normal one.

Backache and a feeling of heaviness in the pelvic region may accompany the condition. Many women complain of a "dragging" sensation. An assortment of complications may involve neighboring organ systems; bleeding and ulceration of the uterus are not uncommon. Coughing and straining can aggravate the symptoms.

Like the various types of hernia, a prolapsed uterus does not improve without treatment but tends instead to worsen gradually. The only permanent treatment is surgical repair. In mild cases, a woman may get relief from symptoms through exercises intended to strengthen the muscles of the pelvic region. Supporting devices,

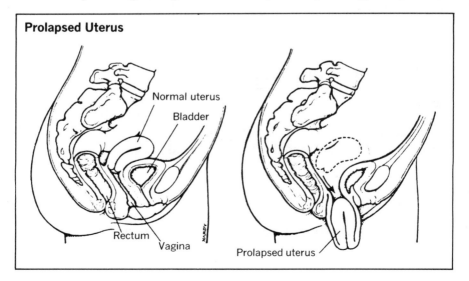

Prolapsed Uterus

Normal uterus
Bladder
Rectum
Vagina
Prolapsed uterus

such as an inflatable, doughnut-shaped pessary, are available as temporary methods of correcting a prolapse. Preventive exercises may be recommended for childbearing women who want to avoid weakened muscles and ligaments leading to prolapse.

Tipped Uterus

The uterus may be out of its normal position without being prolapsed. A malpositioned uterus may be "tipped" forward, backward, or otherwise be out of alignment with neighboring organs. A malpositioned uterus may cause no symptoms, or it may be associated with dysmenorrhea or infertility. If a malpositioned uterus causes pain, bleeding, or other problems, the condition can be corrected surgically, or a pessary support may relieve the symptoms. Displacement of the uterus occasionally is the result of a separate pelvic disease that requires treatment.

Hernias of the Vaginal Wall

The wall of the vagina may be ruptured in childbirth, especially in a mul-

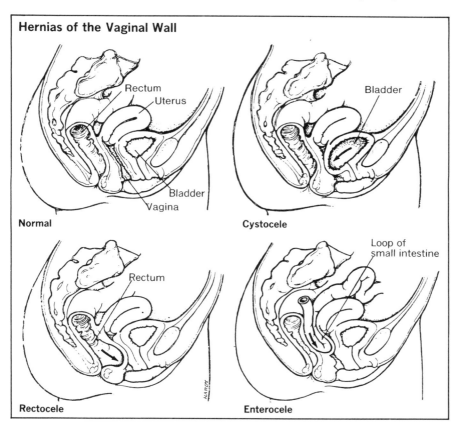

Hernias of the Vaginal Wall

Normal — Rectum, Uterus, Bladder, Vagina

Cystocele — Bladder

Rectocele — Rectum

Enterocele — Loop of small intestine

tiple delivery or birth of a larger-than-average baby. The kind of hernia depends on the exact site of the rupture and what organ happens to lie against the vaginal wall at that point. The condition may be further complicated by a prolapsed uterus. Careful examina-tion of the patient and X-ray pictures may be necessary to determine whether just one or several of the urinary, reproductive, and gastrointestinal organs in the pelvic cavity are involved.

Cystocele

Cystocele is a hernia involving the bladder and the vagina. Structurally, part of the bladder protrudes through the wall of the vagina. The symptoms, in addition to a feeling of pressure deep in the vagina, may be urinary difficulties, such as incontinence, a frequent urge to urinate, and inability to completely empty the bladder. Residual urine in the bladder may contribute to infection and inflammation of the bladder. Treatment includes surgery to correct the condition, pessaries if needed to support the structures, and medications to control infection.

Rectocele

A hernia involving the tissues separating the vagina and the rectum, behind the vagina, is called a *rectocele*. The symptoms are a feeling of fullness in the vagina and difficulty in defecating. Enemas or laxatives may be needed to relieve constipation be-cause straining, or even coughing, can aggravate the condition. Surgery is the only permanently effective treatment. Special diets, laxatives, and rectal suppositories may be prescribed pending surgery.

Enterocele

A herniation of the small intestine into the vagina is called an *enterocele*. Some of the symptoms are similar to those of other hernias involving the vaginal wall, and in addition, a patient with an enterocele may experience abdominal cramps shortly after eating. An enterocele can be dangerous, as well as uncomfortable, because a segment of the small bowel can become trapped and obstructed, requiring emergency surgery.

Varicose Veins

Varicose veins of the vulva, vagina, and neighboring areas are another possible effect of pregnancy, although the legs are more often affected. Obesity, reduced physical activity during pregnancy, and circulatory changes associated with pregnancy can contribute to the development of varicose veins. The symptoms generally are limited to discomfort, although there can be bleeding, particularly at the time of childbirth. Varicose veins that occur in the vulva and vagina during pregnancy and cause discomfort can be treated surgically during the early months of pregnancy. Some drugs and supportive therapy can be used to help relieve symptoms. But many physicians recommend that surgical stripping of veins be delayed until after the pregnancy has been terminated. A complication of untreated varicose veins can be development of blood clots in the abnormal blood vessels. For a discussion of varicose veins of the legs during pregnancy, see "Leg Cramps and Varicose Veins" in Ch. 4, *The Beginning of a Family.*

Benign Neoplasms

The word *neoplasm* refers to any abnormal proliferation of tissue that serves no useful function. There are numerous kinds of neoplasms but just two main groups—cancerous, or *malignant;* or noncancerous, or *benign.* In ordinary speech the word *benign* suggests some positive benefit, but a benign neoplasm, though noncancer-

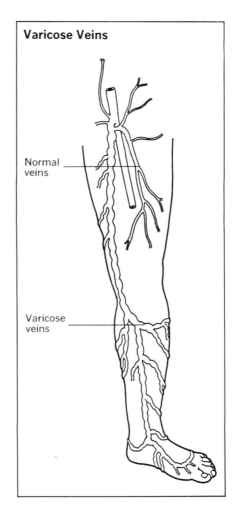

Varicose Veins

Normal veins

Varicose veins

ous, may in fact be harmful to health or at least worrisome. Benign neoplasms that are of particular concern to women are discussed below.

Cysts

A *cyst* is a sac containing a gaseous, fluid, or semisolid material. (Certain normal anatomical structures, like the urinary bladder, are technically known as cysts—hence the term *cystitis* for inflammation of the bladder.) Abnormal, or neoplastic, cysts can develop at several sites within the urinary and reproductive systems.

Vaginal Cysts

A cyst may develop in a gland at the opening of the vagina as a result of infection with a venereal or other disease. Such a cyst can block the flow of secretions from the gland and produce swelling and pain. Dyspareunia, or painful intercourse, is sometimes a symptom. A vaginal-gland cyst usually is treated with antibiotics and hot packs. In some cases, it may be necessary for a physician to make an incision to drain the cyst.

Ovarian Cysts

Cysts in the ovaries may be caused by a malfunction of physiological process or by a pathological condition. Some pathological cysts are malignant. The cysts in the ovaries generally are filled with fluid that may range in color from pale and clear to reddish brown, depending upon the source of the fluid. Some cysts are too small to be seen with the naked eye, whereas others may be four or five inches in diameter when symptoms begin to cause discomfort. There are several different kinds of ovarian cysts.

Follicular Cyst

A *follicular,* or *retention,* cyst is a physiological cyst and is one of the most common types. It develops in an old follicle in which an ovum for some reason has failed to break out of its capsule during the ovulation process. Ordinarily, the contents of such a follicle are resorbed, but sometimes a cyst develops. It rarely grows larger than about two inches in diameter. It may rupture but usually disappears after a few months. The symptoms may include pain with some uterine bleeding and dyspareunia. Treatment consists of warm douches, analgesics, and hormone therapy designed to restore normal ovarian activity. If the symptoms persist or the cyst continues to increase in size, or if serious complications occur, the physician may recommend exploratory surgery.

Occasionally such cysts, whether or not they rupture, produce symptoms that mimic those of appendicitis, with severe abdominal pain. The abdomen may become so tender that a physician cannot palpate the organs in order to distinguish between an ovarian cyst and appendicitis, particularly if the right ovary is involved. The symptoms occur at the time that ovulation would be expected. If the physician cannot be certain that the cause of the abdominal pain is indeed a cyst, for which surgery is not needed, he may recommend surgery anyway—just to be on the safe side.

Multiple follicular cysts, involving the ovaries on both sides (*bilateral polycystic ovaries*) can result in a syndrome (or group of symptoms) that includes infertility, obesity, and abnormal growth of body hair. All of these effects are related to a disruption of normal sex-hormone activity; they generally occur in young women, from teenagers to those in their 20s. The therapy includes both medical and surgical efforts to restore normal menstrual function, a diet to control obesity, and the use of various depilatory techniques to remove unwanted body hair.

Corpus Luteum Cyst

This kind of cyst may develop in the ovary following ovulation or during the early part of a pregnancy. The corpus luteum is a small, temporary gland that forms in the empty follicle after the ovum has been released from the ovary. Its function is to produce the hormone progesterone, which is important in preparing the endometrium, the lining of the uterus, to receive a fertilized ovum. The corpus luteum, however, also can be overproductive of a brownish fluid that fills the former follicular space, causing it to swell to a diameter of two or three inches. The cyst causes symptoms of pain and tenderness and may also result in a disruption of normal menstrual cycles in a woman who is not pregnant.

Most corpus luteum cysts gradually decrease in size without special treatment, except to relieve the symptoms. There may, however, be complications, such as torsion, or painful twisting of the ovary, or a rupture of the cyst. A ruptured corpus luteum cyst can result in hemorrhage and peritonitis, requiring immediate surgery.

Chocolate Cyst

So called because of their brownish-red color, chocolate cysts consist of misplaced endometrial tissue growing on the ovary instead of in its normal position lining the uterus. Chocolate cysts are among the largest of the ovarian cysts, ranging up to five or six inches in diameter. They cause symptoms associated with a variety of disorders of the reproductive system, including infertility, dyspareunia, and dysmenorrhea. Surgery usually is a favored method of therapy, the precise procedure depending upon the amount of ovarian tissue involved. A small chocolate cyst can be cauterized, but a large cyst may require removal of a portion of the ovary. See also "Cancer of the Ovary" later in this chapter.

Cysts of the Breast

Cysts are noncancerous tissues masses that may form in the milk glands or the ducts leading from the glands. They are caused by imbalances in ovarian hormones and they tend to develop in women of all ages and tend to disappear once women reach menopause. The cysts tend to fluctuate in size, often enlarging just before or during menstruation. Pain and tenderness are usually present, although painless cysts are sometimes discovered only when a woman examines her breasts for possible lumps. Cysts may be almost microscopic in size or as large as an inch or more in diameter. It is not uncommon for more than one cyst to occur at the same time in one breast or both.

A medical examination is recommended when any kind of lump can be felt in the breast tissue. This is particularly important for women who have passed menopause. The physician frequently can determine whether a lump is a result of a cyst or cancer by the patient's history and by physical examination, especially when repeated at intervals of several weeks. Mammography and ultrsound are used to confirm the diagnosis.

Women who are troubled by breast cysts may be helped by wearing a good brassiere at all times, even during sleep, to protect tender areas. The only medications available are those that relieve pain and discomfort — symptoms that usually subside when the menopause is reached.

Other Noncancerous Masses

A benign lump in the breast can be caused by either a fat deposit or an abscess. A fatty mass frequently forms if an injury to the breast damages adipose tissue. Because of a similarity of the symptoms to those of breast cancer, a biopsy is usually required to distinguish the lesion from a cancer. The involved tissue may in any case be removed surgically.

An abscess of the breast as a result of an infection, although a rare problem, may produce a lump that requires treatment with antibiotic medications or by an incision to drain the pus. Breast infections leading to abscesses are most likely to occur in nursing mothers but can also develop in women who are not lactating. When an infection develops in a breast being used to nurse a baby, nursing has to be discontinued temporarily while the infection is treated. See also "Cancer of the Breast" later in this chapter.

Polyps

A *polyp* is a strange-looking growth, even for an abnormal growth of tissue. It has been described as having the appearance of a tennis racket or a small mushroom. Polyps are found in many parts of the body, from the nose to the rectum. Usually they are harmless. But a polyp can result in discomfort or bleeding and require surgical excision. Although polyps generally are not cancerous, it is standard procedure to have the polyp tissue, like any excised tissue, tested in the laboratory. If malignant cells accompany a polyp, they are usually found at the base of the growth, which means that some of the tissue around the polyp must be excised along with the growth itself. Once a polyp is removed it does not grow again, although other polyps can occur in the same region.

Cervical Polyp

Polyps in the cervix are not uncommon, occurring most frequently in the years between menarche and menopause. A cervical polyp may be associated with vaginal bleeding or leukorrhea; the bleeding may occur after douching or sexual intercourse. In some cases, the bleeding is severe. Cervical polyps can usually be located visually by an examining physician and removed by minor surgery.

Endometrial Polyp

Endometrial polyps, which develop in the lining of the uterus, usually occur in women who are over 40, although they can develop at any age after menarche. They are frequently the cause of nonmenstrual bleeding. They tend to be much larger than polyps that grow in other organs of the body: an endometrial polyp may be rooted high in the uterus with a stem reaching all the way to the cervix. Such a polyp is usually located and removed during a D- and C- procedure. As in the case of a cervical polyp, the growth and a bit of surrounding tissue are studied for traces of cancer cells.

Benign Tumors

Tumors are rather firm growths that may be either benign or malignant. In practice, any tumor is regarded with suspicion unless malignancy is ruled out by actual laboratory tests. Even a benign tumor represents a tissue abnormality, and if untreated can produce symptoms that interfere with normal health and activity.

Fibromas

Among the more common of the benign tumors is the *fibroma*, commonly known as a *fibroid tumor*, composed of fibrous connective tissue. About one of every 20 ovarian tumors is a fibroma, and a similar growth in the uterus is the most common type of tumor found in that organ. Fibromas also occur in the vulva.

Ovarian Fibroma

Ovarian fibromas are usually small, but there are instances in which they have grown to weigh as much as five pounds. A large fibroma can be very painful and produce symptoms such as a feeling of heaviness in the pelvic area, nausea, and vomiting. The growth may crowd other organs of the body, causing enlargement of the abdomen and cardiac and respiratory symptoms. The only treatment is surgical removal of the tumor, after which there is usually a quick and full recovery.

Uterine Fibroma

Fibroid tumors of the uterus can also grow to a very large size, some weighing many pounds. Like ovarian fibromas, they can press against neighboring organs such as the intestine or the urinary bladder, producing constipation or urinary difficulty. More commonly, there is pain and vaginal bleeding, along with pelvic pressure and enlargement of the abdomen. It is possible in some cases for a fibroid tumor to grow slowly in the uterus for several years without causing serious discomfort to the patient. If the tumor obstructs or distorts the reproductive tract, it may be a cause of infertility.

Treatment of fibroid tumors varies according to their size, the age of the patient and her expectations about having children, and other factors. If the tumor is small and does not appear to be growing at a rapid rate, the physician may recommend that surgery be postponed as long as the tumor poses no threat to health. For an older woman, or for a woman who does not want to bear children, a hysterectomy may be advised, especially if symptoms are troublesome. If the patient is a young woman who wants to have children, the physician is likely to advise a *myomectomy,* a surgical excision of the tumor, since a fibroid tumor of the uterus can cause serious complications during pregnancy and labor. It can result in abortion or premature labor, malpresentation of the fetus, difficult labor, and severe loss of blood during childbirth. While fibroid tumors of the uterus are not malignant, special tests are made of the endometrial tissue as part of any myomectomy or hysterectomy to rule out the possibility that cancer cells may be involved in the disorder.

Endometriosis

Endometriosis is the medical term for a condition in which endometrial tissue, the special kind of tissue that lines the uterus, grows in various areas of the pelvic cavity outside the uterus. Endometrial cells may invade such unlikely places as the ovaries (the most common site), the bladder, appendix, Fallopian tubes, intestinal tract, or the supporting structure of the uterus. The external endometrial tissue may appear as small blisters of endometrial cells, as solid nodules, or as cysts, usually of the ovary, which may be four inches or more in diameter, like the chocolate cysts of the ovaries. Such a mass of sometimes tumorlike endometrial cells is called an *endometrioma.*

The misplaced endometrial tissue causes problems because it goes through menstrual cycles just as the endometrium does within the cavity of the uterus. The endometrial tissue proliferates after ovulation and may cause almost constant pain, wherever it is located, for a few days before the start of menstruation. The symptoms subside after the menstrual flow begins. The effects may include dyspa-

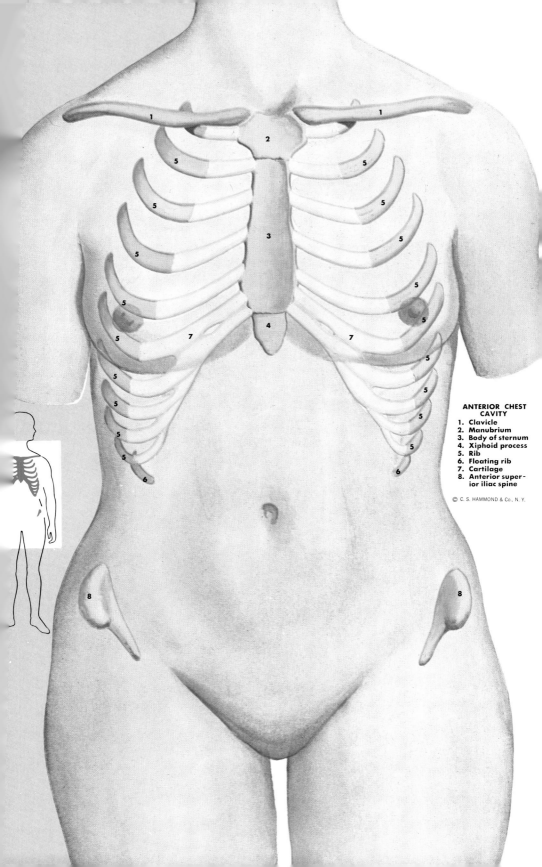

ANTERIOR CHEST
CAVITY
1. Clavicle
2. Manubrium
3. Body of sternum
4. Xiphoid process
5. Rib
6. Floating rib
7. Cartilage
8. Anterior super-
   ior iliac spine

© C. S. HAMMOND & Co., N. Y.

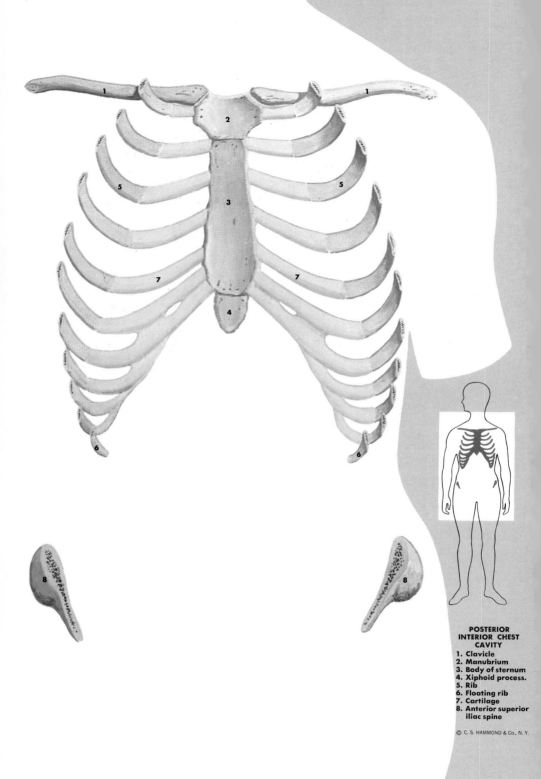

**POSTERIOR
INTERIOR CHEST
CAVITY**
1. Clavicle
2. Manubrium
3. Body of sternum
4. Xiphoid process.
5. Rib
6. Floating rib
7. Cartilage
8. Anterior superior
   iliac spine

© C. S. HAMMOND & Co., N. Y.

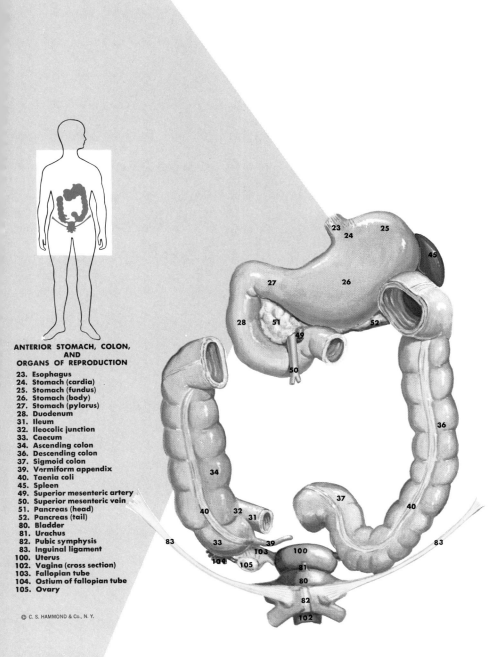

**ANTERIOR STOMACH, COLON,
AND
ORGANS OF REPRODUCTION**

23. Esophagus
24. Stomach (cardia)
25. Stomach (fundus)
26. Stomach (body)
27. Stomach (pylorus)
28. Duodenum
31. Ileum
32. Ileocolic junction
33. Caecum
34. Ascending colon
36. Descending colon
37. Sigmoid colon
39. Vermiform appendix
40. Taenia coli
45. Spleen
49. Superior mesenteric artery
50. Superior mesenteric vein
51. Pancreas (head)
52. Pancreas (tail)
80. Bladder
81. Urachus
82. Pubic symphysis
83. Inguinal ligament
100. Uterus
102. Vagina (cross section)
103. Fallopian tube
104. Ostium of fallopian tube
105. Ovary

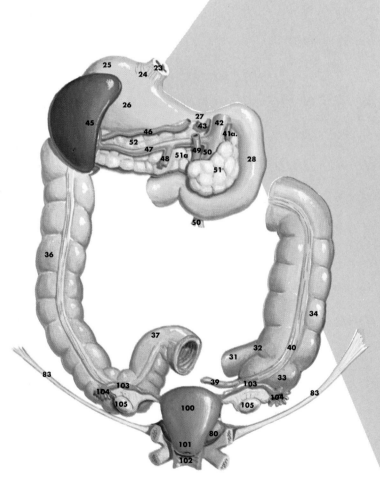

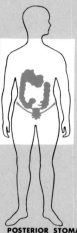

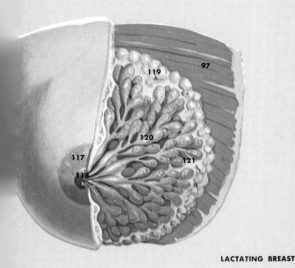
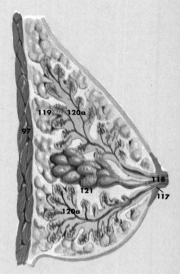

LACTATING BREAST

97.	**Pectoralis major muscle**
117.	**Areola**
118.	**Nipple**
119.	**Fat**
120.	**Lactiferous (milk producing) glands and ducts**
120a.	**Cross section of gland and duct**
121.	**Tissue separating and supporting glandular tissue**

STRUCTURE OF THE MAMMARY GLANDS

The mammary glands are composed of three major elements:
1. Their skin covering and special structures (nipple, areola).
2. The lactiferous glands or functional units of the breast.
3. The supporting structures, the connective tissue "ligaments" and the fat tissue that makes up the mass of the breast.

The breast is supported by the "suspensory ligaments." These are anchored to the sheet of connective tissue surrounding the pectoralis major muscle, and extend in a complex network separated by the fat tissue outward to the skin. The lactiferous glands are buried in the supporting tissues and empty outward onto the surface of the nipple. These glands at first are very small and clustered just beneath the nipple and areola. In pregnancy they enlarge and push downward into the mass of the breast causing it to enlarge in turn. The enlargement continues through the period of breast feeding, following which the glands gradually grow smaller and the entire breast returns to normal size.

S. HAMMOND & Co., N. Y.

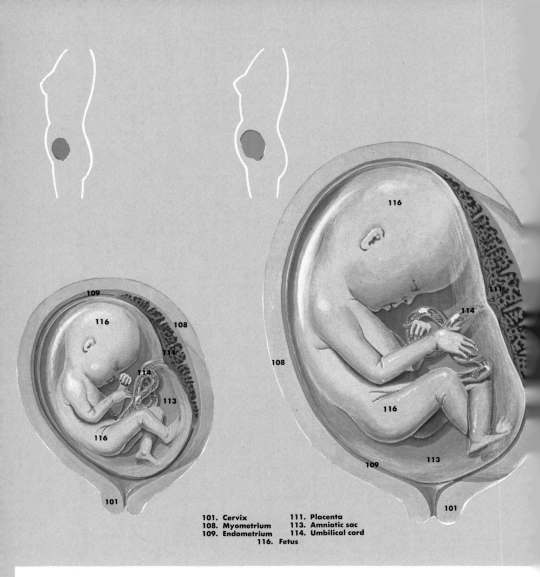

101. Cervix
108. Myometrium
109. Endometrium
111. Placenta
113. Amniotic sac
114. Umbilical cord
116. Fetus

THE FETUS AT 3 1/2 AND 6 MONTHS

Most of the definitive development of the fetus occurs during the first 3½ months, and the remaining 5½ months is primarily concerned with gradual increase in size and maturation of organs already begun. The fetus receives all of its nourishment through the placenta and umbilical cord. There is no direct contact between fetal and maternal blood in the placenta. During its entire development, the fetus floats in a fluid (amniotic fluid) contained within a sac (the amniotic sac) attached to the placenta. This sac is in turn surrounded by the uterine cavity, the endometrium and the muscle or myometrium of the uterus.

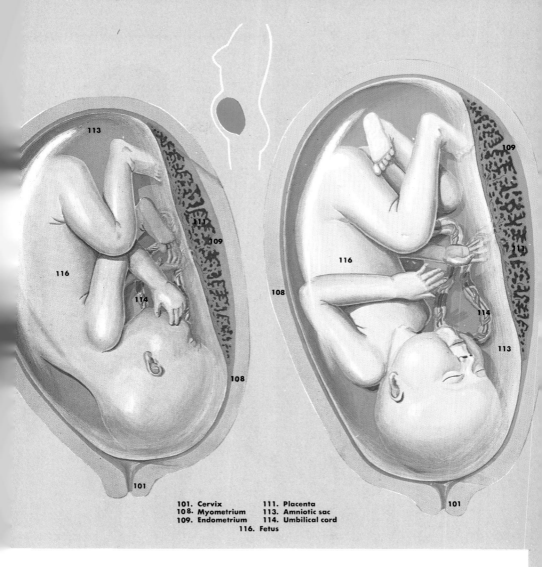

101. Cervix	111. Placenta
108. Myometrium	113. Amniotic sac
109. Endometrium	114. Umbilical cord
116. Fetus	

THE FETUS AT 8 AND 9 MONTHS

Until birth, the fetus is surrounded by the amniotic sac and fluid, and attached to the placenta by the umbilical cord. The fetus continues to increase in size and the uterus stretches to accommodate it. Usually before the eighth month the fetus assumes a head-downward position. At birth, the amniotic sac ruptures, the fluid escapes, and the child is slowly pushed out of the uterine cavity by the contractions of the myometrium. Shortly after birth of the child, the placenta is similarly expelled having been detached from the endometrium.

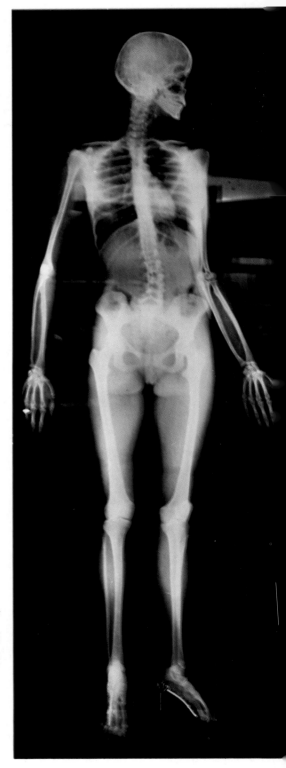

X-RAY OF THE HUMAN BODY
SHOWING THE
BONE STRUCTURE

reunia, rectal bleeding, backache, and generalized pain in the pelvic region as sensitive tissues throughout the pelvic cavity are irritated by monthly cycles of swelling and bleeding.

Because infertility is associated with endometriosis, which can become progressively worse, young women who want to bear children are sometimes encouraged to begin efforts to become pregnant as early as possible if they show signs or symptoms of the disorder. Treatment includes hormone medication and surgery to remove the lesions of endometriosis or the organ involved. For patients with extensive spread of endometrial tissue outside the uterus,

the physician may recommend removal of one or both ovaries. Destruction of the ovaries surgically or by radiation therapy may be employed to eliminate the menstrual cycle activity that aggravates the symptoms of endometriosis. These procedures cause sterility and premature menopause, but some women prefer this to the discomfort of endometriosis. The hormone therapy inhibits the ovulation phase of the menstrual cycle. Without ovulation, the endometrial tissue does not proliferate. For this reason, pregnancy often eliminates or eases the symptoms of endometriosis during parturition and for a period of time thereafter.

Dyspareunia

Dyspareunia, or painful intercourse, is often associated with endometriosis and is attributed to irritation of nerve fibers in the area of the cervix from the pressure of sexual activity. There are many other possible causes of painful intercourse, some functional and some organic in nature. In addition to endometriosis, the problem may be owing to a vaginal contracture, a disorder involving the muscles of the pelvic region, inflammation of the vagina or urethra, prolapsed or malpositioned uterus, *cervicitis* (inflammation of the cervix), or a disorder of the bladder or rectum. A cause

of dyspareunia in older women may be a degeneration of the tissues lining the vagina, which become thin and dry. Temporary therapy for dyspareunia may include water-soluble lubricants, anesthetic ointments, steroid hormones, analgesics, and sedatives. In appropriate cases, surgery is effective in correcting an organic cause of painful sexual intercourse. Functional or psychogenic (of psychological origin) causes of dyspareunia usually require psychological counseling for the patient and her sexual partner.

Backache

Still another effect of endometriosis that can suggest other disorders is backache. When endometrial tissue invades the pelvic region, there may

be a fairly constant pain in the back near the tailbone or the rectum. Usually the backache subsides only after the cause has been eliminated. Temporary measures include those advised for other kinds of backache: sleeping on a firm mattress, preferably reinforced with a sheet of plywood between springs and mattress; application of dry heat or warm baths; sedatives to relieve tension, and analgesics to relieve the pain.

A backache that radiates down the back and into a leg, following the path of a sciatic nerve, can be the result of a disorder of the ovaries or uterus. An ovarian cyst or infection of the Fallopian tubes can produce a backache that seems to be centered in the lumbosacral area of the spinal column. Such backaches, sometimes called gynecologic backaches, tend to occur most frequently during a woman's childbearing years and more often affect women who have had several children than women who have not been pregnant. Tumors also can produce backache symptoms. X-ray pictures, myelograms, and laboratory studies may be required in order to rule out the possibilities that the back pain may be caused by a tumor, a herniated or "slipped" disk, or a deformity of the spinal column that might have been aggravated by one or more pregnancies. Most backaches, however, relate to poor posture or muscle tension. Anxiety or other kinds of emotional stress can aggravate the symptoms. See also "Backaches" in Ch. 23, *Aches, Pains, Nuisances, Worries,* and "Back Pain and Its Causes" in Ch. 25, *Women's Health.*

Cancers of the Reproductive System

Cancer of the Cervix

The cervix of the uterus is the ninth most common site of cancers affecting women. As compared with all cancers of the reproductive organs of women, it rates third, after uterine cancer and ovarian cancer. It has been estimated that about 13,000 cases of cervical cancer are found among American women each year, and approximately 4,500 deaths every year are a result of this disease.

The number of cases of pre-invasive cervical cancer is down because of the increased number of women who undergo regular gynecological examination. When cancer is diagnosed early, the survival rate increases tremendously for the patient.

The actual causes of cervical cancer are still unknown. Current medical thinking suggests that there is no causal relationship between cervical cancer and the use of oral contraceptives.

Preinvasive Stage

The earliest signs of cervical cancer tend to appear between the ages of 25 and 45. At this early, *preinvasive* stage, the cancer is described as *in situ*—confined to its original site. If the cancer is not treated at this stage, the disease spreads and becomes a typical invasive cancer within five to ten years. Signs of bleeding and ulceration usually do not appear until this has occurred. However, because of the relatively slow growth of cervical cancer in the early stage, the disease usually can be detected by a Pap smear test before it becomes invasive.

Invasive Cancer

Cancer that has spread beyond the cervix is far more difficult to treat. Surgery, radiation or chemotherapy, and regular examinations to catch any recurrence of cancer will probably be necessary. It is unusual for anyone to develop invasive cancer without knowing it, if she has undergone regular, routine pelvic exams.

Diagnostic Methods

Pap Smear Test

The *Pap smear* test (named for Dr. George Papanicolaou, who developed the technique in 1928) is a quick and simple method of detecting cancerous cells in secretions and scrapings from mucous membrane. It requires the collection of small samples of cells from the surface of the cervix and from the cervical canal. Such samples are obtained by inserting a plastic spatula or a brush-tipped tube into the vagina, into which a speculum has been placed previously. The device is scraped gently over the area of the cervix. The physician may collect also a sample of vaginal secretions, which may contain possibly cancerous cells not only from the cervix but from the ovaries and uterus as well. (This is the only way a Pap smear test can be done if a woman has had a complete hysterectomy and has no cervix.) All cell samples are placed (smeared) on microscope slides and treated with a chemical preservative. The slides are sent to a laboratory for study and a report is made to the examining physician, usually within a few days, on the findings.

Results from the Pap smear are reported as: normal, inadequate sampling, showing infection, or showing cell abnormalities. Except for the normal results, Paps will be done again to ensure accuracy. No one should wait more than six months for a follow-up reading on an infectious diagnosis and treatment. For all others, follow-up should be immediate. Cell abnormalities are divided into at least three categories: low-grade lesions (non-cancerous), high-grade lesions (noncancerous), and cancer.

Other Diagnostic Tests

When a report of positive findings is returned by the laboratory, the physician immediately arranges for further studies. These involve examination of the cervix visually by a special microscopic technique known as *colposcopy,* and the removal of small tissue samples. These studies are usually done in a physician's office. In some cases a biopsy is necessary. The biopsy sample is taken when possible from the same location on the cervix as the Pap smear that resulted in positive findings. The Loop Electrosurgical Excision Procedure (LEEP) is a method of combining the biopsy and the excision of the diseased tissue. An electrified loop removes the abnormal tissue from the cervix. The small circle that is removed can then be examined for signs of cancer. The electrical charge of the loop cauterizes the cut to prevent infection and bleeding. Treatment ordinarily is not started until all of the studies have verified that there is cancer in the tissues of the cervix; other disorders, such as cervicitis, venereal infection, and polyps, can mimic symptoms of cervical cancer.

Therapy

The kind of treatment recommended for a case of cervical cancer generally depends upon several factors, such as the stage of cancer development and the age and general health of the patient. For a young woman who wishes to have children despite cancer *in situ,* which is limited to the cervix, surgeons may excise a portion of the cervix and continue watching for further developments with frequent Pap smears and other tests. The treatment of choice for cervical cancer in the early stage, however, is surgical removal of the body of the uterus, as well as of the cervix—a procedure called a *total hysterectomy.* This is the usual treatment for women over the age of 40 or for those who do not wish to have children. Sometimes more extensive surgery is necessary.

Radiation treatment may be advised for women who are not considered to be good surgical risks because of other health problems. Radiation may be recommended along with surgery for women with advanced cervical cancer in order to help destroy cancer cells that may have spread by metastasis to other tissues.

The five-year cure rate for cervical cancer is about 99 percent when treatment is started in the early, preinvasive stage. The chances of a cure drop sharply in later stages, but the five-year cure rate is still as high as 65 percent if treatment is started when the cancer has just begun to spread to the vagina or other nearby tissues.

Cancer of the Body of the Uterus

Cancer of the body of the uterus, or *endometrial cancer,* is more common than cancer of the cervix. Uterine cancer is the most common type of cancer of the reproductive organs. Cervical cancer primarily affects women before middle age; uterine cancer occurs more frequently among women beyond the menopause, with its highest rate occurring among women between the ages of 50 and 70. Survival rate for cancer of the uterus is high, with 82 percent living 5 years after diagnosis. Risk factors for uterine cancer include obesity, diabetes, and ovarian cysts. Other potential risks are for women who have taken estrogen-only pills for menopausal symptoms and women who have taken tamoxifen for breast cancer.

Diagnostic Methods

Early symptoms usually include bleeding between menstrual periods or after menopause, and occasionally a watery or blood-stained vaginal discharge. Most patients experience no pain in the early stages, although pain is a symptom in advanced uterine cancer or when the disease is complicated by an infection. Unfortunately, there is no simple test, like the Pap smear for cervical cancer, that provides a good diagnostic clue to the presence of endometrial cancer. The Pap smear does occasionally pick up cells sloughed off by the endometrium, and laboratory tests can tell if they might be malignant. The best chance for early diagnosis is for a woman to report to her gynecologist or physician any signs of abnormal bleeding between periods, or post-menopausal bleeding. Unusual bleeding should be followed up by the doctor with examination of the uterine lining.

A physician who is suspicious of symptoms of endometrial cancer must depend upon direct methods to confirm or rule out the disease. The usual method is a dilatation and curettage (D and C), during which a small sample of uterine lining will be removed for biopsy, or a sample may be withdrawn by suction (aspirated) from the uterine cavity. The cervix is dilated (opened) and the uterine lining scraped with a curette. Aspiration can be done in the physician's office with local anesthesia of the cervix or with no anesthesia. There is little or no discomfort following aspiration.

Therapy

If the diagnostic D and C is done when the abnormal bleeding associated with uterine cancer first begins, the chances of a cure are very good. The first step, if the general health of the patient permits surgery, is complete removal of the uterus, ovaries, and fallopian tubes—a procedure called a *radical hysterectomy.* Radiation may also be administered to control the spread of cancer cells.

A hysterectomy should not affect a woman's normal sexual activity. Sexual relations usually can be resumed about six to eight weeks after the operation, or when the incision has healed. If the incision is made through the pubic region or vagina, there should be little or no visible scar. See "Family Planning," in Chapter 4.

Estrogen and Cancer

There is a higher incidence of cancer of the uterus among women who have tumors of the ovary that produce estrogen, as well as among women whose menopause begins later than the usual age (and hence who have produced estrogen naturally for a longer-than-usual period). Because of the statistical associations between uterine cancer and estrogen-producing tumors, as well as other factors, the American Cancer Society has cautioned that physicians should exert "close supervision of women on estrogen, with an awareness that sustained use [of estrogens] may stimulate dormant factors in the body and lead to development of endometrial cancer." For women who are prescribed estrogen for menopause, it is recommended that the estrogen be given in combination with a synthetic progestin. Unopposed estrogen increases the growth of cancerous tumors already present, and is suspected of increasing the risk of new cancer growths.

Among the conditions for which estrogen has been prescribed for women of middle age and beyond are uncomfortable effects of menopause, such as itching and irritation caused by dryness of the vagina, and what is commonly referred to as "hot flashes." See *The Middle Years,* Ch. 5, "Menopause" for more information.

Diethylstilbestrol

An estrogenlike synthetic compound has definitely been implicated in the development of a type of cancer, *adenocarcinoma,* which primarily affects epithelial tissue. The synthetic hormone known chemically as *diethylstilbestrol* (DES) or stilbestrol was taken for the most part in the late 1940s and through the 1960s by pregnant women for the treatment of such complications as bleeding and threatened miscarriage. Around 1971, physicians became aware that some of the daughters whose mothers had taken DES during their pregnancy had developed an unusual cell formation in vaginal tissue, vaginal and cervical cancers, and some anatomical abnormalities. Cancers have been discovered in daughters as young as seven years of age. An unknown but substantial number of women in the United States alone received DES while pregnant, but approximately 1 in 1000 have been found to be afflicted with cervical or vaginal cancers. The National Cancer Institute has urged that all mothers and daughters who may have been exposed to DES during the mother's pregnancy arrange to be examined by a physician for possible effects of the drug.

The use of DES for pregnant women has been discontinued, although the compound is still available for treating certain cases of breast cancer and menopausal symptoms in nonpregnant women.

Cancer of the Ovary

Ovarian cancer is the fifth most common type of cancer in women, with an average of 21,000 new cases each year. It is second to uterine cancer in the number of cases of cancer of the reproductive system. It has, however, a much lower survival rate. Because of the difficulty in diagnosing ovarian cancer, the cancer is more likely than other forms to go unchecked until it has spread to other areas of the body. Less than 2 in 5 women will survive five years after diagnosis. There are several different kinds of malignant tumors of the ovary; some originate in the ovaries and others are caused by cells that have metastasized from a cancer at some other site, such as the uterus.

There are no age limits for cancer of the ovary, although most cases are detected in women between 50 and 70. A physician at a routine pelvic examination may notice a lump or other abnormal growth in the abdominal region. The symptoms reported by patients usually include abdominal discomfort or digestive problems, possibly because ovarian cancers often grow large enough to press on neighboring organs and cause urinary difficulties, constipation, or other digestive disorders. A clue is given in some cases by endometrial bleeding as a result of abnormal hormone production by the affected ovary. However, the more common kinds of ovarian cancers do not produce hormones. Occasionally, cancer cells from an ovarian tumor will be found in a Pap smear sample. But there are no direct, simple tests for cancer of the ovary.

Treatment for ovarian cancer varies with the individual case. As with cancer at other sites, surgery is generally necessary. The extent of the surgery depends upon the type of lesion and other factors. In an advanced case of an older woman, total hysterectomy along with removal of the ovaries and fallopian tubes would be the treatment of choice. But if the patient is a young woman and the cancer is not extensive, the surgeon may excise the affected ovary and leave the remainder of the reproductive system intact. Radiation and chemotherapy are commonly applied in addition to surgery. The most important risk factor is having relatives who have had ovarian cancer. If a mother, grandmother, or sibling have been diagnosed with ovarian cancer, then the woman is recommended to undergo regular blood tests to check for malignancy. Let your doctor know if you have a family history of ovarian cancer.

Cancer of the Breast

B reast cancer remains the most common of cancers affecting women, killing more women that any other kind of cancer, except lung cancer. About 150,000 women in the United States develop breast cancer each year, and 35 percent die of the disease. The cause of breast cancer is still unknown.

Prevention

The best prevention is education, mammography screening, self-examinations, and the monitoring of high-risk patients. Women whose female relatives have had breast cancer are more likely to be victims than women from families in which breast cancer is not present. Two genes, BRCA1 and BRCA2, have accounted for at least 80 percent of the breast cancer in women with a significant family history of the disease, but 80 percent of the women who develop breast cancer have no family history. High risk patients are defined as women who do not have children or who do not have them before their 30s; women who reach menopause later than normal; women who began menstruating earlier in life than normal. It should be noted that the increased risk is minimal. Also, women with ovarian tumors and women who use supplementary estrogen have been shown by some studies to be at increased risk, while the process of having many children and nursing them, which suppresses estrogen hormone activity, is associated with a decreased risk of developing breast cancer. However, 55 percent of the diagnosed cases are for women who have no known risk factors.

Cancer of the breast is generally not found before the age of 30 and the incidence peaks around the age of 55. There is a second period after the age of 65 when the incidence of breast cancer rises again.

Breast cancer usually begins in the ducts of the milk glands or lobules of the breast. The first noticeable sign is a lump in the breast. The lump may occur anywhere in the breast, but the most common site is the upper, outer quadrant. Most lumps are not usually cancerous, but a biopsy must be performed to check the tissue involved.

A small tumor half an inch in diameter is large enough to be detected during careful self-examination. The lump generally causes no pain; pain is rarely associated with early breast cancer. If the tumor is allowed to grow unchecked, it may cause pulling of the skin from within. The breast may flatten or the skin may dimple or the nipple may sink, tilt, or flatten. Less frequently, the tumor begins in a duct near the nipple, causing irritation of the skin of the nipple and a moist discharge. In such cases a scab eventually forms at that site. In time, cancer cells spread to the nearby lymph nodes and the danger of metastasis to any part of the body becomes very serious.

Detection of Breast Cancer

Fortunately, breast cancer can be treated effectively if it is detected early enough. Some 95 percent of breast cancers are discovered by the patient when she notices a lump. In all too many cases the discovery is made by chance and the lump may be quite large.

The cure rate for breast cancer could be greatly improved if all women made a routine of monthly self-examination and then consulted a physician immediately if they found the least indication of a thickening or a lump. Most such lumps are benign, but it is most important that the ones that are malignant be identified without delay.

The American Cancer Society and the National Cancer Institute recommend that every woman follow a prescribed method of self-examination just after the menstrual period, continuing every month after the menopause. The procedure (see illustration) should only take a few minutes and consists of carefully looking at and feeling the breasts. For more information, contact the American Cancer Society at (800) ACS-2345.

In recent years, methods of early detection have been refined to the point that tumors once undetectable can now be detected before any lump becomes palpable. As many as 80 percent of women diagnosed with early stages of breast cancer can be treated with a lumpectomy, the removal of underarm lymph nodes, radiation, and perhaps chemotherapy.

Mammography

Mammography is a low-dose X ray developed specifically for examination of breast tissue. A tumor shows up on a mammogram as an opaque spot because of mineral concentrations associated with the growth. However, mammography cannot determine whether a tumor is benign or malignant or if the opaque spot on the film is because of some other mineral-rich tissue rather than a tumor. Physicians use mammography and ultrasound as diagnostic tools.

Recommendations for when to seek clinical breast examinations and mammograms are as follows:

- Women 20 years of age and over should perform a breast self-examination every month.

- Women between 20 and 39 years of age should have a physical examination of the breast every three years, performed by a physician, physician assistant, nurse, or nurse-practitioner.

- Women 40 and over should have a physical examination of the

Self-examination of the Breasts

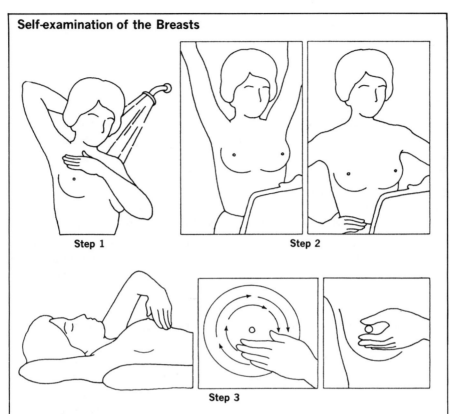

Step 1

Step 2

Step 3

Self-examination of the breasts as recommended by the American Cancer Society. *(Step 1)* Examine breasts during a shower or bath; hands glide easier over wet skin. With fingers flat, move the left hand gently over every part of the right breast, then the right hand over the left breast. Check for any lump, hard knot, or thickening. *(Step 2)* Before a mirror, inspect the breasts with arms at the sides, then with arms raised. Look for any changes in the contour of each breast, a swelling, dimple of skin, or changes in the nipple. Then rest palms on hips and press down firmly to flex the chest muscles. Left and right breasts will not match exactly — few women's breasts do. But regular inspection will show what is normal for you. *(Step 3)* While lying down with a pillow or folded towel under the right shoulder and with the right hand behind the head, examine the right breast with the left hand. With fingers flat, press gently in small circular motions around an imaginary clock face. Begin at 12 o'clock, then move to 1 o'clock, and so on around back to 12. A ridge of firm tissue in the lower curve of each breast is normal. Next, move in an inch toward the nipple and keep circling to examine every part of the breast, including the nipple. This requires at least three more circles. Then repeat the procedure slowly on the left breast with the pillow under the left shoulder and left hand behind the head. Notice how the breast structure feels. Finally, squeeze the nipple of each breast gently between thumb and index finger. Any discharge, clear or bloody, should be reported to a physician immediately.

breast every year, performed by physician, physician's assistant, nurse, or nurse-practitioner.

- Women 40 years of age and older should have a mammogram every year.

Most insurance companies will pay for yearly mammograms; others pay for biannual mammogram exams. Some states require insurance companies by law to pay for at least one exam. Check with your insurance company about their policy. Medicare covers mammograms for women over the age of 65.

Screening Mammograms

Screening mammography is performed on women with no symptoms in order to detect the very early stages of breast cancer. Screening mammography for women in their forties has been shown to reduce breast cancer deaths in that age group by as much as 44 percent.

Diagnostic Mammograms

Diagnostic mammograms are performed on women who currently have a breast problem such as a lump or nipple discharge, a history of breast cancer, or an area of concern seen in a previous screening mammogram. This diagnostic X ray looks more closely at the problem in the breast by utilizing a wide variety of X-ray views.

Scheduling a Mammogram

If you have regular periods, you should consider scheduling your mammogram seven to ten days after the beginning of your period, when the breasts are less tender. If your periods are irregular, you can schedule a mammogram at any time of the month. Bringing along any previous mammogram films as comparisons between your old films and your current exam will facilitate early detection of the disease.

Ultrasound

Ultrasound depends on sound waves that vibrate at frequencies beyond the range of human hearing; transmitted into the breast, ultrasound can distinguish between lumps that are cystic and fluid-filled—and therefore benign—and those that are solid. Small calcium deposits, which are one of the first signs of breast cancer, are not visible by ultrasound.

Biopsy

When a physician believes there is good evidence of a cancer in a breast as a result of mammography or ultrasound, the next step is a biopsy study. An entire nodule of breast tissue is removed for microscopic examination of the cells. The methods for extraction depend entirely upon the size of the tumor or lesion—whether or not it is large enough to be felt, and also on whether or not the entire tumor or lesion is to be removed. If, for example, the lesion is palpable, that is, the physician can feel it, and it is known to be cancerous, then the patient undergoes what is called a *surgical biopsy*. The patient is transferred to a surgery room where the physician surgically removes the entire lesion. Like most surgical procedures, some scarring is to be expected. If the lesion is viewable only by mammogram or ultrasound, then the radiologist performs a *needle localization*. Using a mammogram or ultrasound as a guide, the radiologist inserts a wire into the breast precisely where the lesion or tumor is located. The patient is transferred to a surgery room where the surgeon extracts the tumor, using the wire as his guide.

If the physician merely wants to sample either breast cells or tissue, several methods are available. In a *stereotactic core biopsy*, usually performed by a radiologist, a specially designed needle is used to draw out a tissue sample. Potentially cancerous cells are sampled in a similar procedure known as *fine needle* aspiration, which is routinely performed by both physicians and radiologists. Scarring is minimal, if at all, in both of these methods.

In each of the procedures discussed above, microscopic examination of the extracted specimen follows.

The Two-Step Procedure

Because of the psychological and physical problems associated with breast cancer, the test and operation can take place in two separate stages. In many cases, though, it may be necessary or more expedient to perform both operations on the same day.

Presurgical Staging involves the administration of various tests that are carried out before any breast surgery. These tests show whether or not the cancer has already spread (or metastasized) to parts of the body other than the breast and local lymph node regions. Staging is widely regarded as a necessary procedure in all cases of breast cancer.

A two-step procedure involves other choices. Where the biopsy is to be carried out separately, the patient may ask to have it done under local anesthesia, as an outpatient. If a general anesthetic appears preferable, the patient may have to spend a night in the hospital. But the *diagnostic biopsy*—involving removal of the tumor or portions of it—and any breast surgery can still be performed separately. After a biopsy specimen is removed, the specimen may be subjected to an estrogen-receptor assay. The assay tells the surgeon whethor or not the cancer depends on the female hormone estrogen for its growth. That information provides a clue to possible future treatment.

Following the biopsy, the pathologist reports on whether or not the specimen is positive or negative for cancer. If the finding is positive, precise information will usually be given on the type of cancer and where it is located in the breast. The patient may want to obtain a second opinion on the permanent-section pathology report and slides from another pathologist.

Breast Cancer Surgeries

Until recently, radical mastectomy was the usual procedure for breast

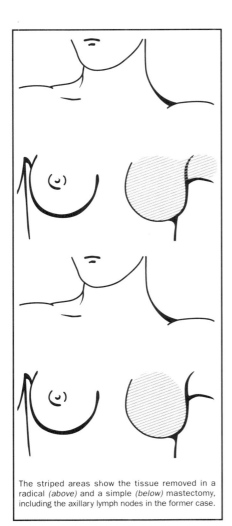

The striped areas show the tissue removed in a radical *(above)* and a simple *(below)* mastectomy, including the axillary lymph nodes in the former case.

tissue and tissue from around the breast area.

A *lumpectomy*, also known as *segmental mastectomy*, is the solution to a great percentage of breast cancer cases, particularly those that are diagnosed early. In a lumpectomy, only the cancer and surrounding tissue are removed. Generally, no reconstructive surgery is necessary and a lumpectomy is usually followed by some combination of radiation therapy and chemotherapy. A common misconception is that radiation and chemotherapy are "either/or" treatments. In general, a patient must have radiation and may or may not undergo chemotherapy.

Other types of breast surgeries include the following:

- Modified radical mastectomy: the underlying muscle stays intact while the breast, lymph nodes and surrounding muscle are removed.

- Simple mastectomy: the breast tissue is removed, but the surrounding muscles and lymph nodes remain.

- Radical mastectomy: the breast, lymph nodes and surrounding muscle are entirely removed. Studies indicate it was no more successful than a lumpectomy or a modified radical mastectomy, yet left the patient deformed and with a very high risk of developing lymphodema (severe arm swelling).

cancer treatment. Today, it's rarely performed. The type of surgery is determined by the type and size of the cancerous growth, the risk of further growth, and other factors. Depending upon the seriousness of the case and the procedure recommended by the surgeon and the pathologist, the patient may decide to remove just the breast tissue, leaving the skin (with the exception of the nipple) for reconstructive surgery, to remove the skin tissue as well, or to remove breast

Survival rates depend as much on timely use of pre- and postoperative radiotherapy and postoperative chemotherapy as on the type of operation, but the surgery type can determine the length of the recovery period.

Some surgeries allow reconstruction of the breast either during or after a mastectomy, usually using artificial material to create a breast to match the natural one.

Radiation

Radiation is used in conjunction with breast-sparing surgery or with large tumors that were treated by mastectomy. It is also used in cases where the cancer recurred or metastasized and as a pain-reliever for patients suffering pain to the bone. Treatments are typically given five days a week for five to seven weeks. A "booster" treatment may follow completion of the initial series of treatments. Consult your physician for a complete list of expected side effects.

Chemotherapy

Adjuvant (auxilliary) chemotherapy is given in addition to surgery and radiation. Typically, chemotherapy is administered if a patient has a large tumor, or if the patient's lymph nodes are involved, or if the patient is in the high-risk category for recurrence or distant metastasis. The preference is to avoid treating a postmenopausal patient with chemotherapy, but there are many instances in which chemotherapy is unavoidable. Postmenopausal women may be given tamoxifen, an antiestrogen drug, or may undergo chemotherapy, anyway.

Hormone therapy

Less toxic than chemotherapy, hormone treatments are normally given to those women whose cancer has not spread to the underarm nodes and whose tumors were hormone-dependent. This is especially the case if a patient is postmenopausal. For these women tamoxifen would also be a standard treatment if the cancers had spread to the lymph nodes.

Prophylactic Mastectomy

A *prophylactic*, or preventive, mastectomy is the removal of an entire breast, or both breasts (total mastectomy), when there is no known breast cancer. In this case, it is not necessary to remove any lymph nodes. Prophylactic mastectomy is an *elective* surgery (that is, while you may choose to have it done, it is not *required*). A woman might consider this option to lessen the risk of developing breast cancer if she has a strong family history of breast cancer or if certain forms of benign breast problems have lead to several biopsies, but it is considered drastic and by many, unnecessary.

Prophylactic mastectomy is controversial because there is no guarantee that it will prevent breast cancer. In rare cases, breast cancer has developed in the scar of the mastectomy. Most doctors prefer to closely observe high-risk patients rather than perform such drastic surgery.

Before taking this irreversible step, women should discuss the mastectomy, reconstructive surgery, possible complications, and post-operative care with their physician and the plastic surgeon who will perform the reconstructive surgery. A second medical opinion, and consultation with a genetic counselor, who, through testing, may be able to provide new or more complete information concerning their risk for breast cancer, is also advised. Patients should also be mindful that reconstructed breasts will not have the same physical appearance as normal breasts.

Women opting for prophylactic mastectomies need to be aware that they will be second-guessed by friends, health care advocates, and even some physicians, who consider this type of mastectomy senseless and barbaric. Many women who have the surgery feel that their decision has allowed them to live a life less crippled by fear, worry, and frequent medical tests and procedures.

Breast implants

Breast implants for reconstruction are the same types used for cosmetic breast enlargement. There are two basic types: silicone-gel and saline filled. The saline sacs duplicate the natural breast's shape. The sac is inserted under the skin and then filled slightly larger than the final size. After the skin has adjusted to the enlarged sac, some of the liquid is drained to give the breast a natural sag, in most cases closely matching the remaining breast.

Although silicone-gel implants have been widely discouraged for cosmetic use since 1992, they are still considered an important rehabilitation option for women with breast cancer or women with premalignant conditions requiring mastectomies, according to the American Cancer Society. The silicone implant is carefully inserted under the skin tissue and the body forms a scar tissue seal around the sac.

Reactions to silicone-gel implants may include side effects such as hardening of scar tissue around the implant, ruptured silicone sacs, and obscured diagnostic X rays. The link between silicone and diseases of the immune system is still under study. In addition, implants also may block the results of mammographic X rays. However, studies show that implants do not increase the risk of breast cancer or cancer in other parts of the body.

According to the United States Food and Drug Administration, women should only consider removing implants if they are experiencing difficulties. Women should have periodic exams to check for ruptures. Those who want implants for cosmetic purposes should know the importance of detecting early cancer through mammography and the

chance of having results obscured by implants.

Preventing and Surviving Rape

Precautions

Although the majority of rape attacks take the victim by surprise, there are precautions that women may take to avoid potentially dangerous situations.

Precautions on a Date

- Make sure you tell someone where you are going and what time you expect to be back.

- Don't become intoxicated, since your reaction to any potentially dangerous situation will be slower.

- Be aware of drugs known as date-rape drugs. They cause disorientation, unconsciousness, and memory loss, allowing the person who has given you the drug to rape you. And, because they are odorless and have no taste, you should take precautions against anyone slipping the drug into your drink.

- Don't bring a man home or go home with him, or go to a secluded spot with him.

- Don't depend solely upon him for a ride home. Be prepared to call a cab, friend, or relative for a ride in case you feel uncomfortable being with him.

- Even if you have known someone for a while, you should still be cautious about any indications of extreme jealousy, possessiveness, or anger.

Overall Precautions

- Keep all entrances to your home well lit. All doors and windows should be locked. Keep your window shades down at night.

- Use a peephole to confirm the identity of all visitors before opening a door.

- Walk assertively, maintaining a brisk stride and upright posture. Stay alert. Be ready to react, if necessary.

- Many schools, businesses, apartment buildings, and parking facilities will provide you with a security guard or other escort. Request an escort if you are uneasy about going alone.

- When possible, avoid deserted areas. Park in well-lit areas. When walking, use well-lit routes.

- Have your keys out and ready to use, before you reach your car or home. Once there, get in and lock the doors immediately.

- If you are being followed, go into the nearest place of business or ring the nearest doorbell. If you are in your car, try to drive to the nearest police station or a well-lit, populated area.

Most importantly, heed your own instincts. Many victims of crime report having "gut feelings" that something was wrong just prior to being attacked. If you feel uneasy or in danger, try to remove yourself from a situation before anything happens.

Surviving the Rape Attack

- Talk to the rapist: this may allow you to stall for time until someone else comes by, or you might be able to calm your attacker and avoid rape.

- Tell the rapist you are meeting someone or expecting someone to come by soon.

- Try to disgust your attacker by inducing yourself to vomit, urinate, defecate, or expel gas.

- Scream. Yell "fire" since many potential rescuers are hesitant to respond to a cry for "police." If there is a fire alarm nearby, set it off.

- Use any sharp object you have available—keys, a pen or pencil, your fingernails—and aim for the attacker's eyes, Adam's apple, ears, or temples.

- Kicking or hitting the attacker's groin or throat may disable him temporarily and provide you with time to escape.

If a Rape Occurs

A woman who has been raped may face a long period in which recovery and normal living seem impossible. Authorities say that what a victim does after experiencing rape may make the transition to normal living easier while also protecting her against recurring health problems.

Talk With Someone

Sharing the events of the rape with a friend, relative or counselor will be painful and difficult, but talking about it will help you cope with the many levels of pain and fear you will probably experience. Rape counselors are among the persons best equipped to handle the emotional needs of a woman who has been raped. The person confided in should be able to go to the police station with you, provide support, make sure your rights are protected, and listen sympathetically to your story.

If you have been raped, and do not have anyone close to turn to, contact one of the Rape Crisis Centers listed at the end of the chapter.

Going to the Hospital

A person that has been raped should go as soon as possible to a hospital and undergo the pelvic and other examinations that physicians administer in such cases. If the woman goes to the hospital immediately, she should not wash herself or change clothes. A shower can remove valuable medical evidence. The pelvic examination is designed to find evidence of abrasions or internal damage, and for collection of any semen left by the rapist. Physicians will also examine for any of the rapist's hair, blood, skin, or semen. Any such evidence may be important in court later, if opting to file a police report.

The hospital visit has other purposes. A physician can also administer preventive injections for sexually transmitted diseases and, if desired, an antipregnancy medication. The latter medication must be taken within three days if it is to be effective.

Reporting to the Police

Failure to report a rape immediately or after a few days probably means the rapist will not be apprehended, unless the identity of the rapist is known. Even so, many rapes go unreported simply because most victims cannot face the added trauma of being questioned in detail. The woman who does report to the police should do so as soon as possible. But reporting late is better than not reporting at all. Reporting a rape does not mean that the victim has to press charges later.

Rape Crisis Centers

Rape crisis centers operate in most communities. Staffing at the centers often include rape victims who devote time to helping other victims. To find help, you can call the Rape, Abuse & Incest National Network (RAINN): 1-800-656-HOPE. It is a national 24-hour toll-free hotline for survivors of sexual assault. By reading the area code and prefix of the caller's telephone number, the hotline automatically routes the call to the rape crisis center nearest the caller. Each call is confidential. Every center participating in the network provides counseling and support.

26

Physicians and Diagnostic Procedures

Many people dislike going to the doctor; many fear going to the hospital. And many are overwhelmed by the enormity of the health care industry; much of its costs and procedures seem incomprehensible to us and out of control. Too often, these people put off seeing a doctor until they develop a debilitating problem. Yet many people overlook the one very important way they can alleviate some of their anxiety over their own medical care: choosing a doctor. Having a doctor you trust and with whom you can communicate well not only makes it more likely that you will make appointments for regular checkups, tests, and immunizations, but you will feel comfortable reporting any symptoms that may be the first signs of serious illness, many of which, when diagnosed early, can be treated successfully.

Your Primary Care Physician

Your primary care physician is your regular doctor, the person you see for checkups, and the first person you call when signs of illness appear. More than likely, he or she will be a *general practitioner* or a *family practitioner,* but may also be an *internist* or other specialist (see below). In selecting a primary care physician you should try to get a few recommendations from other patients, doctors, nurses, or hospital workers. Don't hesitate to make an appointment for an informational interview to meet the doctor in person and ask any questions about his or her methods, background, and philosophy that may be important to you.

Another important thing to check is the doctor's training—how much and from where. Check the American Medical Association's *The Directory of Medical Specialists* and other such directories in the library to find out whether the doctor has graduated from a fully accredited medical school and where he or she received further training.

In addition, remember that good communication is often the key to good health care. Make sure your doctor understands your questions and concerns and make sure you understand your doctor's answers and instructions. Don't hesitate to ask why you're being given a particular medication, or what the purpose is of any tests that are recommended. There are alternatives to some medications, and many tests are very expensive and not always necessary. If you are ever uncomfortable with what your doctor has ordered, seek a second opinion; your doctor should be happy to recommend someone. If not, find out why.

General Practitioner

All doctors must complete four years of schooling at an approved medical school, receive one year of postgraduate training in a supervised clinical setting, and pass a state board examination to become licensed to practice medicine. At this point in his or her training a doctor qualifies as a *general practitioner*. Like the stereotypical old-time country doctor, they treat just about everything from warts to measles, set broken bones, deliver babies, and dispense antibiotics and painkillers.

Family Practitioner

The general practitioner has largely been replaced by the *family practitioner*. Family practitioners must complete a three-year residency that covers certain aspects of internal medicine, pediatrics, obstetrics, and orthopedics, and then pass an exam. They treat the same things that general practitioners treat.

Osteopath

A doctor of osteopathy (D.O.) or *osteopath* has similar qualifications as a doctor of medicine. Osteopathy was founded by Andrew Taylor Still (1828-1917) on the principle that the body possesses a natural ability both to defend itself against disease and to heal itself. Osteopaths place great emphasis on the importance of normal body mechanics and on the use of the hands for detecting and correcting problems.

Medical Specialties

Among the major specialties are the following:

Allergy and Immunology: *Allergists* and *immunologists* specialize in the treatment of allergic and immunologic diseases.

Anesthesiology: An *anesthesiologist* decides which type of anesthesia will be used, administers it during surgery, and monitors its effects after surgery.

Dermatology: A *dermatologist* diagnoses and treats diseases of the skin, hair, and nails.

Emergency Medicine: An *emergency medicine specialist* practices emergency medicine in a trauma center.

Family Practice: The role of the *family practitioner* is discussed above.

Gastroenterology: A *gastroenterologist* diagnoses and treats disorders of the digestive system and of the liver.

Internal Medicine: An *internist* specializes in the diagnosis and nonsurgical treatment of diseases. Subspecialties of internal medicine include: *cardiology,* the study of diseases of the heart; *endocrinology,* the study of diseases of the glands; *gastroenterology; hematology,* the study of blood and blood-forming tissues; *infectious diseases; medical oncology,* the study of tumors; *nephrology,* the study of disorders of the kidneys; *pulmonary diseases,* the study of disorders of the lungs and respiratory system; and *rheumatology,* the study of connecting and supporting tissues.

Neurological Surgery: The *neurological surgeon* deals with the diagnosis, treatment, and surgical management of disorders and diseases of the brain, spinal cord, and nervous systems.

Neurology: A *neurologist* diagnoses and treats disorders of the brain and nervous system as well as of the muscles.

Nuclear Medicine: The *nuclear medicine specialist* is concerned with the use of radioactive material in the diagnosis and treatment of disease.

Obstetrics and Gynecology: An *obstetrician* specializes in the treatment of pregnant women and delivers babies. A *gynecologist* specializes in the treatment of women and their particular diseases, especially the reproductive system. Often, physicians specialize in both areas.

Ophthalmology: An *ophthalmologist* specializes in the medical and surgical treatment of the eye. Ophthalmologists also treat eye diseases.

Orthopedic Surgery: An *orthopedist* diagnoses, treats, and surgically corrects disorders and injuries of the bones, joints, muscles, cartilage, and ligaments.

Otorhinolaryngology: An *otorhinolaryngologist* treats disorders of the ears, nose, and throat.

Pathology: A *pathologist* investigates the course and causes of diseases.

Pediatrics: A *pediatrician* specializes in all medical aspects of child care. Subspecialties of pediatrics include: *pediatric cardiology, pediatric endocrinology, pediatric hematology/oncology, neonatal/perinatal medicine,* and *nephrology.*

Physical Medicine and Rehabilitation: A *physiatrist* deals with restoring either the full or partial use of body parts that have been injured or diseased, or have been defective at birth.

Plastic Surgery: A *plastic surgeon* repairs defects of the skin and underlying tissue. The plastic surgeon also performs surgery sought purely for cosmetic reasons.

Psychiatry: A *psychiatrist* treats behavior disorders, often with psychotherapy, but also with drugs.

Radiology: A *radiologist* specializes in the use of radiant energy such as X rays to diagnose and treat disease.

Surgery: A *general surgeon* specializes in the diagnosis and surgical treatment of a wide range of diseases, although most surgeons choose to specialize further.

Urology: A *urologist* diagnoses and treats disorders of the urinary-tract organs, and in men, problems of the reproductive system.

The Physical Examination

One of the first questions many people have about the physical exam is "How often should I have one?" Visits for infants from birth to 18 months are typically scheduled at 2, 4, 6, 15, and 18 months. Visits for children from 2 to 18 are typically scheduled once a year. Visits for individuals aged 19 to 65 are recommended every 1 to 3 years, for most people beginning on the low side (every 3 years) and progressing to every year as one approaches age 65. After age 65 annual visits are recommended.

A typical physical examination will include a careful health appraisal by an examining physician, including a detailed health history of the patient and study of the patient's body appearance and functions.

The patient's *medical history* is important because the physician needs to know any medical problems the pa-

tient may have had in the past, including operations or pregnancies, medications the patient is allergic to or is currently taking, and any incidence of family illnesses that may make the patient more susceptible to such things as heart disease or cancer.

After the medical history has been recorded or updated, the physician may begin a general inspection of the patient's body, beginning with the head and neck and working down to the feet. The physician looks for possible deformities, scars or wounds, pulsations, or throbbing areas. Bruises, areas of skin peeling or flaking, areas of heavy skin pigmentation or loss of pigmentation, hair distribution, perspiration or goose bumps, firmness or slackness of the skin, warts, calluses, and other features are noted.

The physician usually checks the

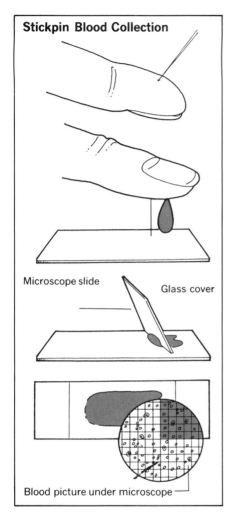

Stickpin Blood Collection

Microscope slide

Glass cover

Blood picture under microscope

physician some information about the condition of the lungs. A related technique, *auscultation,* involves listening to sounds within the body through a stethoscope. During percussion, the physician listens for changes in sounds that range from resonance over hollow spaces to dullness over solid or muscular areas. Lack of resonance over a normally resonant area of the lung might indicate fluid, pneumonia, or perhaps an abnormal mass. Percussion may also give the first sign of enlargement of organs, such as the liver, heart, or spleen. During auscultation, the physician listens for abnormal breathing sounds as the air rushes in and out of the lungs. Abnormal breathing sounds can indicate specific aberrations in lung function. In auscultation of the heart, the physician listens for extra heartbeats, rubbing sounds, the rumbling noises of a heart murmur, or the sounds of normally functioning heart valves opening and closing.

The physician may also use the stethoscope to listen to sounds beyond the chest area. He or she may listen to the sounds of blood flowing through vessels of the neck, bowel sounds through the wall of the abdomen, and the subtle noises made by joints, muscles, and tendons as various limbs are moved.

Weight, height, blood pressure, and pulse rate are also checked as part of any routine examination. There can be a wide variation in these readings from individual to individual, but drastic changes for a given person may signal a health disorder.

exterior of the body by a method known as *palpation,* which means feeling with the fingers and hands. Rough vibrations from a disorder in the respiratory system, the trembling sensation of blood encountering an obstruction, or the grating feeling of a bone deformity can be detected during palpation. In addition to palpation, the physician may apply *percussion,* or tapping, of certain body areas. Tapping the chest, for example, gives the

Common Screening Tests

A variety of tests may be given in a routine physical exam, depending on the patient's age, family history, and current state of health. Some of the following tests will be done each time the patient visits the doctor and some are necessary only when specific complaints or concerns are raised or when an individual reaches a certain age or risk category. Your doctor should explain any new test to you.

Blood Pressure and Pulse Rate

The patient's blood pressure and pulse rate are checked on every office visit. Blood pressure is measured with a *sphygmomanometer* and a stethoscope. The sphygmomanometer is attached to an inflatable cuff, which is wrapped around the upper arm; a rubber bulb is used to inflate the cuff and increase pressure in it so that it can control the blood flow in the arm. The physician locates the pulse with the stethoscope and increases the cuff pressure until the pulse (heartbeat) can no longer be heard. Then the physician slowly deflates the cuff and lets the reading on the gauge fall gradually until he hears the first beat of the heart. The reading on the gauge at that point is recorded as the *systolic pressure*. The physician continues to relax the pressure in the cuff and watches for the reading at the point where the thumping of the heart disappears again. That number is recorded as the *diastolic pressure*.

The doctor checks a patient's pulse rate to find out if the heart is beating normally. The pulse is the rhythmic expansion of the arteries that takes place after each heart beat. The pulse rate is the number of pulsations of an artery per minute. The normal pulse rate for a person at rest varies from as little as 50 for elderly people to as much as 100 for children.

Eyes, Mouth, and Ears

Inspection of the eyes is usually done with the aid of an *ophthalmoscope,* with which the physician can see the retina at the back of the eye. Distended retinal veins may be a sign of a variety of disorders, including diabetes or heart disease; signs of hardening of the arteries also may be observed in the eyes before other indications are found elsewhere. The condition of retinal blood vessels may also signal the development of hypertension.

A device called an *otoscope* is inserted in the outer ear to examine the external auditory canal and eardrum. The condition of the tongue, teeth, and gums can reveal much about the health of the individual.

Cholesterol Measurement

An elevated blood cholesterol level is an important risk factor for coronary artery disease. For most people a blood cholesterol level above 200 mg/dl should be cause for concern, indicating a need for further tests and perhaps a change in life-style.

Blood cholesterol levels are meas-ured by withdrawing a small amount of blood—usually from the arm—to be analyzed in a lab. The result is given in terms of milligrams of cholesterol per deciliter of blood. It's a good idea to have your blood cholesterol checked at age 25 and then once every 3 to 5 years thereafter.

Blood Tests

Complete Blood Count

A Complete Blood Count (CBC) provides the physician with more information than any other single laboratory screening procedure. Four common measurements are taken from it:

Hemoglobin concentration. Hemoglobin is the chemical substance that transports oxygen through the bloodstream to all the cells of the body. This measurement determines the amount of hemoglobin per unit volume of blood.

Red blood cell count. This test measures the number of red cells per cubic millimeter of blood. A low red blood cell count may indicate anemia, as well as be a potential early warning sign for leukemia, kidney malfunction, internal bleeding, or sickle cell anemia.

Hematocrit. The hematocrit measures the ratio of red blood cells to the plasma in the blood. Like the hemoglobin concentration and the red blood cell count, the hematocrit can indicate anemia, and all three tests are generally given in order to help diagnose the specific type and cause of anemia.

White blood cell count. This test measures the number of white cells per cubic millimeter of blood. A high white blood cell count can indicate an infection, a major injury, or even leukemia. A low count can be a sign of poor diet, certain infections, or another type of leukemia. If taken in the presence of a fever, the white blood cell count can help distinguish between a bacterial and a viral infection.

Blood Glucose

The glucose test determines the amount of sugar in the blood. Individuals who experience symptoms of diabetes mellitus (such as excessive thirst or urination), hypoglycemia (lightheadedness or fainting), or who are pregnant will most likely be given a blood glucose test. A very high level of blood sugar can indicate diabetes, while a very low level can indicate hypoglycemia. In either case or in border-line cases an *oral glucose tol-*

erance test is given. This test requires that the individual fast for 12 to 14 hours before the test. The patient is then given a concentrated sugar so-lution to drink, and blood is drawn at regular intervals over the next several hours. This test has replaced the urine test for sugar.

Blood Urea Nitrogen (BUN) and Blood Creatinine

Blood urea and creatinine are prod-ucts of protein metabolism. A high level of either in the blood means that the kidneys are not filtering them properly from the blood, possibly be-cause of kidney damage.

Blood Electrolytes

The four blood electrolytes are so-dium, potassium, chloride, and bicar-bonate, and they play important roles in the blood pH, the cells' water bal-ance, and kidney function. Most often this test is given to patients who are taking diuretics, those with liver, kid-ney, or heart disease, or those who may be experiencing dehydration or excessive vomiting or diarrhea.

Urinalysis

The urinalysis is a simple and impor-tant test that can indicate much about a person's overall health and identify potential problems, such as kidney disease, diabetes, and urinary tract in-fections. For a routine urinalysis a sample can be taken at any time of day, although the physician may spec-ify the first morning's urine, or may give special instructions about food and water intake before taking the urine sample.

Urinalysis includes a specific grav-ity test (a test to measure the extent to which solids are concentrated in the urine as an indication of how well the kidneys are conserving the body's fluids) and a pH test (a test to mea-sure the acidity of the urine as an in-dication of how well the kidneys are able to remove acid wastes).

There are also tests for the pres-ence of glucose (sugar), protein, blood, and bilirubin (a substance pro-duced in the liver from the break-down of old blood cells); none of these substances is normally found in the urine. The presence of glucose is an indication of diabetes; protein in the urine is associated with diabetes, hypertension, and other diseases; blood in the urine can indicate many problems including kidney stones, cysts, infection, and cancer; the pres-ence of bilirubin suggests a problem in the liver or bile ducts. The pres-ence of bacteria or of a large number of white blood cells is typically an in-dication of a urinary tract infection.

Routine blood work and a urinaly-sis are simple, common tests that can catch many potential problems early. When abnormalities exist, other, more specific—and often more expensive—tests are required for confirmation before treatment can be-gin. Given the fact that any test can give a false result, whether through human error or through individual variations, the question of whether or

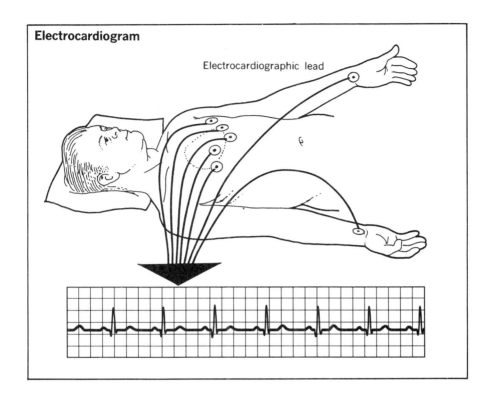

Electrocardiogram

Electrocardiographic lead

not individuals should have these tests is a much-debated point in the medical community and one best discussed with one's primary care physician.

Electrocardiogram

The electrocardiogram (ECG or EKG) measures heart activity by detecting the electrical activity in the heart. Electrodes attached to the chest, neck, arms, and legs record the pathway of electrical impulses through the heart muscle and record these impulses as tracings on special graph paper. The test is simple and safe, and takes five to ten minutes to perform.

The purpose of the EKG is to detect heart disorders or blockages in the coronary arteries. A normally beating heart produces basically the same pattern of waves in all people. Variations in this pattern can indicate a number of potential problems: irregular heart rhythms, damage to the heart muscle, enlargement of the heart's chambers, mineral imbalances in the blood. The EKG can also reveal whether the patient has had, or is having, a heart attack.

This test is not foolproof, however, and can produce false results. Some people with normal EKGs have heart trouble, and the graph may show abnormalities where none exists.

EKGs are usually a routine part of a physical checkup after age 40; before that age, patients are recommended to have at least one EKG to use for comparison later.

Cancer Screening Test

Carcinoembryonic antigen (CEA), a substance normally found only in fetuses, may indicate the presence of certain cancers when found at elevated levels in adults. This test is typically used in patients who have been treated for such cancers as colon/rectal, breast, lung, ovarian, pancreatic, and stomach to check for possible recurrence of the disease.

Mammogram

A *mammogram* is an X ray of the breast done to locate breast tumors and cysts. To date, it is the only screening exam that can find small tumors before they can be felt and when they have the greatest chance of being cured. It is estimated that yearly mammograms for women over 40 could lead to a one-third reduction in the number of deaths from breast cancer.

The patient must remove all clothing from the waist up and stand with the breast placed on a small shelf that extends out from the machine. The patient is then guided forward so that the edge of the shelf presses into the chest just below the breast. A compression device is brought down onto the breast, and pressure is applied for less than 30 seconds. This is the most uncomfortable part of the test, as much pressure is necessary in order to get the most detailed picture possible and use the least amount of radiation. Eliminating caffeine and foods that tend to cause water retention two weeks prior to the exam makes the breasts less sensitive.

The American Cancer Society recommends that women aged 40 and older have a mammogram every year.

For more information and a comparison of diagnostic and screening mammograms, see *Women's Health*, Ch. 25, "Cancer of the Breast."

Pap Smear

The *pap smear* tests for cervical cancer by the microscopic examination of cells from the vaginal walls and cervix. Although it is not infallible this test detects 95 percent of cervical cancers; it is an important aid in the detection of this disease at a stage when it is often without symptoms and it is still curable.

The procedure can be done any time except during the menstrual period. The patient undresses from the waist down and lies down on her back with her legs spread apart and her feet in special stirrups. The physician inserts a lubricated *speculum* into the vagina and opens it to expose the cervix and its os (mouth). The doctor then inserts a small applicator through the speculum and rubs it gently against the cervix and sometimes the os. The applicator is removed and rubbed onto a glass slide (the smear). The speculum is then removed.

The first pap smear should be done when a woman turns 18 or becomes sexually active (whichever occurs first), and should be followed by pap smears for 2 consecutive years. Providing these tests are negative and there are no risk factors present, tests can be done less frequently at the discretion of one's doctor, although an annual pap smear for women between 25 and 60 is common.

Prostate Tests

Cancer of the prostate is a leading cause of death in men over 50. If detected early, prostate cancer can usually be cured. It can often be detected by digital rectal examination (DRE), a routine procedure in which the doctor inserts a gloved finger into the rectum and feels the prostate gland. Another test measures blood levels of the prostate-specific antigen (PSA), a protein produced in the prostate that may be elevated when cancer is present.

Occult Blood Test

Colon cancer is the second most common form of cancer in the United States. An early warning sign of colon cancer is blood in the stool. It is called *occult,* or hidden, blood because it cannot be detected by sight. It is recommended that everyone over age 50 be tested for occult blood annually.

Usually, stools are tested for occult blood at home with the help of a self-test kit. The test calls for smearing cards with stool samples collected over several days. The samples are sent to a lab to be tested for hidden blood. If blood is detected, further diagnostic tests, including a colonoscopy (a visual examination of the entire colon), may be ordered.

Sigmoidoscopy

Another procedure for detecting colon cancer is *sigmoidoscopy,* the use of a tubular scope called a sigmoidoscope to examine the lower segment of the large intestine. The purpose of this test is to detect tumors in the rectum and colon. To ensure a clean lower bowel, the patient must follow a special diet—typically an all-liquid diet—for several days prior to the test, use laxatives the night before, and take an enema on the day of the test. The patient puts on a hospital gown and lies on the left side with the knees drawn up to the chest. A thin, lubricated tube is inserted into the rectum and slowly advanced along the large intestine. The tube contains optical filaments through which light can pass and transmit images to a microscope or monitor for the doctor to view. It may also contain small instruments that enable the doctor to take tissue samples. Air may be forced through the tube to expand the intestine, which can cause a feeling of discomfort. The procedure takes from 15 to 30 minutes. The American Cancer Society recommends a baseline sigmoidoscopy for everyone at age 50 (or 40 if there is a family history of colon cancer) and once every three years after that.

Sexually Transmitted Diseases

The prevalence of sexually transmitted diseases (STDs), such as syphilis, gonorrhea, chlamydia, genital herpes, and AIDS makes regular tests for these diseases in sexually active people who are not in monogamous relationships vitally important. Tests are typically blood tests or swab tests and should be done every year or two.

Tuberculosis

Tuberculosis is normally tested for with a simple *skin test*. The forearm is either pricked with a small device with four prongs or a subcutaneous injection is used. In either case, the patient is asked to check the area after 48 to 72 hours for signs of redness, raised bumps, or swelling.

Stress Test

Stress tests are often given to older people who are about to begin an exercise program. During this test, the heart's activity is monitored with an electrocardiogram (EKG) while the patient exercises on a treadmill or stationary bicycle. The procedure is usually done in a physician's office or a local hospital. It is a trouble-shooting test designed to reveal problems that a resting EKG does not. At rest, an EKG may indicate that the heart is receiving sufficient oxygen; but with exertion, as the heart's workload increases, the exercise stress test may reveal signs of an inadequate oxygen supply to certain areas of the heart muscle. The most common cause of this condition is a narrowing of coronary arteries due to a buildup of plaque. Thus the stress test can help identify an abnormality that might otherwise go undetected until a person is exercising and unexpectedly experiences chest pain. A routine stress test is often recommended at age 45, and as early as 35 if the patient has at least one risk factor for coronary artery disease. Risk factors include smoking, obesity, hypertension, and elevated cholesterol levels.

Chest X ray

The *chest X ray* was once a routine part of the physical exam. Its expense, potential danger, and limited results in the absence of symptoms has made it less popular. (An individual X ray in and of itself is not harmful, but because exposure to radiation is cumulative throughout your life, a series of

X rays over a lifetime can result in increased risk of cancer.) A chest X ray produces a picture that includes the heart and lungs. It can be useful in identifying certain heart problems, and is also used to detect lung cancer.

If you are advised to have a chest X ray, you will be asked to remove all clothing from the waist up and to wear a gown. Depending on the particular area to be X rayed, you will either sit, stand, or lie down. Generally two or three exposures are taken for each area targeted.

Immunizations

Nearly everyone knows the importance of having their children immunized, but many people may not realize that it is important for adults to have regular immunizations as well. When a patient is immunized, he or she receives a shot of modified microbes (bacteria or viruses) or toxins. Although not strong enough to actually give the patient the disease, the dose of microbes does stimulate the patient's own immune system to build up antibodies against the disease, thus making him or her immune to future exposures. Vaccines do wear off, however, and it is best to keep a record of all immunizations and receive scheduled booster shots.

Diphtheria

Diphtheria is spread by airborne bacteria that release toxins that can attack the heart and other internal organs. Adults should receive a booster shot every ten years.

Tetanus

Tetanus is spread by bacteria that enter the body through a contaminated wound. Adults should receive a booster shot (often combined with the diphtheria shot) every ten years. If you sustain a contaminated wound, your doctor may recommend a tetanus booster is you have not had one in 5 years.

Influenza

The risk of death from the *flu* increases with age, and people over 65 are strongly advised to receive annual flu shots in the fall. In 1976 about 500 cases of a rare paralytic condition called Guillain-Barre syndrome were associated with a swine flu vaccine. No influenza vaccines since have been associated with the development of Guillain-Barre.

Pneumococcal Pneumonia

A vaccine is available that offers protection against the 23 strains of bacteria that cause about 80 percent of pneumococcal diseases in the United States. All adults age 65 and older should receive the pneumonia vaccine on an annual basis, as should younger adults with chronic cardiopulmonary disorders, diabetes, renal disease, liver disease, blood diseases, cancers, and diseases that suppress immunity such as HIV infection.

Those at risk of death from influenza should also be immunized with the pneumonia vaccine, but only once. Because it may increase adverse side effects, repeat or booster shots of the vaccine are not recommended.

Measles and Mumps

Many people born after 1957 have not had and have not been immunized against *measles* and *mumps* and thus are particularly susceptible to these diseases. In addition, those vaccinated between 1963 and 1967 may have gotten a short-lasting killed-virus vaccine and should be revaccinated.

Anyone born between 1957 and 1967 should be revaccinated unless 1) they had a case of measles confirmed by a physician's diagnosis, 2) they are immune, as demonstrated by a blood test, 3) they have a record of receiving live vaccine no earlier than their first birthday.

Hepatitis A

Hepatitis is an inflammation of the liver, usually caused by a virus infection. Hepatitis A is the most common form of the disease. It is transmitted mainly by contaminated food or water. Symptoms include fever, nausea, vomiting, and jaundice.

There is a safe and effective vaccine available to people at high risk for the disease and to travelers to countries where hepatitis A is endemic.

Hepatitis B

Like the HIV virus that causes AIDS, hepatitis B is spread through blood contact with virus-infected body fluids; the most common form of transmission is sexual contact. However, hepatitis B is much more contagious than the HIV virus and is the leading cause of cirrhosis and cancer of the liver. Half of those infected with hepatitis B never develop symptoms, and thus become unwitting chronic carriers of it. Vaccination is strongly recommended, especially for those with a high risk of infection, such as health care workers, sexually active persons with multiple partners, intravenous drug users, hemodialysis patients, newborns with infected mothers, and residents and staff of institutions for the mentally retarded.

Children

The standard immunizations for children are 1) combined vaccines for diphtheria, pertussis, and tetanus (DPT); 2) a series of polio vaccinations combining inactivate poliovirus vaccine (IPV) followed by oral, attenuated poliovirus vaccine (OPV); 3) vaccines for measles, mumps, and ru-

bella (MMR); 4) hemophilus influenza type B conjugate vaccine (HIB). The Centers for Disease Control recommends the following schedule:
- 2 months: DPT, IPV, HIB
- 4 months: DPT, IPV, HIB
- 6 months: DPT and HIB

- 12 months: DPT, OPV, HIB, TB test, MMR

- 4 to 6 years: DPT, MMR, and OPV

Hepatitis B and chicken pox vaccines are also available.

Other Diagnostic Tests

If a definite diagnosis cannot be made on the basis of the medical history, preliminary physical exam, and routine diagnostic tests, more specialized tests may be required. What follows is a description, grouped by body system, of some of the other diagnostic tests.

Tests for Mental Disorders

When a physician suspects that a patient has a mental disorder, the physician must first rule out the possibility that the symptoms are caused by a physical illness. After physical disorders have been ruled out, mental-status tests may be administered. These include the Rorschach inkblot test, the Thematic Apperception Test, the Minnesota Multiphasic Personality Inventory, and the Wechsler Adult Intelligence Scale. These tests are used to diagnose various psychological and psychiatric disorders, including depression, paranoia, anxiety, psychopathy, and schizophrenia.

The Skeletal System

The skeletal system includes the bones and cartilage, and the specialist who handles problems of the skeletal system is the orthopedic surgeon. Disorders of the nervous system and joints often overlap skeletal problems and may necessitate tests by a neurologist or rheumatologist.

X rays are the most important diagnostic tool for special investigations of the bones. They can reveal a hairline fracture of a major bone, a bony deposit, or abnormal alignment.

Synovial aspiration, or a *synovial fluid exam,* involves the withdrawal of a tiny amount of synovial fluid with a needle inserted into a joint. The laboratory analysis of the fluid can help diagnose such problems as gout and some forms of arthritis.

MRI, or *magnetic resonance imaging,* is a way of creating an image of a body part by taking advantage of the way protons behave in a magnetic field when exposed to a radio-frequency pulse: the way they line up and the form of the radiowave that they emit produces the image. The patient lies down on a table, and a surface coil is applied. The surface coil

The Human Skeleton

Front view　　　　　　　　　　　**Rear view**

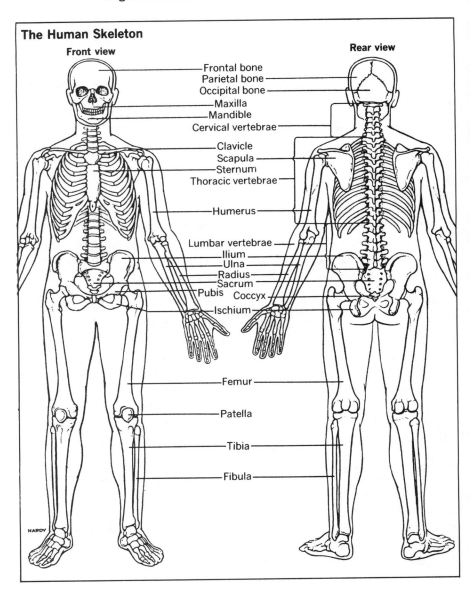

Frontal bone
Parietal bone
Occipital bone
Maxilla
Mandible
Cervical vertebrae
Clavicle
Scapula
Sternum
Thoracic vertebrae
Humerus
Lumbar vertebrae
Ilium
Ulna
Radius
Sacrum
Pubis　Coccyx
Ischium
Femur
Patella
Tibia
Fibula

HARDY

is the device that emits the radio-frequency pulse. The patient's heartbeat and respiration are monitored, usually by a small band placed around a finger. Next, the table moves the patient so that the area to be examined

is inside the magnet. The magnet is in the form of a tunnel and may make some people feel claustrophobic. At this point the noise level increases and may be uncomfortable. Several images are taken, with the table moving slightly between each. MRI is safer than X rays because there is no exposure to ionizing radiation; however, pregnant women and people with implanted stimulatory devices, such as pacemakers, should not have MRI performed.

Nuclear imaging involves the injection, swallowing, instillation, or inhalation of a *radioactive isotope* (a marker, or tracer) of a substance that is naturally absorbed by the organ or tissues that need observation. A camera sensitive to the radiation emitted by the isotope is then used to create an image that shows the location of the material within the body. Two uses of this technique for skeletal exams are the bone scan and the bone density test. These tests are more sensitive than X rays and can often identify a problem months before it shows up on the X ray. They are used when the X ray comes back normal, but symptoms persist.

In the *bone scan* the patient receives an injection of an isotope that is taken up by bone tissues. Scanning begins two to four hours later. Either the entire body or just the part under observation is imaged. Injuries, infections, and tumors can all be located with this technique.

The *bone density test* is used to diagnose osteoporosis, the decrease in bone density that is the major cause of fractures in the elderly. The most accurate bone-density test is dual-energy X-ray absorptiometry (DXA), which uses low doses of radiation— less than is used in an X ray—to measure bone density. The test is painless and safe and can be performed in 5 to 15 minutes.

Ultrasonography is most often employed in skeletal exams to determine whether a "lump" or "bump" is solid or fluid-filled. Ultrasonography follows the same principle that applies to sonar: Sound waves emitted by a transducer are directed at a particular part of the body; they bounce back, and are translated into an image. Tissues, bones, water, air— all vary consistently in the way they reflect the sound wave, thus making possible the interpretation of the reflected image.

Arthroscopy is a way of seeing inside the body by using an arthroscope, an optical instrument equipped with lenses and lights that is inserted in a small opening. The area most often studied by this method is the knee.

The Muscles and Joints

The human body has more than 600 muscles of various sizes and shapes, all of them attached to the skeletal system. They enable us to move as they contract. The joints are the spaces between two coupled bones that allow the bones to move in more than one direction. Muscles and joints are the domain of the rheumatologist.

The synovial fluid exam, X rays, MRI, nuclear imaging, and ultrasonography described under the skeletal system are used to examine the muscles and joints as well. When there is a problem with muscle control, inability to relax a muscle, or weakness in commonly used muscles, another test that may be ordered is the *electromyogram*. This test measures a muscle's electrical potential, which should be zero if the muscle is relaxed. An electrode is attached to the skin over the target muscle and another electrode, in the form of a small needle, is inserted in the muscle. Lead wires from the two electrodes are attached to a monitor, and measurements of the muscle's electrical activity are made while the patient contracts and relaxes it. This test helps determine whether the problem is with the muscle itself or with the nerves controlling it (in which case an electroneurogram is in order).

Joints are prone to stiffness and damage from swelling of the surrounding bursa and tendons. X rays and MRIs will detect damage to the bursa and tendons.

Skin

The dermatologist specializes in treating skin disorders. Many problems specific to the skin can be diagnosed by physical examination and questioning of the patient.

Skin tests are commonly done on allergy sufferers to determine what they are allergic to. In a *prick test* the forearm is cleansed and a drop each of up to 35 different solutions is placed in rows on the arm. The doctor then takes a small needlelike object and pricks the center of each drop. After 15 minutes any of the solutions to which the patient is allergic will produce a slight swelling much like a mosquito bite. A *scratch test* is similar; a small scratch is made on the arm and the drop is applied. In the *intradermal test* the solution is injected. A *patch test* is done when the patient has a rash, probably caused by something that touches the skin. Patches of possible allergens are placed on the back, and the patient returns in two days for a reading.

Sores that refuse to heal; changes in the shape, color, and texture of warts or moles; and blemishes that bleed or itch are all considered symptoms of skin cancer and should be checked by your doctor. These skin eruptions are usually removed entirely and a biopsy is performed on the tissue. They can be cut out (excised) or removed with an electric needle or laser.

The Nervous System

The brain, spinal cord, and network of nerves make up the nervous system. The neurosurgeon and the neurologist are the specialists.

In a *spinal tap,* or *spinal fluid exam,* the doctor inserts a needle into the lower back and removes a small amount of spinal fluid, which is then examined in the lab. The test may cause severe headaches; it is used to diagnose infections, brain hemorrhages, tumors, polio, meningitis, and other conditions. *Myelography* is a similar study, much more painful, in

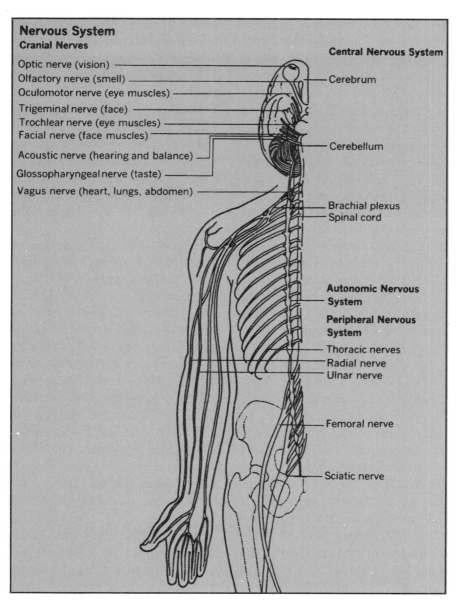

Nervous System

Cranial Nerves

Optic nerve (vision)
Olfactory nerve (smell)
Oculomotor nerve (eye muscles)
Trigeminal nerve (face)
Trochlear nerve (eye muscles)
Facial nerve (face muscles)
Acoustic nerve (hearing and balance)
Glossopharyngeal nerve (taste)
Vagus nerve (heart, lungs, abdomen)

Central Nervous System

Cerebrum
Cerebellum
Brachial plexus
Spinal cord

Autonomic Nervous System

Peripheral Nervous System

Thoracic nerves
Radial nerve
Ulnar nerve
Femoral nerve
Sciatic nerve

which a small amount of spinal fluid is removed, dye injected in its place, and X rays are taken while the patient lies on a table. Slipped disks, some types of arthritis, and different types of tumors are commonly diagnosed this way, although the use of MRI (see skeletal system) and computerized axial tomography (CT) are also used and are often done first.

The CT exam is a noninvasive procedure that produces a series of X-ray images showing "slices" of the targeted body part. For the exam, the patient lies on a table (called a gantry) which is then moved into the machine. Several exposures are taken, with the table moving slightly between each. For some studies it is necessary to inject a special dye, which can cause mild discomfort. Some people experience a claustrophobic reaction while inside the machine. CT is about 100 times more sensitive than conventional X rays and is used to detect calcium deposits, tumors, cysts, and abscesses. Because of its sensitivity to tissue density, it can sometimes distinguish benign from malignant tumors.

The *brain scan* continues to be an important diagnostic tool. This radioisotope study of the brain is used to detect tumors, hemorrhages, stroke, or blood vessel abnormalities.

The brain scan involves the injection in the arm of a radioactive isotope and the scanning of the brain by either a single-photon emission computed tomography camera (SPECT) or a positron emission tomography camera (PET). The SPECT scanner uses gamma rays to create images and the PET scanner uses positrons (a type of subatomic particle found in the nucleus of an atom) to create images. The PET scan is able to read through different depths of tissue, so problems deeply buried in the brain can be detected without surgery.

When the blood supply to the brain is limited by the blocking of the carotid arteries (a condition known as transient ischemic attack, or TIA), momentary loss of brain function can occur and can eventually lead to a stroke. Thus examining the carotid arteries is important if the patient has symptoms or significant risk factors. This can be done by X ray or by ultrasound. In the ultrasound test two techniques are generally used. The first creates images (called duplex) and the second measures the rate and quality of blood flow (called Doppler). Both involve the gentle movement of the transducer slowly over each side of the neck. The procedure takes about 30 minutes.

Patients who have experienced TIA, stroke, or vertigo may undergo *ocular plethysmography* (OPG) to detect narrowing of the ophthalmic artery. The patient is seated in a chair with a headrest, blood pressure is taken in each arm, and EKG leads are placed on the chest. Anesthetic drops are placed in each eye. The technologist then places tiny plastic cups into the corner of each eye. The cups are attached to wire leads connected to the machine. The patient is instructed to keep the eyes wide open. The machine then produces a slight suction on each eye and measures its pressure.

When epilepsy is suspected, following certain head injuries, or when the patient is experiencing confusion, sleep problems, and even impotence, an *electroencephalograph* (EEG) may be ordered. The patient sits in a chair while a technologist attaches 16 to 22 electrodes to his or her head. EKG leads are also placed on the chest. The patient then lies down and may even fall asleep. The technologist may instruct the patient to open and close both eyes while a strobe light flashes. The test takes about two hours.

The electromyogram was discussed under the section on muscles. If the muscle is not the problem, the nerves connected to it may be and a *nerve conduction study,* or *electroneurogram,* is ordered. This test measures the speed of the electrical impulse across a nerve and the speed of the muscle's response to it. Elec-trodes are affixed to the skin over the target muscle. The target nerve is then given a mild electric shock. The electrode over the muscle measures both the time between the shock and the response (the muscle will twitch) and the intensity of the response. The corresponding nonaffected muscles are also tested for comparison. There is no hazard, and the shock feels like a mild sting or burn.

The Circulatory System

The cardiologist specializes in diseases of the heart and circulatory system. Coronary artery disease is the most common form of heart disease and involves the blocking of the arteries to the heart. There can also be problems with the heart muscle itself, problems with the heart valves, or congenital problems resulting from birth defects.

The electrocardiogram and the stress test have already been discussed. Nuclear imaging, ultrasound, and X rays are also used to detect coronary artery disease. In order to detect exactly how blocked the arteries are and determine the necessary correctional procedure, an *angiograph,* or *angiogram,* is done.

The angiograph begins with the insertion of a special needle in a major artery (usually in the groin). A sudden spurt of blood indicates correct positioning. A wire is then inserted through the needle, which stops the bleeding. The wire is advanced to the target area, and the needle is removed. A catheter is then slid over the wire and is advanced to the target area. The wire is then withdrawn. The next step is the injection of a special dye to the target area. To prevent its being diluted it must be injected at high velocity and in large quantity. For most people the injection is extremely uncomfortable, with some reporting severe pain, a feeling of heat, headache, chest pain, or dizziness. The next step involves the rapid imaging of the target area, usually by a series of X-ray pictures. Often different views are needed of the targeted area, which means that the catheter must be repositioned and the dye reinjected. Once the pictures are finished the catheter is slowly removed and pressure is applied to the hole to seal the artery. The pressure involved is intense and lasts for 10 to 15 minutes. Because it is necessary for the patient to be conscious during the procedure, the entire process may cause extreme anxiety, which in turn increases the risk of heart attack. The patient is normally given a sedative to help relieve the anxiety. An overnight stay in the hospital following the procedure is routine. *Venography* is a sim-

The Circulatory System

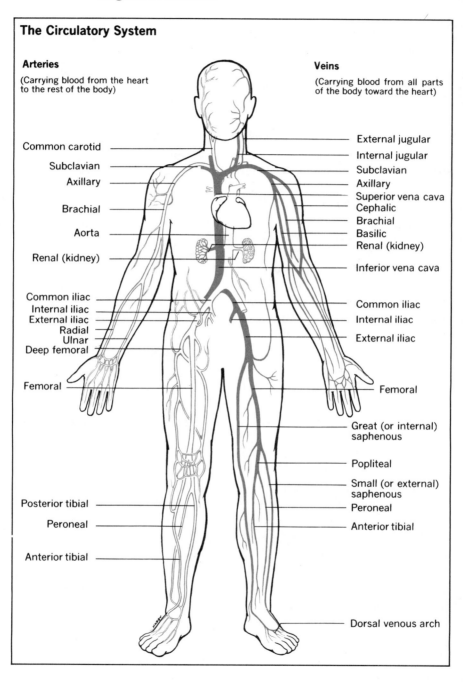

Arteries

(Carrying blood from the heart
to the rest of the body)

Common carotid
Subclavian
Axillary
Brachial
Aorta
Renal (kidney)
Common iliac
Internal iliac
External iliac
Radial
Ulnar
Deep femoral
Femoral
Posterior tibial
Peroneal
Anterior tibial

Veins

(Carrying blood from all parts
of the body toward the heart)

External jugular
Internal jugular
Subclavian
Axillary
Superior vena cava
Cephalic
Brachial
Basilic
Renal (kidney)
Inferior vena cava
Common iliac
Internal iliac
External iliac
Femoral
Great (or internal)
saphenous
Popliteal
Small (or external)
saphenous
Peroneal
Anterior tibial
Dorsal venous arch

ilar study of the veins.

Not all people who experience sudden and severe chest pain are having a heart attack. A technique called *infarct detection* can confirm the diagnosis of heart attack. Normally per-

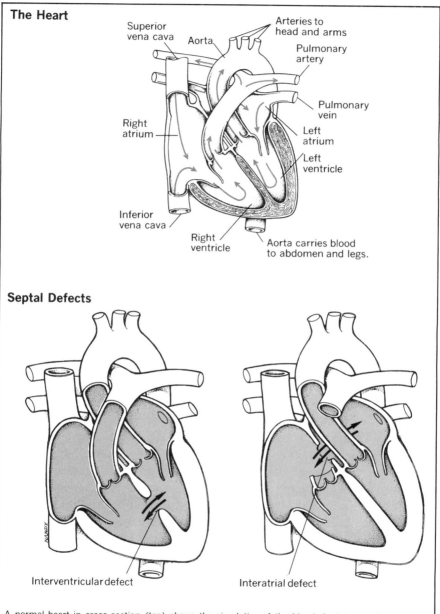

The Heart

Superior vena cava

Aorta

Arteries to head and arms

Pulmonary artery

Pulmonary vein

Right atrium

Left atrium

Left ventricle

Inferior vena cava

Right ventricle

Aorta carries blood to abdomen and legs.

Septal Defects

Interventricular defect

Interatrial defect

A normal heart in cross section *(top)*, shows the circulation of the blood. An interventricular defect *(bottom left)* allows blood to pass directly between the left and right ventricles. An interatrial defect *(bottom right)*, with the aorta seen in cross section over the left atrium, allows blood to pass freely between the two atria. Any septal defect interferes with the effectiveness of the pumping action of the heart.

formed within the first 12 to 24 hours after the onset of the pain, the test in- volves the injection of an isotope (thallium-201) into a vein. The patient is then positioned under a gamma-ray camera and an image is created of the heart that will make evident any occluded (blocked) vessels. A similar nuclear imaging process is used to obtain information about the heart's *wall motion* (how well the muscle relaxes and contracts) and *ejection fraction* (how much blood leaves a chamber of the heart when it contracts). Both tests give valuable information about the heart's health.

While X rays provide more detail, nuclear imaging can also be used to check *circulatory integrity,* or how open the veins and arteries are. Again, a radioactive isotope is injected into a vein near the target area and images are produced via a gamma-ray camera.

Evaluation of the ejection fraction, valve function, and pericardial fluid (found in the pericardial membrane that surrounds the heart) can also be done with ultrasound. In a process similar to that described earlier for the carotid arteries, *echocardiography* produces an image of the working heart.

The Digestive System, the Liver, and the Pancreas

The gastroenterologist specializes in disorders of the digestive system and the liver.

As in many other systems, X rays are the traditional diagnostic tool for gastrointestinal problems. Nuclear imaging, however, may be used for some specific complaints. For example, if you're having trouble with heartburn an *esophageal reflux* test may be done to determine whether or not you have a hiatus hernia. The patient eats nothing the night before the exam. A small balloon is placed over the stomach, held in place by a special inflatable belt. The patient then stands in front of a gamma-ray camera and drinks a glass of orange juice to which a radioactive isotope has been added. Pictures are taken as the fluid moves to the stomach. The patient then lies down on a table and the cuff is inflated, causing the balloon to apply pressure to the stomach. Pictures are taken to see if this pressure causes the liquid in the stomach to back up into the esophagus. If it does, a hiatus hernia is the diagnosis.

In a gastrointestinal examination, X rays are usually taken first, and an endoscopy is done if a tissue sample is needed for biopsy. Endoscopy gives the physician a direct view of the gastrointestinal tract. The endoscope is a flexible tube with a light source, a camera, and instruments for taking tissue samples. The patient eats nothing the night before the exam. After undressing and putting on a gown, the patient lies down and drinks a bitter-tasting local anesthetic to inhibit the gag reflex. A mild sedative is also administered.

The patient lies on his left side with the mouth open. The endoscope is then put in the mouth and advanced down toward the stomach. Photographs are commonly taken, and samples of tissue or gastric juice may also be taken. The exam takes about

The Digestive System

Salivary glands
Salivary glands secrete saliva, containing enzymes that act on carbohydrates. The saliva also moistens the food for swallowing.

Pharynx
The pharynx connects the mouth to the esophagus.

Epiglottis

Trachea (windpipe)

Esophagus
The esophagus carries the food to the stomach.

Liver
The liver produces bile that is carried to the digestive tract by the bile duct.

Gallbladder
The gallbladder stores excess bile.

Pyloric sphincter

Bile duct

Duodenum

Transverse colon

Small intestine
The small intestine secretes enzymes that act on proteins and carbohydrates. Digested food is absorbed by the small intestine.

Ascending colon

Vermiform appendix

Anus

Nasal cavity

Teeth
Teeth break up food into a soft, pulpy mass that can be swallowed.

Tongue
The tongue helps to move the food between the teeth. It also contains the taste receptors.

Cardiac sphincter

Stomach
The stomach secretes gastric juices that help break down proteins and fats by enzyme action.

Pancreas
The pancreas produces digestive juices that help break down starches, proteins, and fats. These juices are carried to the intestine by the pancreatic duct.

Pancreatic duct

Large intestine

Sigmoid colon

Rectum
The rectum stores feces until elimination.

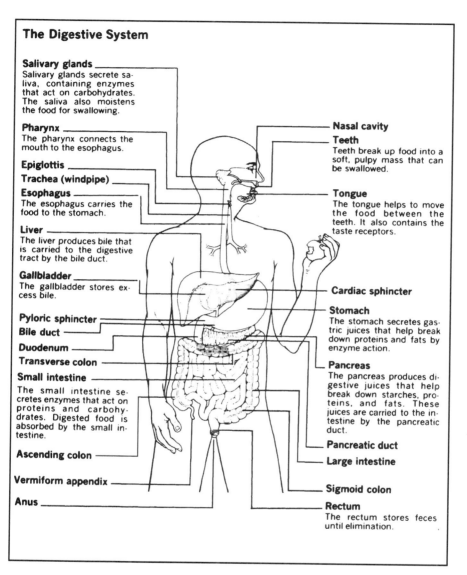

2 to 3 hours.

An *upper GI* may be in order if your doctor suspects an ulcer or tumor. No food is allowed for 8 hours before the test. An injection of glucagon (which may cause nausea or dizziness) is normally given to slow down the movements of the stomach. Next, the patient swallows a small cupful of granular material which produces gas and causes the stomach to distend. Finally, the patient is given a glass of barium and stands with his back to the X-ray table. A fluoroscopic screen is positioned in front of the patient, and the radiologist instructs him to take small swallows of the barium. A series of pictures are taken, with the patient changing position several times. If the entire small intestine is being studied, the patient is next taken to a waiting area and returns every 15 to 30 minutes for more pictures. A stomach—duodenum study takes about a half hour. The longer study takes from 1 to 3 hours.

A *lower GI,* often called simply a *barium enema,* is much more involved. It is used when there is a suspicion of diverticulitis, bowel obstruction, colon polyps, colitis, or other intestinal disorders. A strict diet is prescribed, along with laxatives, for several days before the test. Two enemas are given on the morning of the study. For this exam the patient lies down on the X-ray table. The doctor inserts a lubricated, gloved finger into the patient's rectum to make sure there are no obstructions and then inserts the enema tip. The tip has a built-in balloon that can be inflated if the patient feels unable to retain the enema. Like the upper GI, an injection of glucagon is often given to counteract the feeling of "fullness" experienced by most people. The fluoroscope is then positioned and the technologist begins the enema: a solution of barium is pumped into the rectum until it fills the large intestine. Air may then be pumped into the rectum for greater contrast. Both the enema and the air can cause a feeling of fullness and discomfort. The patient retains the enema and the air until all the pictures are taken.

There is a breath test used to detect the bacterium *Helicobacter pylori,* which is thought to be the cause of many ulcers. The patient simply blows into a small plastic bag, then drinks a glass of clear, tasteless liquid. The liquid consists of substances that will be broken down by any *H. pylori* in the stomach. Thirty minutes later, the patient exhales into another plastic bag. Both bags are sent to a laboratory to be tested for *H. pylori.* The breath test for *H. pylori* bacterium is about 95 percent accurate.

The gall bladder, an organ in the upper right abdomen responsible for storing the bile necessary for fat digestion, is a frequent site of infection and may also develop stones. Examination of the gall bladder can be done with X rays, ultrasound, or nuclear imaging. Most routine gall bladder studies are done with ultrasound. An 8-hour fast is required before the test. The patient is given a gown to wear, may be asked to drink a white liquid, and then lies down on the couch. The doctor applies a special lubricant to the abdominal area and moves the transducer over it. The patient can watch the results on a monitor.

If stones develop in the gall bladder and block the flow of bile, infection results—a condition called acute cholecystitis. Nuclear imaging is considered the most specific diagnostic tool for this disorder. The patient fasts for 4 hours before the exam. An isotope is injected and the patient lies down under a gamma-ray camera. Pictures are taken every 5 to 10 minutes for a half hour and then every 15 minutes for one and a half hours.

The liver makes the bile needed for fat digestion, and the pancreas makes the enzymes necessary for fat digestion. Neither the entire liver nor the entire pancreas can be seen with X rays. X rays of the blood supply and ductal structures, however, enable the skilled specialist to make accurate assumptions about the condition of either. CT imaging can give a full picture of both organs and is safer than X rays. Ultrasound is also useful.

If the results of lab tests suggest liver disease or if the organ is enlarged, a special *needle biopsy* may be done. The patient is normally asked to avoid eating the night before the test. Medication by mouth or injection may be given. The gastroenterologist feels the lower edge of the liver, selects a spot, and injects a small amount of local anesthetic under the skin. Next a larger needle with a syringe is inserted. There will be pressure and even a dull pain. The plunger of the syringe is pulled back, and liver cells are extracted. The needle is then removed and pressure is applied to the puncture site.

The Respiratory System

The respiratory system includes the pharynx, trachea, bronchi, and the lungs.

A chest X ray (described earlier) is usually the first test done when symptoms indicate a possible problem in the respiratory system. When the bronchi must be seen in more detail, a *bronchogram* may be done. This requires the suppression of the "coughing reflex" by spraying a local or topical anesthetic in the patient's mouth and back of the throat. Then a thin metal tube shaped like a candy cane (a cannula) will be placed in the mouth with the curved end over the back of the tongue. Anesthetic is injected into the cannula, which runs down the back of the throat into the bronchi. A rubber tube (catheter) is passed through the patient's nose, down the back of the throat, through the larynx, the trachea, and then into the bronchi of one or both lungs. A special dye is then instilled into the catheter, which runs down and fills the tubes. The dye highlights the bronchi, making it easier to see blockage and tight areas on the X ray.

A *bronchoscopy* may be in order if X rays or CT reveal potential problems and the physician needs a closer look or a tissue sample. The physician inspects the larynx, trachea and bronchi through a flexible fiber-optic tube called a bronchoscope. Miniature instruments are fed through the bronchoscope to collect tissue samples.

A group of tests called *pulmonary function tests* help the physician determine if certain symptoms may be due to either restrictive or obstructive lung disease. These tests measure how much air can be forcibly exhaled after inhaling as deeply as possible, how much air remains in the lungs after a forcible exhalation, and how much air is expired with each normal breath. They evaluate how well the lungs stretch with each breath inhaled and how well they collapse with each breath exhaled.

The Respiratory System

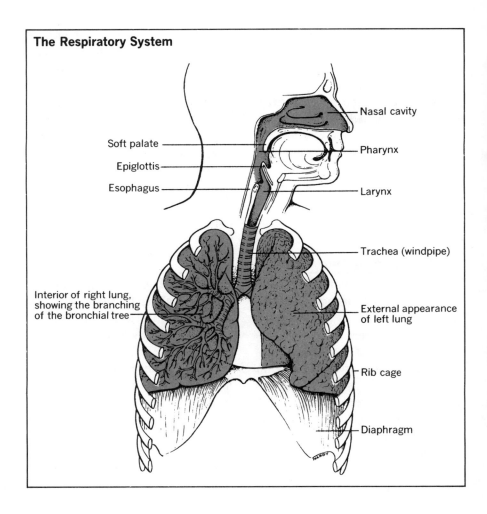

Nasal cavity

Soft palate

Pharynx

Epiglottis

Esophagus

Larynx

Trachea (windpipe)

Interior of right lung, showing the branching of the bronchial tree

External appearance of left lung

Rib cage

Diaphragm

The patient is put in a pressurized plexiglass cabin called a body box, which looks like a large phone booth. The patient's nose is closed off with a nose clip and a special mouthpiece is inserted in the mouth. Then, the patient performs a series of breathing maneuvers by exhaling into the mouthpiece, which is attached to monitoring equipment. The tests take 15 to 45 minutes.

The Endocrine System

There are 7 endocrine glands that make up the endocrine system: pituitary, thyroid, parathyroids, adrenals, pancreas, ovaries (women), and testicles (men). The glands secrete hormones that produce a specific effect or regulate a certain action of other body organs. Laboratory tests of blood and urine are important diagnostic tools for the glands, and all can be visualized with X rays, CT, nuclear imaging, and ultrasound if lab tests indicate a potential problem. Some tests may necessitate the injection of a special dye to highlight the target area.

The Kidneys and the Urinary System

Laboratory tests of the urine are the most obvious way of beginning a diagnosis of kidney or urinary system problems. A resting EKG may also be done as well as nuclear imaging, ultrasound, and X rays. If a kidney biopsy is needed, the patient is normally given an anesthetic to induce drowsiness and is then instructed to lie face down on a table. The procedure is similar to that of the liver biopsy. First the anesthetic is injected, then the aspirating needle is inserted. This takes only a minute or so. An overnight stay is required for observation. Patients may experience a dull backache for several days after the biopsy.

An *intravenous urography* is a common test for urinary tract problems. Colon cleansing (strict diet, laxative, enemas) is often done before the test. Dye is injected into the patient's arm (or may drip in gradually from a diluted bottle of fluid). X rays are taken at timed intervals. A compression cuff (like a large blood pressure cuff) may be put around the abdomen to apply pressure just below each kidney, and more pictures are taken. The patient is then told to void his or her bladder; another X ray is taken, and the test is over.

Ears, Nose, and Throat

The otorhinolaryngologist specializes in treating problems of the ears, nose, and throat. Difficulty in hearing, faulty balance or vertigo, earache, and ringing in the ears (tinnitus) are common ear complaints. Congestion, discharge from the nose, postnasal drip, itching and sneezing, headaches over the eyes, pain over the upper teeth, and unexplained fever are complaints associated with the nose and sinuses. Laryngitis, sore throat, or difficulty in swallowing are common throat complaints.

An *audiogram* evaluates and measures hearing. The patient is seated in a booth and earphones are placed over the ears. A series of tones that vary in loudness are played through the earphones and the patient uses hand signals to indicate hearing a tone. Each ear is tested separately.

A *tympanogram* measures vibrations of the eardrum. A rubber plug is inserted in one ear and mild pressure is applied. The tympanogram reveals the type of hearing loss caused by a perforated eardrum, by an eardrum that has become thickened from an infection, or by an obstruction in the middle ear.

Patients who experience dizziness may be given an *electronystagmogram,* a series of neurological tests that rec-

A Guide to Some Home Medical Tests

Kind	Function	How It Works	Time Required
Blood glucose monitoring	Measures the level of glucose (a kind of sugar) in blood	Wash your hands thoroughly. Prick a finger or earlobe to obtain a drop of blood, then follow instructions.	1 to 2 minutes
Ovulation monitoring	Measures the quantity of luteinizing hormone (LH) in urine	A chemically treated strip is dipped in urine specimen and compared with a color guide.	20 minutes to 1 hour
Pregnancy	Detects human chorionic gonadotropin, produced by a developing placenta, in urine	Chemicals are mixed with a urine specimen in a small test tube. A ring formation or color change indicates pregnancy.	20 minutes to 2 hours
Urinary tract infections	Detects nitrite in urine	Chemically treated test strip is dipped in urine specimen on three consecutive mornings.	30 to 40 seconds
Occult fecal blood	Detects hidden blood in stools	A color change, appearing when stool specimen is brought into contact with peroxide and guaiac, indicates hidden blood.	30 seconds to 16 minutes
Gonorrhea	Detects the bacteria causing gonorrhea in the specimen of pus from the penis	Specimen, collected on a slide, is allowed to air-dry. Then follow directions.	Several days
Blood pressure	Measures the pressure of blood on the walls of the arteries	The center of a cuff is placed on the pulse point of the upper arm. With or without a microphone, the user listens for artery sounds.	2 to 5 minutes
Impotence	Detects, measures the rigidity of erections during sleep	Soft fabric band or stamps are placed around the penis before the subject goes to bed at night. The strips break at different degrees of pressure.	Overnight
Vision	Screens for visual acuity problems	Using three different tests, you read special eye charts.	2 to 3 minutes

ord eye movements. Abnormal movements of the eye can indicate a problem with the balance mechanism (vestibular system). The technician tapes a small metal disk under each eye and on the bridge of the nose. These sensors are attached by lead wires to a graph machine. The patient is then instructed to follow a slowly moving target with the eyes as eye movements are recorded. In the next test the patient, with eyes closed, lies down and turns to one side. Eye movements are recorded as water is placed into the external ear canal. This procedure often produces dizziness or nausea that persists for several hours.

Smears and cultures are the common lab tests for nose and throat complaints. X ray examinations may also be done. In some cases a biopsy may be necessary. For the nose, a needle aspiration is the common method, either through the nose or upper gum of the mouth. A local anesthetic is given first. An excisional biopsy may be necessary, in which case a small piece of tissue is removed. For the throat an excisional biopsy is commonly done, normally under general anesthesia, and an overnight stay in the hospital may be required. A laryngoscope is used to obtain the sample. The throat remains sore for several days afterwards.

The Eyes

Opthalmologists are certified doctors of medicine who specialize in medical and surgical care of the eye. As such, they have the greatest range of expertise among eye-care specialists. In addition to testing vision and prescribing corrective lenses, opththalmologists diagnose and treat all eye disorders, from minor infections to conditions such as glaucoma that can lead to blindness.

Optometrists diagnose vision problems and prescribe lenses, screen for glaucoma, and identify and treat other disorders. They are not physicians, but they have completed two years of study in an approved college followed by four years at a school of optometry.

Opticians fit and sell corrective lenses prescribed by an opthalmologist or optometrist.

The common eye exam includes tests for visual acuity, color blindness, and muscle integrity. Other tests are the slit-lamp exam, tonometry, and retinal exam.

The Snellen visual acuity chart is used to measure visual acuity. Letters, numbers, or symbols are arranged in rows, each row formed by characters of the same size. The top row contains large characters, with each succeeding row formed by smaller characters. The patient is asked to stand or sit 20 feet from the chart and identify the figures line by line from top to bottom until the figures are no longer recognizable. The doctor will check each eye individually while the patient covers the alternate eye; then both eyes are tested together. This test detects errors of vision such as nearsightedness, farsightedness, and astigmatism, which are the result of defects in the size and shape of the eye. Continuing the test, the opthalmologist fits the patient with a series of corrective lenses of different strengths. The patient looks through each sample lens and reads the Snellen chart again, identifying those lenses that help him see the letters or symbols most clearly.

Color blindness is the inability to recognize one or more colors. Various charts are used to detect color blindness. One commonly used chart contains patterns of colored dots. A color blind person will not be able to distinguish between dots of certain colors and therefore will not be able to discern a design defined by these dots.

The muscle integrity exam tests eye movement to determine if both eyes can focus together. The movement of the eye toward any desired direction is controlled through the coordinated action of six muscles at-

Focusing

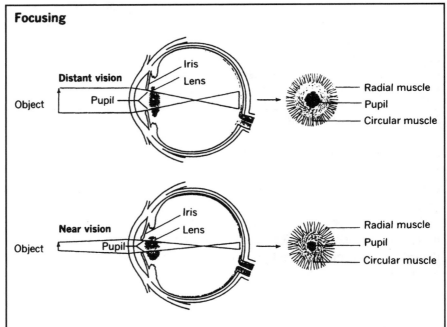

When viewing a distant object (more than 20 feet away), the lens flattens and the pupil dilates, allowing more light to enter the eye. The pupil is dilated by the action of the outer radial muscles of the iris, which contract and thus stretch the previously contracted circular muscles. When viewing a near object, the lens becomes more oval and the pupil contracts as more light enters the eye. This prevents overstimulation of the retina. The pupil is reduced in size by the contraction of the inner circular muscles, which serve to stretch the previously contracted radial muscles.

tached to the eyeball under the conjunctiva. For an object to be perceived properly, the eye muscles must work in unison to focus the image on the center of the retina at the back of the eye. In the muscle integrity exam, the patient is asked to look in various directions. Both eyes will move together if the muscles are working properly.

The slit-lamp microscope is used to obtain a magnified view of structures at the front of the eye—the sclera, iris, conjunctiva, cornea, and lens—which are carefully checked for signs of injury or disease. A common disorder detected by slit-lamp examination is the cataract, the clouding of the nor-

mally clear lens. The standard treatment for cataracts is surgical removal of the lens, which, in most cases, is then replaced with an artificial lens. Alternatives to an artificial lens include contact lenses or thick-lensed eyeglasses.

Glaucoma is a disease caused by inadequate drainage of the fluid within the eyeball. The resulting increase in the pressure of the fluid damages the optic nerve, leading to a gradual narrowing of the field of vision and, eventually, blindness. Glaucoma is the leading cause of blindness in the United States. An instrument called a tonometer is used to measure the pressure of fluid within the eyeball.

The tonometer is placed on the pupil after a drop of anesthetic has been applied to the eye, and a gauge records the resistance of the eye to the slight pressure applied. It is recommended that this painless procedure be done for those 40 and over every 2 to 3 years, or annually if there is a family history of glaucoma.

The final test in the general eye exam is the retinal exam. The room is darkened, and the doctor uses an ophthalmoscope to look through the pupil into the back of the eye.

A common disease of the retina is macular degeneration, an age-related disorder that causes increasingly blurred central vision in the elderly. A leading cause of blindness in the United States is diabetic retinopathy, a deterioration of the blood vessels of the retina brought on by diabetes.

Diagnostic Tests and the Patient's Rights

As medical costs continue to rise, questions about the necessity of various diagnostic tests will continue to be raised. For the healthy individual, it makes little sense to undergo more than the few routine screening tests necessary for his particular age group; there is always the chance of an error that may lead to additional tests at even greater expense, not to mention the emotional trauma that a false positive could cause.

For the patient experiencing particular symptoms, or those in high risk categories, the number and kind of diagnostic tests are a concern. Batteries, or sets, of tests are a particular cause for concern. The batteries can be complex, and the physician may not take the time to explain each one in detail so that the patient thoroughly understands what they mean in terms of discomfort, risk, and cost. The value of a particular test must also be weighed against its results. Expensive CT and MRI tests are the "study of choice" for many problems, but for others, the less expensive X ray might do just as well or better. When presented with the need for diagnostic tests, then, the patient should endeavor to become as informed as possible about what is necessary. As already mentioned, having a physician with whom you can converse easily and understand is an important factor in the quality of the medical care you receive.

27

Nutrition and Weight Control

Just as it was for our earliest ancestors, food is an integral part of our daily lives. Not only is food essential for survival, but oftentimes the way in which we structure our lives—our work habits, our recreational activities—revolves around how, when, and where we get food and eat it.

Ironically, however, because most of us live a much faster-paced lifestyle than we did even twenty years ago, we spend less time choosing, preparing, and eating food. We grab breakfast on the run (if we eat it at all), hurry through lunch, and rarely take time to plan and prepare a lei-surely, well-balanced dinner. Often everyone in the family is on a different schedule, with the result that all too often we rely on prepackaged microwave dinners or take out fast food. Consequently, many of us are not eating properly, spending money on expensive vitamins to make up for poor nutrition, starving ourselves to lose weight, or gaining extra pounds by filling up on empty calories.

Practicing good eating habits may take a little more time and planning than we think we can afford, but its benefits will pay off in the long run in a healthier, happier way of life.

Basic Nutritional Requirements

The process by which food is converted into useful energy is called *metabolism*. It begins with chemical processes in the gastrointestinal tract which change plant and animal food into less complex components so that they can be absorbed to fulfill their various functions in the body — growth, repair, and fuel. Different foods have different energy values, measured in calories. An ideal diet for the average healthy individual provides the highest nutritional benefits from the fewest number of calories. Information on the protein, fat, and carbohydrate content in specific foods, as well as the number of calories, may be obtained by consulting the tables "Nutrients in Common Foods." The Metric Equivalents table converts spoon and cup measures into metric measures.

Protein

Of the several essential components of food, *protein* is in many ways the most important. This is so not only because it is one of the three principal sources of energy, but also because much of the body's structure is made up of proteins. For example, the typical 160-pound man is composed of about 100 pounds of water, 29 pounds of protein, 25 pounds of fat, 5 pounds of minerals, 1 pound of carbohydrate, and less than an ounce of vitamins. Because the muscles, heart, brain, lungs, and gastrointestinal organs are made up largely of protein, and since the protein in these organs is in constant need of replacement, its importance is obvious.

The recommended dietary allowance for protein is 0.8 g/Kg of body weight per day for persons aged 15 and up and 1 g/Kg of body weight for children under 15. (To convert your weight from pounds to kilograms, divide by 2.2. Thus a woman weighing 130 pounds weighs about 59 kilograms and needs about 47 grams of protein a day. A man weighing 175 pounds needs about 64 grams of protein a day.) Most Americans, however, eat about twice the amount they need, and while more may sound better, too much is too much. Your body uses only what it needs. Some excess protein is excreted as urine; the rest is converted to fat.

Chemically, proteins are varying mixtures of amino acids that contain various elements, including nitrogen. There are 22 different amino acids that are essential for the body's protein needs. Nine of these must be provided in the diet and are thus called *essential* amino acids; the rest can be synthesized by the body itself.

Meat, fish, poultry, eggs, and milk or milk products are the primary protein foods and contain all of the necessary amino acids; they are therefore called *complete* proteins. Grains and vegetables are partly made up of protein, but more often than not, they do not provide the whole range of amino acids required for proper nourishment. When properly combined, however, vegetable proteins, too, can be complete. For example, mixing rice and dried beans provides the same quality of protein as a steak (with a lot less fat).

One gram of protein provides four calories of energy.

Carbohydrates

Carbohydrates are another essential energy source. Called *starches* or *sugars,* they are present in large quantities in grains, fruits, and nuts. As *complex carbohydrates,* or *polysaccharides,* they are found in the foods named and particularly in breads, breakfast cereals, flours, pastas, barley, legumes, rice, and starchy vegetables. *Simple carbohydrates,* or mono- or disaccharides, are found in such foods as table sugars, candy, pastries, and soft drinks.

Complex carbohydrates are primary sources of calories, nutrients, and fiber—for such purposes as muscle contraction, weight reduction, and control of sodium and cholesterol. Simple carbohydrates, on the other hand, are pure sources of calories and contain little nutritional value. It is for this reason that they are often termed "empty" calories. Lack of adequate carbohydrates means the body will begin to convert body fat or protein into sugar.

Although there is no absolute dietary requirement for carbohydrates, it is generally recommended that more than half the energy requirement beyond infancy be provided by complex carbohydrates. One gram of carbohydrate provides four calories of energy. Thus the average man consuming about 2,900 calories per day should consume about 360 grams of carbohydrate. The average woman consuming about 2,200 calories per day should consume about 275 grams of carbohydrate.

Fats

Fats are a chemically complex food component composed of *glycerol* (a sweet, oily alcohol) and fatty acids. Fats exist in several forms and come from a variety of sources. One way to think of them is to group them as visible fats, such as butter, salad oil, or the fat seen in meat, and as invisible fats, which are mingled, blended, or absorbed into food, either naturally, as in nuts, meat, or fish, or during cooking. Another way is to think of them as solid at room temperature (fats), or as liquid at room temperature (oils).

Saturated and Unsaturated

Fats are also classified as *saturated* or *unsaturated.* This is a chemical distinction based on the differences in molecular structure of different kinds of fat. If the carbon atoms in a fat molecule are surrounded or boxed in by hydrogen atoms, they are said to be saturated. This type of fat tends to be solid at room temperature, and high consumption of it increases the cholesterol content of the blood, which can lead to heart disease. *Unsaturated* fats, such as those found in fish and vegetable oils, contain the least number of hydrogen atoms and do not add to the blood cholesterol content. They are either *monounsaturated* or *polyunsaturated.* In general, fats in foods of plant origin are more unsaturated than in those of animal origin (except for coconut and palm oils, which are highly saturated). It is recommended that you consume no more than 30 percent of your daily calories from fats; 10 percent of each of the three types, or, for our average man, about 32 grams total; for our average woman, about 24 grams total.

Fats play several essential roles in the metabolic process. First of all, they provide more than twice the number of calories on a comparative weight basis than do proteins and carbohydrates (one gram of fat contains nine calories). They also can be stored in the body in large quantities (in adipose tissue) and used as a later energy source. They serve as carriers of the fat-soluble vitamins A, D, E, and K, and—of no little importance—they add to the tastiness of food.

Vitamins

Vitamins, which are present in minute quantities in foods in their natural state, are essential for normal metabolism and for the development and maintenance of tissue structure and function. In addition to the fat-soluble vitamins noted above, there are a number of B vitamins, as well as vitamin C, also called *ascorbic acid.* If any particular vitamin is missing from the diet over a sufficiently long time, a specific disease will result.

Vitamin A

Vitamin A is essential for vision, growth, cell growth and development, reproduction, a strong immune system, and healthy hair, skin, and mucous membranes.

Vitamin A is fat soluble and is therefore stored by the body (in the liver). It comes in two forms: retinol, found only in animal foods (chiefly liver), and beta-carotene, found in fruits and vegetables (chiefly deep green or orange ones like spinach and sweet potatoes). Retinol is instantly available for bodily use, while beta-carotene must be converted by the body into retinol before it can be used. (Because the body will not convert excess beta-carotene into retinol, there is no danger of overdosing on this form of vitamin A. Retinol, however, can be extremely toxic at high levels.)

Symptoms of vitamin A deficiency include dry rough skin, slow growth, night blindness, thickening of bone, and increased susceptibility to infection. Vitamin A deficiency is rare in the United States.

Formerly measured in International Units (IU), vitamin A content is now expressed retinol equivalents (RE). One RE equals 10 IU of beta-carotene and 3.33 IU of retinol. The Recommended Daily Allowance (RDA) for vitamin A for adult males is 1000 RE and for adult women, 800 RE.

Modified Calorie/Weight Reduction Diet

Sample Menus

	1,500 Calories	**1,800 Calories**	**2,000 Calories**

Breakfast	1 serving fruit/juice
	1 slice toast
	1 serving egg or
	  substitute
	1 serving margarine
	1 cup skim milk
	coffee/tea
		1 serving fruit/juice
		1 slice toast
		1 serving egg or
		  substitute
		1 serving cereal
		1 serving margarine
		1 cup skim milk
		coffee/tea
			1 serving fruit/juice
			1 slice toast
			1 serving egg or
			  substitute
			1 serving cereal
			1 serving margarine
			1 cup skim milk
			coffee/tea

Lunch	2-3 ounces meat
	1 serving potato or
	  substitute
	1 serving bread
	vegetables
	salad/non-fat
	  dressing
	2 servings fruit
	1 serving margarine
	coffee/tea
		2-3 ounces meat
		1 serving potato or
		  substitute
		1 serving bread
		vegetables
		salad/non-fat
		  dressing
		2 servings fruit/juice
		1 serving margarine
		coffee/tea
			2-3 ounces meat
			1 serving potato or
			  substitute
			1 serving bread
			vegetables
			salad/non-fat
			  dressing
			2 servings fruit/juice
			1 serving margarine
			1 cup skim milk
			coffee/tea

Dinner	2-3 ounces meat
	1 serving potato or
	  substitute
	1 serving bread
	vegetables
	salad/non-fat
	  dressing
	1 serving fruit
	2 servings margarine
	coffee/tea
		2-3 ounces meat
		1 serving potato or
		  substitute
		1 serving bread
		vegetables
		salad/non-fat
		  dressing
		2 servings fruit/juice
		2 servings margarine
		coffee/tea
			2-3 ounces meat
			2 servings potato or
			  substitute
			1 serving bread
			vegetables
			salad/non-fat
			  dressing
			1 serving fruit/juice
			2 servings margarine
			coffee/tea

Snack	3 graham crackers
	1 cup skim milk
		1 ounce meat
		1 slice bread
		1 serving reduced-fat
		  mayonnaise
		1 cup skim milk
			1 ounce meat
			1 slice bread
			1 serving reduced-fat
			  mayonnaise
			non-alcoholic
			  beverage

From the *Clinical Center Diet Manual*, Clinical Center Nutrition Department, National Institutes of Health, Department of Health and Human Services.

Vitamin D

Vitamin D is essential for proper metabolism of calcium, which is primarily responsible for the healthy growth of bones and teeth.

Vitamin D is fat soluble and therefore excessive intake can be toxic. It is consumed chiefly as an addition to milk and is also manufactured by the body by a reaction of sunlight on sterols present in the skin.

The major deficiency disease of vitamin D in children is rickets (deformation of the skeleton) and in adults excessive bone loss and fractures. The RDA for adults over 24 is 5 micrograms.

Vitamin E (tocopherol)

Vitamin E is essential for healthy nerve function and reproduction.

Vitamin E is found principally in plant oils, particularly wheat germ oil and nuts. It is fat soluble, but there is little danger of toxicity because absorption by the body is inefficient.

Vitamin E is measured in tocopherol equivalents (TE). The RDA for adult males is 10 TE and for adult women 8 TE. Deficiencies in a normal diet are rare.

Vitamin K

Vitamin K is essential for proper clotting of the blood.

Vitamin K is fat soluble and is found primarily in green leafy vegetables. Another form of the compound is synthesized by intestinal bacteria. Like vitamin E, there is little danger from ingesting too much vitamin K, and most diets provide an adequate supply.

The RDA for adult males over age 24 is 80 micrograms and for adult women 65 micrograms.

Vitamin C (ascorbic acid)

Vitamin C is essential for healthy skin, bones, teeth, and muscles, for producing and maintaining collagen, and for fighting infection.

Vitamin C is water soluble and therefore must be ingested every day. It is widely available in a variety of colorful fruits and vegetables, such as peppers, broccoli, cabbage, oranges, strawberries, and tomatoes. Unfortunately, vitamin C is also the most unstable of all vitamins and minerals: it is easily destroyed by heat and oxygen, and thus care should be taken in cooking and storing of fruits and vegetables.

The classic vitamin C deficiency disease is scurvy, typified by the wasting away of muscles, wounds and bruises that don't heal, and bleeding, deteriorating gums. Milder forms of vitamin C deficiency produce milder versions of these symptoms. Vitamin C deficiency has also been linked to such health problems as the common cold, anemia, atherosclerosis, asthma, cancer of the stomach and esophagus, infertility in males, rheumatoid arthritis, and cataracts.

Vitamin C is measured in milli-

Average Daily Calorie Consumption

Men	Calories
Sedentary	2,500
Moderately active	3,000
Active	3,500
Very active	4,250
Women	**Calories**
Sedentary	2,100
Moderately active	2,500
Active	3,000
Very active	3,750

Guidelines for average daily calorie consumption by men and women. With increasing use of labor-saving devices, most Americans fall into the sedentary category.

Calorie Consumption for Some Activities

Type of Activity	Calories Per Hour
Sedentary: reading, sewing, typing, etc.	30–100
Light: cooking, slow walking, dressing, etc.	100–170
Moderate: sweeping, light gardening, making beds, etc.	170–250
Vigorous: fast walking, hanging out clothes, golfing, etc.	250–350
Strenuous: swimming, bicycling, dancing, etc.	350 and more

Table 1

Desirable Weights for Men and Women Aged 25 and Over[1]
(in pounds by height and frame, in indoor clothing)

MEN (in shoes, 1-inch heels)				WOMEN (in shoes, 2-inch heels)			
Height	Small Frame	Medium Frame	Large Frame	Height	Small Frame	Medium Frame	Large Frame
5' 2"	112–120	118–129	126–141	4' 10"	92– 98	96–107	104–119
5' 3"	115–123	121–133	129–144	4' 11"	94–101	98–110	106–122
5' 4"	118–126	124–136	132–148	5' 0"	96–104	101–113	109–125
5' 5"	121–129	127–139	135–152	5' 1"	99–107	104–116	112–128
5' 6"	124–133	130–143	138–156	5' 2"	102–110	107–119	115–131
5' 7"	128–137	134–147	142–161	5' 3"	105–113	110–122	118–134
5' 8"	132–141	138–152	147–166	5' 4"	108–116	113–126	121–138
5' 9"	136–145	142–156	151–170	5' 5"	111–119	116–130	125–142
5' 10"	140–150	146–160	155–174	5' 6"	114–123	120–135	129–146
5' 11"	144–154	150–165	159–179	5' 7"	118–127	124–139	133–150
6' 0"	148–158	154–170	164–184	5' 8"	122–131	128–143	137–154
6' 1"	152–162	158–175	168–189	5' 9"	126–135	132–147	141–158
6' 2"	156–167	162–180	173–194	5' 10"	130–140	136–151	145–163
6' 3"	160–171	167–185	178–199	5' 11"	134–144	140–155	149–168
6' 4"	164–175	172–190	182–204	6' 0"	138–148	144–159	153–173

[1]Adapted from Metropolitan Life Insurance Co., New York. New weight standards for men and women. *Statistical Bulletin* 40:3.

Table 2

Average Weights for Men and Women[1]
(in pounds by age and height, in paper gown and slippers)

	MEN						
Height	18–24 Years	25–34 Years	35–44 Years	45–54 Years	55–64 Years	65–74 Years	75–79 Years
5' 2"	137	141	149	148	148	144	133
5' 3"	140	145	152	152	151	148	138
5' 4"	144	150	156	156	155	151	143
5' 5"	147	154	160	160	158	154	148
5' 6"	151	159	164	164	162	158	154
5' 7"	154	163	168	168	166	161	159
5' 8"	158	168	171	173	169	165	164
5' 9"	161	172	175	177	173	168	169
5' 10"	165	177	179	181	176	171	174
5' 11"	168	181	182	185	180	175	179
6' 0"	172	186	186	189	184	178	184
6' 1"	175	190	190	193	187	182	189
6' 2"	179	194	194	197	191	185	194
	WOMEN						
4' 9"	116	112	131	129	138	132	125
4' 10"	118	116	134	132	141	135	129
4' 11"	120	120	136	136	144	138	132
5' 0"	122	124	138	140	149	142	136
5' 1"	125	128	140	143	150	145	139
5' 2"	127	132	143	147	152	149	143
5' 3"	129	136	145	150	155	152	146
5' 4"	131	140	147	154	158	156	150
5' 5"	134	144	149	158	161	159	153
5' 6"	136	148	152	161	164	163	157
5' 7"	138	152	154	165	167	166	160
5' 8"	140	156	156	168	170	170	164

[1]Adapted from National Center for Health Statistics: Weight by Height and Age of Adults, United States. *Vital Health Statistics*. PHS Publication No. 1000—Series 11, No. 14.

grams (mg). The RDA for adults is 60 mg. Megadoses of vitamin C are often recommended to fight colds or as a general preventive measure against disease, although the body only uses as much as it needs; the rest is excreted in the urine. Toxicity is rarely a problem.

Thiamin (vitamin B$_1$)

Thiamin is essential for the proper metabolism of carbohydrates and for a healthy nervous system.

Thiamin is water soluble and is found primarily in cereals, wheat germ, pork, and nuts. It is strongly susceptible to destruction during cooking. Deficiency is not common among the general population, but studies have shown heavy drinkers, pregnant women, and the elderly to be more deficient. Severe thiamin deficiency results in beriberi, a disease that weakens the body, disables the mind, and permanently damages the heart. Symptoms of deficiency include loss of appetite, nausea, vomiting, constipation, depression, fatigue, poor eye-hand coordination, irritability, headaches, and anxiety.

Thiamin is measured in milligrams. The RDA for adult males is 1.5 mg and for adult women 1.1 mg. Danger of toxicity is rare as excess thiamin is excreted in urine.

Riboflavin (vitamin B₂)

Riboflavin is essential for growth and repair of tissues and aids in DNA synthesis. It helps metabolize proteins, fats, and carbohydrates.

Most Americans get plenty of this water-soluble vitamin, which is readily found in liver, eggs, and milk products. Studies have found that children in low-income families, however, are less likely to get enough riboflavin. Signs of deficiency include a purplish-colored tongue; cracks at the corners of the mouth; sores and burning of the lips, mouth, and tongue; itchy inflamed eyelids; flaky skin around the nose, ears, eyebrows, or hairline; and light sensitivity of eyes. Deficiency in riboflavin often means deficiency in other B vitamins as well. Cataracts, birth defects, and anemia have been linked to riboflavin deficiency.

Unlike vitamin C and thiamin, riboflavin is not easily destroyed by cooking, although adding baking soda to vegetables when cooking creates an alkaline solution that destroys it. Risk of toxicity is very low, and excess riboflavin is excreted in the urine.

Riboflavin is measured in milligrams. The RDA for adult males is 1.7 mg and for adult women 1.3 mg.

Niacin (vitamin B₃)

Niacin is essential for the release of energy from carbohydrates, fats, and proteins and for the formation of DNA.

Most Americans get plenty of niacin from their diets; only heavy drinkers are at risk of deficiency. Severe deficiencies of niacin result in pellagra, a disease virtually wiped out in the United States since the 1930s with the advent of fortified flour and cereals with the vitamin.

Niacin is widely available in a variety of plant and animal foods, including fish, liver, turkey, cereals, and peanuts. The body is also able to convert the amino acid tryptophan into niacin, and thus proteins high in tryptophan also provide plenty of niacin.

Niacin is measured in milligrams (60 mg of tryptophan equal 1 mg of niacin). The RDA for adult males is 19 mg and for women 15 mg.

Recommended Dietary Allowances for Fat-Soluble Vitamins					
	Age	Vit. A (mcg RE)	Vit. D (mcg)	Vit. E (mgTE)	Vit.K (mcg)
Infants	0 to .5	375	7.5	3	5
	.5 to 1	"	10	4	10
Children	1 to 3	400	"	6	15
	4 to 6	500	"	7	20
	7 to 10	700	"	"	30
Males	11 to 14	1,000	"	10	45
	15 to 18	"	"	"	65
	19 to 24	"	"	"	70
	25 to 50	"	5	"	80
	51 +	"	"	"	"
Females	11 to 14	800	10	8	45
	15 to 18	"	"	"	55
	19 to 24	"	"	"	60
	25 to 50	"	5	"	65
	51 +	"	"	"	"
Pregnant		"	10	10	"
Nursing	1st 6 months	1,300	"	12	"
	2nd 6 months	1,200	"	11	"

Vitamin B$_6$

Vitamin B$_6$ is essential for fat and carbohydrate metabolism and for the formation and breakdown of amino acids. It also helps regulate blood glucose levels and is needed to synthesize hemoglobin.

Vitamin B$_6$ occurs in three forms: pyridoxine, pyridoxal, and pyridoxamine, which are converted by the body into pyridoxal phosphate and pyridoxamine phosphate. It is most readily found in nuts, kidney, liver, eggs, pork, poultry, dried fruits, and fish.

Although few Americans get the full RDA of vitamin B$_6$, there is no evidence of corresponding overt deficiency symptoms. The following health problems, however, have been linked to B$_6$ deficiency: asthma, carpal tunnel syndrome, cancer (melanoma, breast, and bladder), diabetes, coronary heart disease, premenstrual syndrome, sickle-cell anemia, and aging and dementia.

In moderate doses B$_6$ is not toxic. Although excessive amounts of this water-soluble vitamin are to a great extent flushed out of the body in the urine, high doses have produced neurological disturbances such as numbness in the hands, feet, and mouth.

Vitamin B$_6$ is measured in milligrams. The RDA for adult men is 2 mg and for women 1.6 mg.

Vitamin B$_{12}$

Vitamin B$_{12}$ is important for normal growth, healthy nerve tissue, and normal blood formation.

Most Americans get plenty of B$_{12}$. It is found chiefly in animal foods: meat, fish, eggs, and milk products.

Recommended Dietary Allowances for Water-Soluble Vitamins

	Age	Vit. C (mg)	Thiamin (mg)	Riboflav. (mg)	Niacin (mg)	Vit. B6 (mg)	Folate (mcg)	Vit. B12 (mcg)
Infants	0 to .5	30	0.3	0.4	5	0.3	25	0.3
	.5 to 1	35	0.4	0.5	6	0.6	35	0.5
Children	1 to 3	40	0.7	0.8	9	1	50	0.7
	4 to 6	45	0.9	1.1	12	1.1	75	1
	7 to 10	"	1	1.2	13	1.4	100	1.4
Males	11 to 14	50	1.3	1.5	17	1.7	150	2
	15 to 18	60	1.5	1.8	20	2	200	"
	19 to 24	"	"	1.7	19	"	"	"
	25 to 50	"	"	"	"	"	"	"
	51 +	"	1.2	1.4	15	"	150	"
Females	11 to 14	50	1.1	1.3	"	1.4	180	"
	15 to 18	60	"	"	"	1.5	"	"
	19 to 24	"	"	"	"	1.6	"	"
	25 to 50	"	1.1	"	"	"	"	"
51 +		"	1	1.2	13	"	"	"
Pregnant		70	1.5	1.6	17	2.2	400	2.2
Nursing	1st 6 months	95	1.6	1.8	20	2.1	280	2.6
	2nd 6 months	90	"	1.7	20	"	260	"

Only strict vegetarians (vegans), who eat none of these foods are in danger of deficiency. Problems for everyone arise with age, however; the stomach may become less able to absorb B_{12} and deficiency may result. Pernicious anemia is the classic B_{12} deficiency disease and may take years to appear. Other health problems that may be linked to B_{12} deficiency include infertility, nervous system disorders, and walking difficulties.

Cooking results in few losses of B_{12}, and toxicity is not a danger. The RDA for B_{12} for adults is 2 micrograms.

Folacin (folic acid, or folate)

Folacin is essential for many metabolic processes, especially cell growth and division.

Women, especially pregnant women, and alcoholics are most likely to be folacin deficient. Signs of deficiency include anemia, weakness, pallor, headaches, forgetfulness, sleeplessness, and irritability. Vitamin B_{12} deficiency can aggravate folacin deficiency because B_{12} is essential to release folacin from bodily storage. Other health problems that may be associated with folacin deficiency include depression, dementia, neuropsychological disorders, toxemia of pregnancy, infections, and fetal damage.

Folacin is widely distributed in fruits and vegetables, but it is easily destroyed during cooking and storage. The RDA for folacin for adult men is 200 micrograms and for women, 180 micrograms.

Biotin

Biotin is essential for overall growth and well-being. It is important in the metabolism of fats and in the utilization of carbon dioxide.

The best sources of biotin are liver, egg yolks, soy flour, cereals, and yeast. It is also produced by intestinal bacteria, although it is not known whether this form is readily absorbed by the body. Deficiencies are most often produced by the ingestion of large amounts of raw egg white, which contains a biotin-binding protein called avidin that prevents the absorption of biotin. Symptoms of deficiency include nausea, vomiting, swelling of the tongue, pallor, depression, hair loss, and dry scaly dermatitis.

The RDA for adults is a wide range: from 30 to 100 micrograms. Toxicity from a normal diet is not a concern.

Pantothenic acid

Pantothenic acid is essential for general growth and well-being. It is an important component in a number of metabolic reactions such as the release of energy from carbohydrates, fats, and proteins and the synthesis of sterols and steroid hormones.

Pantothenic acid is widely distributed among foods, chiefly animal tissues, cereals, and legumes. Evidence of dietary deficiency of pantothenic acid has not been clinically recognized in humans, and there is no specific disease associated with pantothenic acid deficiency.

Pantothenic acid is measured in milligrams. There is no RDA, but daily consumption by adults of between 4 and 7 mg is considered safe. Toxicity from a normal diet is not a concern.

Minerals

Minerals are another component of basic nutritional needs. All living things extract them from the soil, which is their ultimate source. Like vitamins, they are needed for normal metabolism and must be present in the diet in sufficient amounts for the maintenance of good health. The essential minerals include calcium, phosphorus, magnesium, iodine, iron, zinc, selenium, molybdenum, copper, manganese, fluoride, and chromium.

Calcium

Calcium is essential for bone growth, development, and retention as well as for proper nerve conduction, muscle contraction, blood clotting, and membrane permeability.

Dairy products are the primary

sources of calcium, but the mineral is also found in green leafy vegetables and soft bones, such as those of sardines and salmon. Maximum calcium ingestion is extremely important during the years from birth to age 25, when the body reaches its peak bone mass. Deficiencies are most common in women and have been linked to the development of osteoporosis in the later years.

The RDA for calcium for children between the ages of 11 and 24 is 1,200 mg. For adults over 24 the RDA is 800 mg. Ingestion of very large amounts of calcium may inhibit the absorption of iron, zinc, and other essential minerals.

Phosphorus

Phosphorus is a structural component of all cells. It is a part of DNA, and is therefore essential in the growth, maintenance, and repair of all body tissues. It is also critical for energy transfer and production.

Phosphorus is present in nearly all foods, principally cereals and proteins. Deficiency is a serious concern only for premature infants fed exclusively human milk.

The RDA for phosphorus is the same as that for calcium, 800 mg for adults over 24. Toxicity from a normal diet is not a concern.

Magnesium

Like phosphorus, magnesium is a structural component in soft tissue cells and is therefore important in the growth, maintenance, and repair of these tissues. It is also important in energy production, lipid and protein synthesis, the formation of urea, muscle relaxation, and in the prevention of tooth decay.

The best sources of magnesium are nuts, legumes, unmilled grains, and green vegetables. Deficiencies from a normal diet are rare and are related instead to various diseases such as those of the gastrointestinal tract, kidney dysfunction, and malnutrition and alcoholism. Symptoms of deficiency include weakness, confusion, personality changes, muscle tremor, nausea, lack of coordination, and gastrointestinal disorders.

The RDA for adult men is 350 mg and for adult women 280 mg.

Iodine

Iodine is an essential component of thyroid hormone, which is important in cellular reactions, metabolism, and growth and development.

Iodized salt and water are the most common sources, and most animal foods contain adequate supplies depending on the soil quality and the amount of iodine added to animal feeds. Iodine is also added in the processing of bread dough. Deficiencies in the United States are not common. The classic deficiency disease in adults is goiter. Iodine deficient fetuses are at a risk of developing cretinism.

The RDA for iodine for adults is 150 micrograms.

Iron

As an essential component of hemoglobin and myoglobin, iron is necessary for the proper transfer of oxygen to cells and muscles. It is also important for energy production and collagen synthesis.

Many Americans don't get enough iron. Women and very young children get the least, followed by the elderly. Iron deficiency leads to anemia: muscles become weak, and fatigue, listlessness, and a tendency to tire easily set in. Even mild iron deficiency, however, can affect a person's intellectual capabilities, especially children's. Symptoms of deficiency in children include irritability, hyperactivity, learning problems, shortened attention span, poor motivation, and poor intellectual performance.

There are two types of iron, heme and nonheme. Heme comes from animal foods and is much more readily absorbed than nonheme iron, which comes from vegetables. When eaten together, however, the rate of absorption for nonheme iron increases significantly. Also, iron eaten with just a little vitamin C dramatically increases its absorption. Tannins (in tea and red wine) block iron absorption. Iron-rich foods include liver and other organ meats, beef, dried fruits, pumpkin and sunflower seeds, legumes, dark green leafy vegetables, prune juice, and whole grain cereals.

The RDA for adult males is 10 mg and for adult women 15 mg. There is little danger of toxicity from a normal diet, although some people have an inherited defect in regulating iron absorption and can easily get too much.

Zinc

Zinc is essential for cell multiplication, tissue regeneration, sexual maturity, and proper growth. It is also important as a cofactor in more than 20 enzymatic reactions and serves as a binder in many others.

Severe zinc deficiency is not a problem in the United States, but the effects of mild deficiency—common especially in children, women, and the elderly—on overall health are feared to be widespread. Signs of deficiency include loss of appetite, stunted growth in children, skin changes, small sex glands in boys, delayed sexual maturation, impotence, loss of taste sensitivity, white spots on fingernails, delayed wound-healing, and dull hair color.

Animal foods are good sources of

Recommended Dietary Allowances for Minerals

	Age	Calcium (mg)	Phospho. (mg)	Magnesium (mg)	Iron (mg)	Zinc (mg)	Iodine (mcg)	Selenium (mcg)
Infants	0 to .5	400	300	40	6	5	40	10
	.5 to 1	600	500	60	10	"	50	15
Children	1 to 3	800	800	80	"	10	70	20
	4 to 6	"	"	120	"	"	90	"
	7 to 10	"	"	170	"	"	120	30
Males	11 to 14	1,200	1,200	270	12	15	150	40
	15 to 18	"	"	400	"	"	"	50
	19 to 24	"	"	350	10	"	"	70
	25 to 50	800	800	"	"	"	"	"
	51 +	"	"	"	"	"	"	"
Females	11 to 14	1,200	1,200	280	15	12	"	45
	15 to 18	"	"	300	"	"	"	50
	19 to 24	"	"	280	"	"	"	55
	25 to 50	800	800	"	"	"	"	"
	51 +	"	"	"	10	"	"	"
Pregnant		1,200	1,200	320	30	15	175	65
Nursing	1st 6 months	"	"	355	15	19	200	75
	2nd 6 months	"	"	340	"	16	200	"

zinc as are oysters, milk, egg yolks, wheat germ, pumpkin and sunflower seeds, nuts, cheese, dry beans, lentils, and whole grains. Toxicity is rare. The RDA for adults is 12 mg.

Selenium

Selenium functions in a similar way to vitamin E, as an antioxidant helping to protect cells from destruction by toxic agents. Its consumption has also been associated with lower incidences of cancer and heart disease.

Good sources of selenium include whole grains, seafood, liver, kidney, meat, seeds, and nuts. Deficiency may be a problem in areas with selenium-poor soils. Selenium is toxic at higher than trace amounts. The RDA for adult males is 70 micrograms and for adult women 55 micrograms.

Molybdenum

Molybdenum is essential in the function of certain enzyme systems and is also necessary in iron metabolism.

Sources of molybdenum include meats, whole grains, legumes, leafy vegetables, and organ meats. The molybdenum content of vegetables varies widely depending on the content of the soil in which they were grown. Deficiency is not known in humans. Ingesting more than trace amounts is not recommended. The RDA for adults is between 75 and 250 micrograms.

Copper

Copper is important as a cofactor in several enzyme systems and as a catalyst in the synthesis of hemoglobin. It also aids in collagen formation and is involved in the synthesis of phospholipids, which maintain healthy nerve fibers.

Copper deficiency is believed to be more common than once thought, and it has been linked to heart disease, central nervous system disorders, anemia, and bone disorders. Good sources of copper include shellfish, liver, nuts and seeds, meats, and green leafy vegetables. Copper supplements are not recommended because they can interfere with other minerals, and copper is toxic at more than trace amounts. The RDA for copper is 1.5 to 3 mg.

Manganese

Manganese has a variety of functions, some that other minerals can perform in its place. It is known to play a role in such things as collagen formation, urea formation, synthesis of fatty acids and cholesterol, digestion of proteins, normal bone formation and development, and protein synthesis.

Manganese deficiency has not been observed in humans. Sources of manganese include liver, kidney, spinach, whole grain cereals and breads, dried peas and beans, and nuts. Excessive intake of manganese can interfere with iron absorption. More than trace amounts of manganese are not recommended. The RDA is 2 to 5 mg.

Fluoride

Fluoride is essential for the development of healthy teeth and bones and the prevention of tooth decay.

Fluoride deficiency shows up in increased incidences of tooth decay. Fluoridated water is the most common source of fluoride for many people. For those without access to such water fluoride tablets or toothpaste are helpful. Fish, tea, milk, and eggs are also sources of fluoride. The RDA for adults is between 1.5 and 4 mg.

Chromium

Chromium is important for maintaining normal glucose metabolism. It also acts as a cofactor for insulin.

Chromium deficiency can show up in the form of glucose intolerance in malnourished children and in some diabetics. Sources of chromium include whole grains, brewer's yeast, meats, and cheeses. Hard water also contains chromium. Chromium intake should not exceed trace amounts. The RDA for adults is between 50 and 200 micrograms.

Estimated Safe and Adequate Daily Dietary Intakes of Selected Vitamins and Minerals

		Biotin	Pant. acid	Copper	Manganese	Fluoride	Chromium	Molyb.
		(mcg)	(mg)	(mg)	(mg)	(mg)	(mcg)	(mcg)
Infants	0 to 0.5	10	2	0.4-.06	0.3-0.6	0.1-0.5	10-40	15-30
	0.5 to 1	15	3	0.6-0.7	0.6-1.0	0.2-1.0	20-60	20-40
Children/	1 to 3	20	"	0.7-1.0	1.0-1.5	0.5-1.5	20-80	25-50
Adoles-	4 to 6	25	3-4	1.0-1.5	1.5-2.0	1.0-2.5	30-120	30-75
cents	7 to 10	30	4-5	1.0-2.0	2.0-3.0	1.5-2.5	50-200	50-150
	11 +	30-100	4-7	1.5-2.5	2.0-5.0	"	"	75-250
Adults		30-100	"	1.5-3.0	"	1.5-4.0	"	"

Fiber

Fiber in the diet is important for proper elimination. It provides bulk, and its use has been linked to the prevention of many health problems: constipation, appendicitis, colon cancer, diverticular disease, spastic colon, hiatal hernia, varicose veins, hemorrhoids, coronary heart disease, high blood pressure, gallstones, diabetes, obesity, ulcerative colitis, and Crohn's disease.

Fiber is found almost exclusively in plant foods and comes in basically two types: water soluble or water insoluble. Soluble fiber is found primarily in fruits and vegetables and in oat bran in the form of gums and pectin and affects the way the body metabolizes sugars and fats. Insoluble fiber is primarily associated with whole grains, the traditional "bran," such as wheat bran and rice bran, and is the fiber we think of when we think of laxatives. Generally, the less processed the food, the higher it is in either kind of fiber.

Fiber in high doses can affect the absorption of other vitamins and minerals as well as cause flatulence, bloating, nausea, diarrhea, and impaction or rupture of the bowel. Daily consumption of 35 to 40 grams of fiber is recommended for optimum health and safety.

Water

Water is not really a food in the fuel sense, but it is in many ways a crucial component of nutrition: the body's need for water is second only to its need for oxygen. It makes up from 55 to 65 percent of the body's weight, and is constantly being eliminated in the form of urine, perspiration, and expired breath. It must be replaced regularly, for while a person can live for weeks without food, he can live for only a few days without water.

Normally, the best guide to how much water a person needs is his sense of thirst. The regulating mechanism of excretion sees to it that an excessive intake of water will be eliminated as urine. The usual water requirement is on the order of two quarts a day in addition to whatever amount is contained in the solids which make up the daily diet.

Basic Daily Diets

Everyone should have at least the minimal amount of basic nutrients for resting or basal metabolism. The specific needs of each individual are determined by whether he is still growing, and by how much energy is required for his normal activities. All those who are still growing—and growth continues up to about 25 years of age—have relatively high food needs.

For Infants

That food needs of an infant are especially acute should surprise no one. The newborn baby normally triples in weight during the first year and is very active in terms of calorie expenditure.

For the first six months, breast milk or formula, or a combination of the two, fills the baby's nutritional needs. A baby needs about two and a half ounces of milk per pound of body weight. This provides 50 calories per pound, and in the early months is usually given in six feedings a day at four-hour intervals.

If the baby appears healthy and is gaining adequate weight, and if the stomach is not distended by swallowed air, appetite is normally a satisfactory guide to how much the baby needs to eat. The formula-fed baby should get a supplement of 35 milligrams of ascorbic acid and 400 international units of vitamin D if the latter has not been added to the milk during its processing.

Solid Foods

Between two and six months of age, the baby should begin to eat solid foods such as cooked cereals, strained fruits and vegetables, egg yolk, and homogenized meat. With the introduction of these foods, it is not really necessary to calculate the baby's caloric intake. Satisfaction of appetite, proper weight gain, and a healthy appearance serve as the guides to a proper diet.

By one year of age, a baby should be getting three regular meals a day, and as the baby's teeth appear, food no longer needs to be strained. By 18 to 24 months, baby food should no longer be necessary. For more information, see Ch. 2, *The First Dozen Years*.

Basic Food Groups

The recommended daily amounts of food for people over the age of two have been established with reasonable accuracy, but they always contain a fairly generous safety factor.

The Four Group Division

In general, foods are divided into four major groups:

- Meat, fish, eggs
- Dairy products
- Fruits and vegetables
- Breads and cereals

The Seven Group Division

For purposes of planning daily requirements, a more detailed way of considering food groupings is the following:

- Leafy green and yellow vegetables
- Citrus fruits, tomatoes, and raw cabbage

Fats, oils, sweets:
Use sparingly

Milk, yogurt, and cheese:
2–3 servings

Meat, poultry fish, dry beans, eggs, and nuts:
2–3 servings

Vegetables:
3–5 servings

Fruits:
2–4 servings

Bread, cereal, rice, and pasta: 6–11 servings

Derived from the U.S. Department of Agriculture's "Eating Right Pyramid."

* Potatoes and other vegetables and fruits

* Milk, cheese, and ice cream

* Meat, poultry, fish, eggs, dried peas, and beans

* Bread, flour, and cereals

* Butter and oils

The "Daily Food Guide" table can be used as a general guide to planning nutritionally balanced meals for pre-teens, teens, and adults of any age.

The Six Group Division (The Food Guide Pyramid)

Very similar to the seven group division, the six group division puts all vegetables into one group. The pyramid chart is meant to convey three key points: eat less fat, eat a variety of foods, and eat the recommended number of servings from each group.

The Years of Growth

A proper diet is crucial during the years from 2 to 18, since this is a period of tremendous growth.

Children should also learn about balanced diets, learn decent manners at the table, and develop a sense of timing about when to eat and when not to eat.

Creating a Pleasant Atmosphere at Mealtime

* Children should never be bribed with candy, money, or the promise of special surprises as a way of getting them to eat properly.

* They should not be given the idea that dessert is a reward for finishing the earlier part of the meal.

* Relatively small portions should be served and completely finished before anything else is offered.

* Between-meal snacks should be discouraged if they cut down on the appetite at mealtime.

* From time to time, childern should be allowed to choose the foods that they will eat at a meal.

Parents should keep in mind that the atmosphere in which childern eat and the attitudes instilled in them toward food can be altogether as basic as the nourishment for their bodies.

Teenage Diet

From the start of a child's growth spurt, which begins at age 10 or 11 for girls and between 13 and 15 for boys, and for several years thereafter, adolescent appetites are likely to be unbelievably large and somewhat outlandish. Parents should try to exercise some control over the youngster who is putting on too much weight as well as with the one who is attracted by a bizarre starvation diet.

Adult Nutrition

The average American adult experiences slow but steady weight gain. For some, this develops into an obesity problem. Since being even moderately overweight can pose health risks, weight gain as an adult should be viewed as a hazard that could jeopardize health. A sensible diet is recommended.

For Older People

People over 60 tend to have changes in their digestive system that are related to less efficient and slower absorption. Incomplete chewing of food because of carelessness or impaired teeth can intensify this problem. Avoiding haste at mealtimes ought to be the rule.

In cases where a dental disorder makes proper chewing impossible, food should be chopped or pureed.

Food for older people should be cooked simply, preferably baked, boiled, or broiled rather than fried, and menus excessively rich in fats should be avoided. A daily multivitamin capsule is strongly recommended for those over 60.

Eating for Life

The U.S. Department of Agriculture and the U.S. Department of Health and Human Services recommend seven basic guidelines to avoid excess weight and maintain optimum health:

- Eat a variety of foods

- Maintain a desirable weight

- Avoid too much fat, saturated fat, and cholesterol

- Eat foods with adequate starch and fiber

- Avoid too much sugar

- Avoid too much sodium

- If you drink alcoholic beverages, do so in moderation

The guidelines are designed for healthy adult Americans, but are considered especially appropriate for people who may already have some of the risk factors for chronic diseases, including a family history of obesity, premature heart disease, diabetes, high blood pressure, or high blood cholesterol levels.

The U.S.D.A. and the U.S.D.

H.H.S. also recommend the "Choose More Often" approach to healthful eating.

Choose More Often:

Low-fat meat, poultry, fish
Lean cuts of meat trimmed of fat (round tip roast, pork tenderloin, loin of lamb chop), poultry without skin, and fish, cooked without breading or added fat.

Low-fat or Non-fat dairy products
1 percent or non-fat milk, buttermilk; non-fat or low-fat yogurt; lower fat cheeses (part-skim ricotta, fresh parmesan or feta); sherbet.

Dry beans and peas
All beans, peas, and lentils—the dry forms are higher in protein.

Whole grain products
Reduced-fat breads, bagels, and English muffins made from whole wheat, rye, bran, and corn flour or meal; whole grain or bran cereals;

whole wheat pasta; brown rice; bulgur.

Fruits and vegetables
All fruits and vegetables: apples, pears, cantaloupe, oranges, grapefruit, pineapple, peaches, bananas, carrots, broccoli, Brussels sprouts, cabbage, kale, potatoes, tomatoes, sweet potatoes, spinach, cauliflower, turnips, etc.

Fats and oils high in unsaturates
Unsaturated vegetable oils, such as canola oil, corn oil, cottonseed oil, olive oil, and soybean oil, and margarine; reduced-fat and reduced-calorie mayonnaise and salad dressings.

Some tips for following the "choose more often" approach in grocery shopping, food preparation, and eating out:

When Grocery Shopping

Focus on variety. Using the above guidelines, choose a wide selection of low-fat foods rich in fiber. Although the goal is to reduce fat to 30 percent or less, when choosing foods that do contain fat, try to choose ones that contain primarily unsaturated fats.

Read food labels. Nutrition labels on

most packaged foods give information on the nutrients in each serving: total calories and calories from fat; total and saturated fat; cholesterol; sodium; total carbohydrates, including dietary fiber, and sugars; protein; and certain vitamins and minerals. The label also calculates the percent daily value of each of these nutrients, meaning the percentage of the recommended amount of the nutrient that the food provides, based on a 2,000-calorie diet. Choose products that are low in fat—especially saturated fat—and high in fiber.

Beware of sodium. Many processed, canned, and frozen foods are high in sodium. Cured or processed meats, cheeses, soups and condiments (soy sauce, mustard, tartar sauce) are high in sodium. Check labels for salt, onion or garlic salt, and any ingredient with sodium in its name. Compare products and choose the ones with lower levels.

When Preparing Food

Use small amounts of fat and fatty foods when planning meals.
When you do use fat, use it sparingly and allow the full flavor of the foods to dominate, instead of a single element like cheese or butter. Try to use only ½ teaspoon of fat per serving. Gradually introduce nonfat or low-fat alternatives into your diet.

Use less saturated fat. While reducing your total fat intake, substitute unsaturated fat and oils for saturated. Instead of butter, try vegetable oil, margarine or a low-fat cooking spray. To substitute, use equal portions, or less.

Use low-fat alternatives. Substitute 1 percent, skim, or reconstituted nonfat dry milk for whole milk. Use buttermilk, nonfat or low-fat yogurt, or evaporated skim milk in place of cream and sour cream. Try reduced-fat or fat-free mayonnaise, sour cream and salad dressings. Also try using egg whites or egg substitutes in place of eggs, which are extremely high in fat and cholesterol.

Choose lean meat. Trim all visible fat from meat and poultry, including poultry skin. Canned, reduced fat and sodium stocks are now available for making soup.

Use low-fat cooking methods. Bake, steam, broil, microwave, or boil foods rather than frying. Avoid gravies and try vegetable-based instead of cream-based sauces.

Increase fiber. Substitute whole-grain flour for white flour. Have generous servings. Whenever possible, eat the edible fiber-rich skin as well as the rest of the vegetable or fruit.

Use herbs, spices, and other flavorings. For a different way to add flavor to meals, try lemon juice, basil, chives, curry powder, onion, cracked pepper, and garlic in place of fats and sodium. Try low-fat recipes and adjust old ones to reduce fat and sodium.

When Eating Out

Choose the restaurant carefully. Are low-fat, high-fiber items on the menu, like pasta? How are meat, chicken, and fish dishes cooked—broiled, baked, or fried? Avoid fast food places.

Try ethnic cuisines. Italian and Asian restaurants often feature low-fat dishes—though you must be selective and alert to portion size. Try a small serving of pasta or fish in a tomato sauce at an Italian restaurant. Many Chinese, Japanese, and Thai dishes include plenty of steamed vegetables and a high proportion of vegetables to meat. Steamed rice, steamed noodle dishes and vegetarian dishes are good choices, too. Ask for food without soy sauce or salt.

Make sure you get what you want. Be in control when you eat out. Ask how dishes are cooked. Don't hesitate to request that one food be substituted for another. Order a green salad or baked potato in place of french fries or order fruit or sherbet instead of ice cream. Request sauces and salad dressings on the side and use only a small amount. Ask that butter and rolls not be sent to the table. If you're not very hungry, order two low-fat appetizers rather than an entire meal, split a menu item with a friend, get a doggie-bag to take half of your meal home, or order a half-size portion. When you finish, let the waiter clear dishes to avoid post-meal nibbling.

Eat slowly. Don't eat to get your money's worth, eat to sate your hunger. Eating quickly can either leave you still feeling hungry or sick with indigestion. By deliberately slowing down your intake of food, you will more likely feel full earlier in the meal and your body will be able to properly digest your food.

Be reasonable. If you don't eat out very often, one meal won't ruin your health. If you feel like ordering a rich meal or having dessert, simply cut back on the extras; avoid the bread and butter, don't order an appetizer, have one glass of wine instead of two.

Raising Children with Healthy Eating Habits

Children who are raised with healthy eating habits are more likely to continue these habits in their adult life. For example, if dessert is more frequently fresh fruit than ice cream sundaes, a child will not grow up associating a special treat with only rich fatty sweets. The nectarine, pear or apple will seem just as special. Likewise, as an adult the same child will be less likely to overindulge with sweets or other fatty foods.

Malnutrition

The classic diseases of nutritional deficiency, or malnutrition, such as scurvy and pellagra, are now rare, at least in the United States. The chief reason for their disappearance is the application of scientific knowledge gained in this century of the importance of vitamins and minerals in the diet. Thus most bread is fortified with vitamins and minerals, and in ad dition, commercial food processing has made it possible for balanced diets of an appealing variety to be eaten all year round.

Many people do not get an adequate diet, either through ignorance or because they simply cannot afford it. A number of food programs have been created to assist them, but unfortunately, the programs don't reach everyone who needs help.

Metric Equivalents of Traditional Food Measures	
1 teaspoon	= 5 milliliters
1 tablespoon	= 15 milliliters
¼ cup	= 60 milliliters
⅓ cup	= 80 milliliters
½ cup	= 120 milliliters
⅔ cup	= 160 milliliters
¾ cup	= 180 milliliters
1 cup	= 240 milliliters or 0.24 liter

Causes of Malnutrition

Some people, either because of ignorance or food faddism, do not eat a balanced diet even though they can afford to. There are also large numbers of people with nutritional deficiency diseases who can be described as abnormal, at least in regard to eating. Some are alcoholics; others live alone and are so depressed that they lack sufficient drive to feed themselves properly. Combination of any of these factors increase the likelihood of poor nutrition and often lead to health-damaging consequences.

Disease

People can also develop nutritional deficiencies because they have some disease that interferes with food absorption, storage, and utilization, or that causes an increased excretion, usually in the urine, of substances needed for nutrition. These are generally chronic diseases of the gastrointestinal tract including the liver, or of the kidneys or the endocrine glands.

Medications

Nutritional deficiencies can also result from loss of appetite caused by medications, especially when a number of different medications are taken simultaneously. This adverse affect on the appetite is a strong reason for not taking medicines unless told to do so by a physician for a specific purpose.

Most people are not aware of inadequacies in their diet until there are

Nutrients in Common Foods

Food	Food energy	Protein	Fat	Carbohydrate
	Calories	Grams	Grams	Grams
Milk and Milk Products				
Milk; 1 cup:				
Fluid, whole	165	9	10	12
Fluid, nonfat (skim)	90	9	trace	13
Buttermilk, cultured (from skim milk)	90	9	trace	13
Evaporated (undiluted)	345	18	20	24
Dry, nonfat (regular)	435	43	1	63
Yogurt (from partially skimmed milk); 1 cup	120	8	4	13
Cheese; 1 ounce:				
Cheddar or American	115	7	9	1
Cottage:				
From skim milk	25	5	trace	1
Creamed	30	4	1	1
Cream cheese	105	2	11	1
Swiss	105	7	8	1
Desserts (largely milk):				
Custard, baked; 1 cup, 8 fluid ounces	305	14	15	29
Ice cream, plain, factory packed:				
1 slice or individual brick, ⅛ quart	130	3	7	14
1 container, 8 fluid ounces	255	6	14	28
Ice milk; 1 cup, 8 fluid ounces	200	6	7	29
Eggs				
Egg, raw, large:				
1 whole	80	6	6	trace
1 white	15	4	trace	trace
1 yolk	60	3	5	trace
Egg, cooked; 1 large:				
Boiled	80	6	6	trace
Scrambled (with milk and fat)	110	7	8	1
Meat, Poultry, Fish, Shellfish				
Bacon, broiled or fried, drained, 2 medium thick slices	85	4	8	trace
Beef, cooked without bone:				
Braised, simmered, or pot-roasted; 3 ounce portion:				
Entire portion, lean and fat	365	19	31	0
Lean only, approx. 2 ounces	140	17	4	0
Hamburger patties, made with				
Regular ground beef; 3-ounce patty	235	21	17	0
Lean ground round; 3-ounce patty	185	23	10	0
Roast; 3-ounce slice from cut having relatively small amount of fat:				
Entire portion, lean and fat	255	22	18	0
Lean only, approx. 2.3 ounces	115	19	4	0
Steak, broiled; 3-ounce portion:				
Entire portion, lean and fat	375	19	32	0
Lean only, approx. 1.8 ounces	105	17	4	0

Nutrients in Common Foods *(continued)*

Food	Food energy	Protein	Fat	Carbohydrate
	Calories	Grams	Grams	Grams
Beef, canned: corned beef hash; 3 ounces	155	8	10	9
Beef and vegetable stew; 1 cup	220	16	11	15
Chicken, without bone: broiled; 3 ounces	115	20	3	0
Lamb, cooked: Chops; 1 thick chop, with bone, 4.8 ounces: Lean and fat, approx. 3.4 ounces	340	21	28	0
Lean only, 2.3 ounces	120	18	5	0
Roast, without bone: Leg; 3-ounce slice: Entire slice, lean and fat	265	20	20	0
Lean only, approx. 2.3 ounces	120	19	5	0
Shoulder; 3-ounce portion, without bone: Entire portion, lean and fat	300	18	25	0
Lean only, approx. 2.2 ounces	125	16	6	0
Liver, beef, fried; 2 ounces	120	13	4	6
Pork, cured, cooked: Ham, smoked; 3-ounce portion, without bone	245	18	19	0
Luncheon meat: Boiled ham; 2 ounces	130	11	10	0
Canned, spiced; 2 ounces	165	8	14	1
Pork, fresh, cooked: Chops; 1 chop, with bone, 3.5 ounces: Lean and fat, approx. 2.4 ounces	295	15	25	0
Lean only, approx. 1.6 ounces	120	14	7	0
Roast; 3-ounce slice, without bone: Entire slice, lean and fat	340	19	29	0
Lean only, approx. 2.2 ounces	160	19	9	0
Sausage: Bologna; 8 slices (4.1 by 0.1 inches each), 8 ounces	690	27	62	2
Frankfurter; 1 cooked, 1.8 ounces	155	6	14	1
Tongue, beef, boiled; 3 ounces	205	18	14	trace
Veal, cutlet, broiled; 3-ounce portion, without bone	185	23	9	0
Fish and shellfish: Bluefish, baked or broiled; 3 ounces	135	22	4	0
Clams: raw, meat only; 3 ounces	70	11	1	3
Crabmeat, canned or cooked; 3 ounces	90	14	2	1
Fishsticks, breaded, cooked, frozen, 10 sticks (3.8 by 1.0 by 0.5 inches each), 8 ounces	400	38	20	15

Nutrients in Common Foods *(continued)*

Food	Food energy Calories	Protein Grams	Fat Grams	Carbohydrate Grams
Haddock, fried; 3 ounces	135	16	5	6
Mackerel; broiled; 3 ounces	200	19	13	0
Oysters, raw, meat only; 1 cup (13-19 medium-size oysters, selects)	160	20	4	8
Oyster stew: 1 cup (6–8 oysters)	200	11	12	11
Salmon, canned (pink); 3 ounces	120	17	5	0
Sardines, canned in oil, drained solids; 3 ounces	180	22	9	1
Shrimp, canned, meat only; 3 ounces	110	23	1	—
Tuna, canned in oil, drained solids; 3 ounces	170	25	7	0
Mature Beans and Peas, Nuts				
Beans, dry seed: Common varieties, as Great Northern, navy, and others, canned; 1 cup:				
Red	230	15	1	42
White, with tomato or molasses:				
With pork	330	16	7	54
Without pork	315	16	1	60
Beans, dry seed: Lima, cooked; 1 cup	260	16	1	48
Cowpeas or black-eyed peas, dry, cooked; 1 cup	190	13	1	34
Peanuts, roasted, shelled; 1 cup	840	39	71	28
Peanut butter; 1 tablespoon	90	4	8	3
Peas, split, dry, cooked; 1 cup	290	20	1	52
Vegetables				
Asparagus: Cooked; 1 cup	35	4	trace	6
Canned, 6 medium-size spears	20	2	trace	3
Beans Lima, immature, cooked; 1 cup	150	8	1	29
Snap, green: Cooked; 1 cup	25	2	trace	6
Canned; solids and liquid; 1 cup	45	2	trace	10
Beets, cooked, diced; 1 cup	70	2	trace	16
Broccoli, cooked, flower stalks; 1 cup	45	5	trace	8
Brussels sprouts, cooked; 1 cup	60	6	1	12
Cabbage; 1 cup: Raw, coleslaw	100	2	7	9
Cooked	40	2	trace	9
Carrots: Raw: 1 carrot (5½ by 1 inch) or 25 thin strips	20	1	trace	5
Cooked, diced, 1 cup	45	1	1	9
Canned, strained or chopped; 1 ounce	5	trace	0	2
Cauliflower, cooked, flower buds; 1 cup	30	3	trace	6

some dramatic consequences. Nor is it easy to recognize the presence of a disorder that might be causing malnutrition. A physician should be consulted promptly when there is a persistent weight loss, especially when the diet is normal. He should also be informed of any changes in the skin, mucous membranes of the mouth or tongue, or nervous system function, because such symptoms can be a warning of dietary deficiency.

The family or friends of a person with a nutritional deficiency can often detect his condition because they become aware of changes in his eating patterns. They can also note early signs of a deficiency of some of the B vitamins, such as cracks in the mucous membranes at the corners of the mouth, or some slowing of intellectual function.

Correction of Nutritional Deficiencies

Nutritional deficiencies are among the most easily preventable causes of disease. It is important to realize that even mild deficiencies can cause irreparable damage, particularly protein deprivation in young children, which can result in some degree of mental retardation. Periodic medical checkups for everyone in the family are the best way to make sure that such deficiencies are corrected before they snowball into a chronic disease. In most cases, all that is required is a change of eating habits.

Weight

Probably the most important dietary problem in the United States today is obesity. It is certainly the most talked about and written about, not only in terms of self-esteem, but more importantly, in terms of good health.

Physicians, dieticians and other health experts use height and weight tables to calculate an average and these experts should be consulted to insure that the tables are being accurately applied and analyzed. While the notion of an "average" weight may be viewed by some with suspicion, the truth is that Americans are steadily gaining weight. Studies indicate that people who are obese have a higher rate of disease and a shorter life ex-

pectancy than those of average weight. Added weight places an added strain to the body, especially the heart. Obesity causes over 300,000 deaths a year and obese people need health care services more frequently than thinner people. Incredibly, thirty percent of the U.S. population is believed to be obese. Being too fat and being overweight are not necessarily the same, however. Heavy bones and muscles can increase a person's weight, but only an excess amount of fat tissue can make someone obese.

An individual is usually considered obese in the clinical sense if he weighs 20 percent more than the standard tables indicate for his size and age. Too much emphasis on the importance of the height and weight tables can be as destructive as too little emphasis. Increasingly, teenage girls and boys suffer from overly-pessimistic assess-

ments of their weights. Anxiety over acceptance by their peers and subtle, informal pressure from advertising and media sources to be "model-thin," has pushed teens to anorexia and bulimia.

The Pinch Test

Another method of determining obesity is to use the "pinch" test. In most adults under 50 years of age, about half of the body fat is located directly under the skin. There are various parts of the body, such as the side of the lower torso, the back of the upper arm, or directly under the shoulder blade, where the thumb and forefin-

ger can pinch a fold of skin and fat away from the underlying bone structure.

If the fold between the fingers—which is, of course, double thickness when it is pinched—is thicker than one inch in any of these areas, the likelihood is that the person is obese.

The Problem of Overweight

The percentage of overweight people in this country has been increasing steadily, chiefly because people eat more and use less physical energy than they used to. Americans do very little walking because of the availability of cars; they do very little manual labor because of the increasing use of machines. They may eat good wholesome meals, but they have the time for nibbling at all hours, especially when sitting in front of the television screen.

These patterns usually begin in childhood. Youngsters rarely walk to school any more; they get there by bus or car. They often have extra money for snacks and soft drinks, and frequently parents encourage them to

overeat without realizing that such habits do them more harm than good.

Most overweight children remain overweight as adults. They also have greater difficulty losing fat, and if they do lose it, tend to regain it more easily than overweight adults who were thin as children. Many adults become overweight between the ages of 20 and 30. Thus, by age 30, about 12 percent of American men and women are 20 percent or more overweight, and by age 60, about 30 percent of the male population and 50 percent of the female are at least 20 percent overweight. As indicated above, the phenomenon of weight gain while aging does not represent biological normalcy.

Why People Put On Weight

Why does weight gain happen? Excess weight is the result of the imbalance between caloric intake as food and caloric expenditure as energy, either in maintaining the basic metabolic processes necessary to sustain life or in performing physical activity. Calories not spent in either of these ways become converted to fat and accumulate in the body as fat, or *adipose* tissue.

A *calorie* is the unit of measurement that describes the amount of energy potentially available in a given food. It is also used to describe the amount of energy the body must use up to perform a given function.

Counting Calories

If an adult gets the average 3,000 calories a day in his food from the age of 20 to 70, he will have consumed about 55 million calories. About 60 percent of these calories will have been used for his basic metabolic processes. The rest—22 million calories—might have resulted in a gain of about 6,000 pounds of fat, since each group of 3,500 extra calories could have produced one pound of fat.

In some ways, it's a miracle that people don't become more obese than they do. The reason, of course, is that most or all of these extra calories are normally used to provide energy for physical activity. Elsewhere in this chapter are some examples of calorie expenditure during various activities.

A reasonably good way for an adult to figure his daily caloric needs for moderate activities is to multiply his desirable weight by 18 for men and 16 for women. If the typical day includes vigorous or strenuous activities, extra calories will, of course, be required.

Parental Influences and Hereditary Factors

Although there are exceptions, almost all obese people consume more calories than they expend. The reasons for this imbalance are complex. One has to do with parental weight. If the weight of both parents is normal, there is only a 10 percent likelihood that the children will be obese. If one parent is obese, there is a 50 percent probability that the children will be too, and if both are, the probability of obese offspring is 80 percent.

No one knows for certain why this is so. It is probably a combination of diet habits acquired in youth, conditioning during early years to react to emotional stress by eating, the absence of appropriate exercise patterns, and genetic inheritance.

Some obese people seem to have an impairment in the regulatory mechanism of the area of the central nervous system that governs food intake. Simply put, they do not know when to stop eating. Others, particularly girls, may eat less than their nonobese counterparts, but they are considerably less active. Some researchers think that obese people have an inherent muscle rhythm deficiency. In rare cases, a few people appear to have an abnormality in the metabolic process which results in the accumulation of fat even when the balance between calories taken in and expended is negative and should lead to weight loss.

Nutrients in Common Foods *(continued)*

Food	Food energy	Protein	Fat	Carbohydrate
	Calories	Grams	Grams	Grams
Celery, raw: large stalk, 8 inches long	5	1	trace	1
Collards, cooked; 1 cup	75	7	1	14
Corn, sweet:				
Cooked; 1 ear 5 inches long	65	2	1	16
Canned, solids and liquid; 1 cup	170	5	1	41
Cucumbers, raw, pared; 6 slices (⅛-inch thick, center section)	5	trace	trace	1
Lettuce, head, raw:				
2 large or 4 small leaves	5	1	trace	1
1 compact head (4¾-inch diameter)	70	5	1	13
Mushrooms, canned, solids and liquid; 1 cup	30	3	trace	9
Okra, cooked; 8 pods (3 inches long, ⅝-inch diameter)	30	2	trace	6
Onions: mature raw; 1 onion (2½-inch diameter)	50	2	trace	11
Peas, green; 1 cup:				
Cooked	110	8	1	19
Canned, solids and liquid	170	8	1	32
Peppers, sweet:				
Green, raw; 1 medium	15	1	trace	3
Red, raw; 1 medium	20	1	trace	4
Potatoes:				
Baked or boiled; 1 medium, 2½-inch diameter (weight raw, about 5 ounce):				
Baked in jacket	90	3	trace	21
Boiled; peeled before boiling	90	3	trace	21
Chips; 10 medium (2-inch diameter)	110	1	7	10
French fried:				
Frozen, ready to be heated for serving; 10 pieces (2 by ½ by ½ inch)	95	2	4	15
Ready-to-eat, deep fat for entire process; 10 pieces (2 by ½ by ½ inch)	155	2	7	20
Mashed; 1 cup:				
Milk added	145	4	1	30
Milk and butter added	230	4	12	28
Radishes, raw; 4 small	10	trace	trace	2
Spinach:				
Cooked; 1 cup	45	6	1	6
Canned, creamed, strained; 1 ounce	10	1	trace	2
Squash:				
Cooked, 1 cup:				
Summer, diced	35	1	trace	8
Winter, baked, mashed	95	4	1	23
Canned, strained or chopped; 1 ounce	10	trace	trace	2

Nutrients in Common Foods *(continued)*

Food	Food energy	Protein	Fat	Carbohydrate
	Calories	Grams	Grams	Grams
Sweet potatoes:				
Baked or boiled; 1 medium, 5 by 2 inches (weight raw, about 6 ounces):				
Baked in jacket	155	2	1	36
Boiled in jacket	170	2	1	39
Candied, 1 small, 3½ by 2 inches	295	2	6	60
Canned, vacuum or solid pack; 1 cup	235	4	trace	54
Tomatoes:				
Raw; 1 medium (2 by 2½ inches), about ⅓ pound	30	2	trace	6
Canned or cooked; 1 cup	45	2	trace	9
Tomato juice, canned; 1 cup	50	2	trace	10
Tomato catsup; 1 tablespoon	15	trace	trace	4
Turnips, cooked, diced; 1 cup	40	1	trace	9
Turnip greens, cooked; 1 cup	45	4	1	8
Fruits				
Apples, raw; 1 medium (2½ inch diameter), about ⅓ pound	70	trace	trace	18
Apple juice, fresh or canned; 1 cup	125	trace	0	34
Apple sauce, canned:				
Sweetened; 1 cup	185	trace	trace	50
Unsweetened; 1 cup	100	trace	trace	26
Apricots, raw; 3 apricots (about ¼ pound)	55	1	trace	14
Apricots, canned in heavy syrup; 1 cup	200	1	trace	54
Apricots, dried; uncooked; 1 cup (40 halves, small)	390	8	1	100
Avocados, raw, California varieties: ½ of a 10-ounce avocado (3½ by 3¼ inches)	185	2	18	6
Avocados, raw, Florida varieties: ½ of a 13-ounce avocado (4 by 3 inches)	160	2	14	11
Bananas, raw; 1 medium (6 by 1½ inches), about ⅓ pound	85	1	trace	23
Blueberries, raw; 1 cup	85	1	1	21
Cantaloupes, raw, ½ melon (5-inch diameter)	40	1	trace	9
Cherries, sour, sweet, and hybrid, raw; 1 cup	65	1	1	15
Cranberry sauce, sweetened; 1 cup	550	trace	1	142
Dates, "fresh" and dried, pitted and cut; 1 cup	505	4	1	134
Figs:				
Raw; 3 small (1½-inch (diameter), about ¼ pound	90	2	trace	22
Dried; 1 large (2 by 1 inch)	60	1	trace	15
Fruit cocktail, canned in heavy syrup, solids and liquid; 1 cup	175	1	trace	47
Grapefruit:				
Raw; ½ medium (4¼-inch diameter, No. 64's)	50	1	trace	14
Canned in syrup; 1 cup	165	1	trace	44

Nutrients in Common Foods *(continued)*

Food	Food energy	Protein	Fat	Carbohydrate
	Calories	Grams	Grams	Grams
Grapefruit juice:				
Raw; 1 cup	85	1	trace	23
Canned:				
Unsweetened; 1 cup	95	1	trace	24
Sweetened; 1 cup	120	1	trace	32
Frozen concentrate, unsweetened:				
Undiluted; 1 can (6 fluid				
ounces:	280	4	1	72
Diluted, ready-to-serve; 1 cup	95	1	trace	24
Frozen concentrate, sweetened:				
Undiluted; 1 can (6 fluid				
ounces)	320	3	1	85
Diluted, ready-to-serve; 1 cup	105	1	trace	28
Grapes, raw; 1 cup:				
American type (slip skin)	70	1	1	16
European type (adherent skin)	100	1	trace	26
Grape juice, bottled; 1 cup	165	1	1	42
Lemonade concentrate, frozen,				
sweetened:				
Undiluted; 1 can (6 fluid ounces) ...	305	1	trace	113
Diluted, ready-to-serve; 1 cup	75	trace	trace	28
Oranges, raw; 1 large orange				
(3-inch diameter)	70	1	trace	18
Orange juice:				
Raw; 1 cup:				
California (Valencias)	105	2	trace	26
Florida varieties:				
Early and midseason	90	1	trace	23
Late season (Valencias)	105	1	trace	26
Canned, unsweetened; 1 cup	110	2	trace	28
Frozen concentrate:				
Undiluted; 1 can 6 fluid				
ounces)	305	5	trace	80
Diluted, ready-to-serve; 1 cup	105	2	trace	27
Peaches:				
Raw:				
1 medium (2½-inch diameter),				
about ¼ pound	35	1	trace	10
1 cup, sliced	65	1	trace	16
Canned (yellow-fleshed) in heavy				
syrup; 1 cup	185	1	trace	49
Dried: uncooked; 1 cup	420	5	1	109
Pears:				
Raw; 1 pear (3 by 2½-inch				
diameter)	100	1	1	25
Canned in heavy syrup; 1 cup	175	1	trace	47
Pineapple juice; canned; 1 cup	120	1	trace	32
Plums				
Raw; 1 plum (2-inch diameter,				
about 2 ounces	30	trace	trace	7
Canned (Italian prunes, in syrup;				
1 cup	185	1	trace	50

Nutrients in Common Foods *(continued)*

Food	Food energy	Protein	Fat	Carbohydrate
	Calories	Grams	Grams	Grams
Prunes, dried:				
Uncooked; 4 medium prunes	70	1	trace	19
Cooked, unsweetened; 1 cup (17–18 prunes and ⅓ cup liquid	295	3	1	78
Prune juice, canned; 1 cup	170	1	trace	45
Raisins, dried; 1 cup	460	4	trace	124
Raspberries, red:				
Raw; 1 cup	70	1	trace	17
Frozen; 10-ounce carton	280	2	1	70
Strawberries:				
Raw; 1 cup	55	1	1	12
Frozen; 10-ounce carton	300	2	1	75
Tangerines; 1 medium (2½-inch diameter), about ¼ pound	40	1	trace	10
Watermelon; 1 wedge (4 by 8 inches), about 2 pounds (weighed with rind	120	2	1	29
Grain Products				
Biscuits, baking powder, enriched flour; 1 biscuit (2½-inch diameter)	130	2	4	20
Bran flakes (40 percent bran) with added thiamine; 1 ounce	85	3	1	22
Breads:				
Cracked wheat:				
1 pound (20 slices)	1,190	39	10	236
1 slice (½-inch thick)	60	2	1	12
Italian; 1 pound	1,250	41	4	256
Rye:				
American (light):				
1 pound (20 slices)	1,100	41	5	236
1 slice (½-inch thick)	55	2	trace	12
Pumpernickel; 1 pound	1,115	41	5	241
White:				
1–2 percent nonfat dry milk:				
1 pound (20 slices)	1,225	39	15	229
1 slice (½-inch thick)	60	2	1	12
3–4 percent nonfat dry milk:				
1 pound (20 slices)	1,225	39	15	229
1 slice (½-inch thick)	60	2	1	12
5–6 percent nonfat dry milk:				
1 pound (20 slices)	1,245	41	17	228
1 slice (½-inch thick)	65	2	1	12
Whole wheat, graham, or entire wheat:				
1 pound (20 slices)	1,105	48	14	216
1 slice (½-inch thick)	55	2	1	11
Cakes:				
Angel food: 2-inch sector (1/12 of cake, 8-inch diameter)	160	4	trace	36
Butter cakes:				
Plain cake and cupcakes without icing:				
1 square (3 by 3 by 2 inches)	315	4	12	48

Nutrients in Common Foods *(continued)*

Food	Food energy	Protein	Fat	Carbohydrate
	Calories	Grams	Grams	Grams
1 cupcake (2¾-inch diameter)	120	2	5	18
Plain cake with icing: 2-inch sector of iced layer cake (1⁄16 of cake, 10-inch diameter)	320	5	6	62
Rich cake: 2-inch sector layer cake, iced (1⁄16 of cake, 10-inch diameter)	490	6	19	76
Fruit cake, dark; 1 piece (2 by 1½ by ¼ inches)	60	1	2	9
Sponge; 2-inch sector (1⁄12 of cake, 8-inch diameter	115	3	2	22
Cookies, plain and assorted; 1 cookie (3-inch diameter)	110	2	3	19
Cornbread or muffins made with enriched, degermed cornmeal; 1 muffin 2¾-inch diameter)	105	3	2	18
Cornflakes; 1 ounce	110	2	trace	24
Corn grits, degermed, cooked; 1 cup	120	3	trace	27
Crackers: Graham; 4 small or 2 medium	55	1	1	10
Saltines; 2 crackers (2-inch square	35	1	1	6
Soda, plain: 2 crackers (2½-inch square	45	1	1	8
Doughnuts, cake type; 1 doughnut	135	2	7	17
Farina, cooked; 1 cup	105	3	trace	22
Macaroni, cooked; 1 cup: Cooked 8–10 minutes (undergoes additional cooking as ingredient of a food mixture)	190	6	1	39
Cooked until tender	155	5	1	32
Noodles (egg noodles), cooked; 1 cup	200	7	2	37
Oat cereal (mixture, mainly oat flour), ready-to-eat; 1 ounce	115	4	2	21
Oatmeal or rolled oats, regular or quick cooking, cooked; 1 cup	150	5	3	26
Pancakes; baked; 1 cake (4-inch diameter): Wheat (home recipe)	60	2	2	7
Buckwheat (with buckwheat pancake mix)	45	2	2	6
Pies; 3½-inch sector (1⁄8 of 9-inch diameter pie): Apple	300	3	13	45
Cherry	310	3	13	45
Custard	250	7	13	27
Lemon meringue	270	4	11	40
Minced	320	3	14	49
Pumpkin	240	5	13	28
Pretzels; 5 small sticks	20	trace	trace	4

Nutrients in Common Foods *(continued)*

Food	Food energy	Protein	Fat	Carbohydrate
	Calories	Grams	Grams	Grams
Rice, cooked; 1 cup:				
Converted	205	4	trace	45
White	200	4	trace	44
Rice, puffed or flakes; 1 ounce	110	2	trace	25
Rolls:				
Plain, pan (16 ounces per dozen); 1 roll	115	3	2	20
Hard, round (22 ounces per dozen); 1 roll	160	5	2	31
Sweet, pan (18 ounces per dozen); 1 roll	135	4	4	21
Spaghetti, cooked until tender; 1 cup	155	5	1	32
Waffles, baked, with enriched flour: 1 waffle (4½ by 5½ by ½ inches)	215	7	8	28
Wheat, puffed; 1 ounce	100	4	trace	22
Wheat, rolled, cooked; 1 cup	175	5	1	40
Wheat flakes; 1 ounce	100	3	trace	23
Wheat flours:				
Whole wheat; 1 cup, sifted	400	16	2	85
All purpose or family flour: 1 cup, sifted	400	12	1	84
Wheat germ; 1 cup, stirred	245	17	7	34
Fats, Oils, Related Products				
Butter; 1 tablespoon	100	trace	11	trace
Fats, cooking:				
Vegetable fats:				
1 cup	1,770	0	200	0
1 tablespoon	110	0	12	0
Lard:				
1 cup	1,985	0	220	0
1 tablespoon	125	0	14	0
Margarine; 1 tablespoon	100	trace	11	trace
Oils, salad or cooking; 1 tablespoon	125	0	14	0
Salad dressings; 1 tablespoon:				
Blue cheese	90	1	10	1
Commercial, plain (mayonnaise type)	60	trace	6	2
French	60	trace	6	2
Mayonnaise	110	trace	12	trace
Thousand Island	75	trace	8	1
Sugars, Sweets				
Candy; 1 ounce:				
Caramels	120	1	3	22
Chocolate, sweetened, milk	145	2	9	16
Fudge, plain	115	trace	3	23
Hard	110	0	0	28
Marshmallow	90	1	0	23
Jams, marmalades, preserves; 1 tablespoon	55	trace	trace	14
Jellies; 1 tablespoon	50	0	0	13
Sugar; 1 tablespoon	50	0	0	12
Syrup, table blends; 1 tablespoon	55	0	0	15

Nutrients in Common Foods *(continued)*

Food	Food energy	Protein	Fat	Carbohydrate
	Calories	Grams	Grams	Grams
Miscellaneous				
Beverages, carbonated, cola types; 1 cup	105	—	—	28
Bouillon cubes; 1 cube	2	trace	trace	0
Chocolate, unsweetened; 1 ounce	145	2	15	8
Gelatin dessert, plain, ready-to-serve; 1 cup	155	4	0	36
Sherbet, factory packed; 1 cup (8-fluid-ounce container)	235	3	trace	58
Soups, canned, prepared with equal amount of water; 1 cup:				
Bean with pork	168	8	6	22
Beef noodle	140	8	5	14
Bouillon, broth, and consomme	30	5	0	3
Chicken consomme	44	7	trace	4
Clam chowder, Manhattan style	80	2	3	12
Tomato	90	2	3	16
Vegetable beef	80	5	2	10
Vinegar; 1 tablespoon	2	0	—	1

Adapted from *Nutritive Value of American Foods* by Catherine F. Adams. Agriculture Handbook No. 456. U.S. Department of Agriculture, issued November 1975. The cup measure used in the following table refers to the standard 8-ounce measuring cup of 8 fluid ounces or one-half liquid pint. When a measure is indicated by ounce, it is understood to be by weight—1/16 of a pound avoirdupois—unless a fluid ounce is indicated. All weights and measures in the table are in U.S. System units.

Obesity and Health

There are many reasons why obesity is a health hazard. The annual death rate for obese people between the ages of 20 and 64 is half again as high as that for people whose weight is close to normal. This statistical difference is due primarily to the increased likelihood that the obese person will suffer from diabetes mellitus and from diseases of the digestive and circulatory systems, especially of the heart.

One possible reason for the increased possibility of heart disease is that there are about two-thirds of a mile of blood vessels in each pound of adipose tissue. Thus 20 or more pounds of excess weight are likely to impose a great additional work load on the heart.

Obese people are also poorer surgical risks than the nonobese, and it is often more difficult to diagnose and therefore to treat their illnesses correctly.

Permanent loss of excess weight makes the formerly obese person come closer to matching the life expectancy of the nonobese. However, losing and regaining weight as a repeated pattern is even more hazardous in terms of health than consistent obesity.

Psychological Consequences of Obesity

In ways that are both obvious and subtle, obesity often has damaging psychological consequences. This is particularly true for obese children, who tend to feel isolated and rejected by their peers. They may consider themselves victims of prejudice and blame their obesity for everything that goes wrong in their lives. In many cases, the destructive relationship between obesity and self-pity keeps perpetuating itself.

Obese adults are likely to experience the same feelings, but to a somewhat lesser degree. For some, obesity is an escape which consciously or unconsciously helps them to avoid situations in which they feel uncomfortable—those that involve active competition or relationships with the opposite sex.

Avoiding Excess Weight

Clearly, obesity is a condition that most people would like to avoid. Not putting on extra pounds does seem to be easier, in theory at least, than taking them off. One possible explanation for this is that additional adipose tissue consists of a proliferation of fat cells. Shrinking these cells is one thing, eliminating them is another. Our present lack of fundamental knowledge about the regulatory and metabolic mechanisms relating to obesity limits the technique of preventing overweight to recommending a balance between caloric intake and expenditure.

The real responsibility for preventing the onset of obesity in childhood rests with parents. It is important for the parents to set a good example and to instill early on all of the fundamentals of good nutrition and healthy eating habits; these are of the utmost importance in this connection. Caloric expenditure in the form of regular exercise is equally important.

Exercising by Habit

This does not necessarily mean that exercise should be encouraged for its own sake. What it does mean is making a habit of choosing an active way of approaching a situation rather than a lazy way: walking upstairs rather than taking the elevator; walking to school rather than riding; walking while playing golf rather than riding in a cart; running to get the ball that has rolled away rather than ambling toward it. These choices should be made consistently and not just occasionally if obesity is to be avoided. Those people who naturally enjoy the more active way of doing things are lucky. Those who don't should make an effort to develop new patterns, especially if obesity is a family problem.

Anyone with the type of physical handicap that makes a normal amount of exercise impossible should be especially careful about caloric intake.

Weight Reduction

The treatment of obesity is a complicated problem. In the first place, there is the question of who wants or needs to be treated and how much weight should be lost. Except in unusual situations, anyone who wants to lose weight should be encouraged to do so. Possible exceptions are teenagers who are not overweight but who want to be as thin as they can possibly be—the boy who is involved in an athletic event such as wrestling, or the girl who has decided she wants to look like a fashion model.

Crash dieting is usually unwise if the goal is to lose too much weight too rapidly and should be undertaken only after consulting a doctor about its advisability. As for adolescents who have become slightly overweight during puberty, they may be ill-advised to try to take off the extra pounds that probably relate to a temporary growth pattern.

Losing Weight Must Be Self-Motivated

Unless there are compelling medical reasons for not doing so, anyone weighing 20 percent or more over the normal limit for his age and body build should be helped to slim down. It is extremely important, however, for the motivation to come from the person himself rather than from outside pressure.

Unless an overweight person really wants to reduce, he will not succeed in doing so, certainly not permanently, even though he appears to be trying. He must have convinced himself—intellectually and emotionally—that the goal of weight loss is truly worth the effort.

It is very difficult not only for his friends and family but for the person himself to be absolutely sure about the depth of his motivation. A physician treating an overweight patient has to assume that the desire to re-

duce is genuine and will try to reinforce it whenever he can. However, if a patient has made a number of attempts to lose weight over a period of years and has either been unable to reduce to any significant degree, or has become overweight again after reducing, it is probably safe to assume that the emotional desire is absent, or that there are emotional conflicts that stand in the way.

It is very possible that such a person could be harmed psychologically by losing weight, since he might need to be overweight for some deep-seated reason. This can be true for both children and adults. Occasionally it is possible for a psychiatrist or psychologist to help the patient remove a psychological block against losing weight, after which weight reduction can occur if the caloric balance is straightened out.

Effective Planning for Weight Loss

The ultimate key to successful weight reduction is proper eating combined with proper physical activity. This

balance is extremely difficult for many people to achieve because it involves a marked change in attitudes and be-

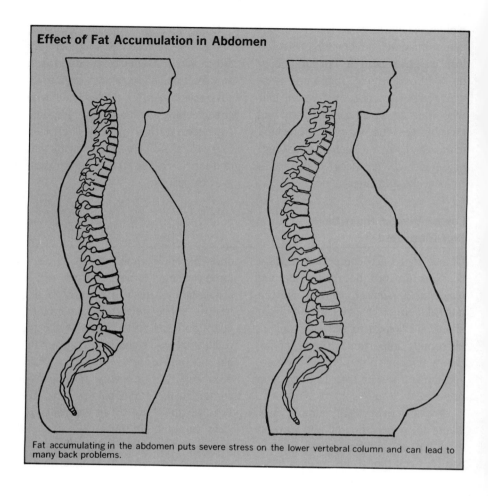

Effect of Fat Accumulation in Abdomen

Fat accumulating in the abdomen puts severe stress on the lower vertebral column and can lead to many back problems.

havior patterns that are generally solidly established and of long duration. Furthermore, once the changes are made, they will have to endure for a lifetime if the weight that has been lost is not to be regained.

It is therefore important that the reducing diet should be somewhat similar to the person's usual eating pattern in terms of style and quality. Intake of fat and calories should be reduced and that of fiber increased, and probably the word "dieting" should not be used to describe the process, since most people don't find the idea of permanent dieting congenial.

Similarly, the increased physical activity that must accompany the new eating style should be of a type that the person enjoys. It is virtually impossible for an overeating person to reduce merely by restricting his caloric intake, or merely by increasing his caloric expenditure. The two must go together.

Cutting Down Step by Step

The first thing to determine when planning to lose weight is the number of pounds that have to go. A realistic goal to set is the loss of about one pound a week. This may seem too slow, but remember that at this rate, fifty pounds can be lost in a year.

Getting Started

Start by weighing yourself on arising, and then for two weeks try to eat in your customary manner, but keep a careful record of everything that you eat, the time it is eaten, and the number of calories it contains. During this period, continue to do your usual amount of physical activity.

When the two weeks are over, weigh yourself again at the same time of day as before. If you haven't gained any weight, you are in a basal caloric state. Then check over your food list to see what might be eliminated each day without causing discomfort.

Pay attention to portion size and try to think in terms of eliminating fats and simple carbohydrates first, because it is essential that you continue to get sufficient vitamins and minerals which are largely found in proteins, complex carbohydrates, fruits, and vegetables. The foods described in the "Food Guide Pyramid" should all continue to be included in your daily food consumption. If you are in the habit of having an occasional drink, remember that there are calories in alcohol but no nutrients, and that most alcoholic beverages stimulate the appetite.

Planning Meals

When you replan your meals, keep in mind that the items you cut down on must add up to between 300 and 400 calories a day if you are going to lose one pound a week.

Your total daily food intake should be divided among at least three meals a day—more, if you wish. If you need to eat more food or to eat more often, try snacking on low-calorie foods such as cabbage, carrots, celery, cucumber, and cauliflower. All of these can be eaten raw between meals.

There is definitely something to be said in favor of having breakfast every morning, or at least most mornings. This may be psychologically difficult, but try to do it, because it will be easier to control your urge to eat too much later in the day.

Increasing Exercise

At the same time that you begin to cut down on your food intake, start to increase your daily exercise in whatever way you find congenial so that the number of calories expended in increased exercise plus the number of calories eliminated from your diet comes to 500 or more. This is your daily caloric loss compared with your so-called basal caloric state.

Daily Food Guide

	Child	Preteen and Teen	Adult	Aging Adult
Milk or milk products (cups)	2–3	3–4 or more	2 or more	2 or more
Meat, fish, poultry, and eggs (servings)	1–2	3 or more	2 or more	2 or more
Green and yellow vegetables (servings)	1–2	2	2	at least 1
Citrus fruits and tomatoes (servings)	1	1–2	1	1–2
Potatoes, other fruits, vegetables (servings)	1	1	1	0–1
Bread, flour, and cereal (servings)	3–4	4 or more	3–4	2–3
Butter or margarine (tablespoons)	2	2–4	2–3	1–2

1. The need for the nutirents in 1 or 2 cups of milk daily can be satisfied by cheeses or ice cream. (1 cup of milk is approximately equivalent to 1½ cups of cottage cheese or 2–3 large scoops of ice cream.)
2. It is important to drink enough fluid. The equivalent of 3–5 cups daily is recommended.
3. The recommended daily serving of meat, fish, and poultry (3 oz.) may be alternated with eggs or cheese, dried peas, beans, or lentils.
4. Iron-rich foods should be selected as frequently as possible by teenage and adult females to help meet their high requirement for this mineral (liver, heart, lean meats, shellfish, egg yolks, legumes, green leafy vegetables, and whole grain and enriched cereal products).

From *Your Age and Your Diet* (1971), reprinted with permission from the American Medical Association.

Achieving Your Goal

You may wish to double your daily caloric loss so that you lose two pounds a week. Do not try to lose any more than that unless you are under close medical supervision.

If you gained weight during your two-week experimental period, you will have to increase your daily caloric loss by 500 for every pound gained per week. Thus, if you gained one pound during the two weeks, you will have to step up your daily caloric loss to 750 to lose a pound a week.

You'll have to keep plugging away to achieve your goal. It will be trying and difficult in many ways. You may get moody and discouraged and be tempted to quit. Don't. You'll probably go on periodic food binges. All this is natural and understandable, so try not to brood about it. Just do the best you can each day. Don't worry about yesterday, and let tomorrow take care of itself.

In many ways it can help, and in some cases it's essential, to have the support and encouragement of family and friends, particularly of those with whom you share meals. You may find it helpful to join a group that has been formed to help its members lose weight and maintain their weight loss. This is a good psychological support.

Maintaining Your Weight Loss

Once you have achieved your desired weight, you can test yourself to see what happens if you increase your caloric intake. Clearly, anyone who can lose weight in the manner described can't stay in a state of negative caloric imbalance indefinitely. But you will have to be careful, or you'll become overweight again. It's a challenge, but people who stick to a disciplined program can be rewarded by success.

Special Problems

If you do not succeed in losing weight in spite of carrying out the program described above, you may need professional help because of some special problem. A qualified physician may try some special diets, or he may even suggest putting you into a hospital so that he can see to it that you have no caloric food at all for as long as three weeks.

Perhaps the situation is complicated by a metabolic abnormality that can be corrected or helped by medication. Although such conditions are rare, they are not unheard of.

Obesity is almost never caused by a "glandular" problem—which usually means an underactive thyroid. Do not take thyroid pills to reduce unless your thyroid has been found to be underactive on the basis of a specific laboratory test.

The indiscriminate use of pills to reduce, even when prescribed, is never helpful in the long run, although it may appear to be at first. The unsupervised use of amphetamines, for example, can be extremely dangerous. See Ch. 29, *Substance Abuse,* for further information about the dangers of amphetamine abuse.

Because so many people are eager to reduce, and because losing weight isn't easy, there are many unethical professionals who specialize in the problem. Avoid them. All they are likely to do for you is take your money and make your situation no better— and often worse—than it was to begin with.

Underweight

Weighing too little is a problem that is considerably less common than weighing too much. In fact, in many cases, it isn't accurate to call it a problem at all, at least not a medical one.

There are some times, however, when underweight may indicate the presence of a disease, especially when a person rather suddenly begins and continues to lose weight, even though there has been no change in his eating habits. This is a situation that calls for prompt medical evaluation. Fortunately, such a person may already be under a physician's care at the time the weight loss is first noticed.

More often, however, underweight is a chronic condition that is of concern to the person who feels his looks would improve if he could only add some extra pounds. This is especially true in the case of adolescent girls and young women.

What To Do About
Weighing Too Little

Chronic underweight is rarely a reflection of underlying disease. It is rather an expression of individual heredity or eating patterns, or a combination of both. Treatment for the condition is the opposite of the treatment for overweight. The achievement of a positive caloric balance comes first; more calories have to be consumed each day than are expended. An underweight person should record his food history over a two-week period in the manner described for an overweight one. Once this has been done, various adjustments can be made.

First of all, he should see that he eats at least three meals a day and that they are eaten in a leisurely way and in a relaxed frame of mind. All of the basic foods should be represented in the daily food intake, with special emphasis on protein and complex carbohydrates. The daily caloric intake should then be gradually increased at each meal and snacks added, so long as the snacks don't reduce the appetite at mealtimes.

Carbohydrate foods are the best ones to emphasize in adding calories. Since the extra food intake may cause a certain amount of discomfort, encouragement and support from family and friends can be extremely helpful. Just as there may be psychological blocks against losing weight, there may well be a complicated underlying resistance to adding it.

Anyone trying to gain weight should remain or become reasonably active physically. Adding a pound or two a month for an adult—and a little more than that for a growing youngster—is an achievable goal until the desired weight is reached. There will probably have to be some adjustments in eating and exercise patterns so that a state of caloric balance is achieved.

How Food Relates
to Disease

Just as proper food is essential in the prevention of some diseases, it is helpful in the treatment of others. It also plays an important role in protecting and fortifying the general health of a patient while a specific illness is being treated.

The components of therapeutic diets are usually prescribed by the physician in charge, but some general principles will be presented here. Remember that diets designed to treat a given disease must supply the patient's basic nutritional requirements.

Ulcers

Special diet is a major treatment consideration in the case of peptic ulcer, whether located in the stomach (gastric) or in the small intestine (duodenal). A major aim of such a diet is the neutralizing of the acidity of gastric juices by the frequent intake of high protein foods such as milk and eggs. Foods which irritate an ulcer chemically, such as excessive sweets, spices, or salt, or mechanically, such as foods with sharp seeds or tough skins, and foods that are too hot or too cold, should be avoided. It is also advisable to eliminate gravies, coffee, strong tea, carbonated beverages, and alcohol, since all of these stimulate gastric secretion. Such a diet is called a *bland* diet. A soft diet is recommended for some forms of gastrointestinal distress and for those people who have difficulty chewing. It is often combined with the bland diet recommended for peptic ulcer patients to reduce the likelihood of irritation. See Ch. 11, *Diseases of the Digestive System,* for further information about ulcers.

Diabetes

As the section on diabetes mellitus indicates (see Ch. 15), the major objectives of the special diet are weight control, control of the abnormal carbohydrate metabolism, and as far as possible, psychological adjustment by the patient to his individual circumstances. To some extent, he must calculate his diet mathematically. First, his daily caloric needs have to be determined in terms of his activities.

If he is overweight or underweight, the total calories per pound of body weight will have to be adjusted downward or upward by about five calories per pound.

After his total daily caloric needs have been figured out, he can calculate the number of grams of carbohydrate, protein, and fat he should have each day: 58 percent of the calories should come from carbohydrates, 12 percent from protein, and 30 percent from fat. One-fifth of the total should be obtained at breakfast and the rest split between lunch and dinner. Snacks that are taken during the day should be subtracted equally from lunch and dinner.

It is important that meals and planned snacks be eaten regularly and that no food servings be added or omitted. Growing children from 1 to 20 years of age who have diabetes will require considerably more daily calories. A rough estimate is 1,000 calories for a one-year-old child and 100 additional calories for each year of age.

Salt-Free Diets

There are a number of chronic diseases which are treated in part by restricting the amount of sodium in the diet. These diseases, which are associated with fluid retention in the body, include congestive heart failure, certain types of kidney and liver diseases, and hypertension or high blood pressure.

The restriction of sodium intake helps to reduce or avoid the problem of fluid retention. The normal daily diet contains about seven or more grams of sodium, most of it in the form of sodium chloride or table salt. This amount is either inherent in the food or added during processing, cooking, or at mealtime. Half the weight of salt is sodium.

For people whose physical condition requires only a small restriction of the normal sodium intake, simply not salting food at the table is a sufficient reduction. They may decide to use a salt substitute, but before doing so should discuss the question with their physician.

A greater sodium restriction, for example, to no more than 5 grams a day, requires the avoidance of such high salt content foods as ham, bacon, crackers, catsup, and potato chips, as well as almost entirely eliminating salt in the preparation and serving of meals. Severe restriction—1 gram or less a day—involves special food selection and cooking procedures, as well as the use of distilled water if the local water has more than 20 milligrams of sodium per quart. In restricting sodium to this extent, it is important to make sure that protein and vitamins are not reduced below the minimum daily requirements. See "Sodium Restricted Diets."

Sodium Restricted Diets

Diets Moderately Restricted in Sodium

If only a moderate sodium restriction is necessary, a normal diet *without added salt* may be ordered. Such an order is interpreted to mean that the patient will be offered the regular salted food on the general selective menu with the following exceptions:

1. No salt will be served on the tray.
2. Soups that are salted will be omitted.
3. Cured meats (ham, bacon, sausage, corned beef) and all salted cheeses will be omitted.
4. Catsup, chili sauce, mustard, and other salted sauces will be omitted.
5. Salt-free gravies, sauces, and salad dressings will be substituted for the regular salted items.
6. Salted crackers, potato chips, nuts, pickles, olives, popcorn, and pretzels will be omitted.

This diet contains approximately 3 grams of sodium or 7.5 grams of sodium chloride, depending on the type and quantity of the food chosen.

Other Diseases Requiring Special Diets

There are several other disorders in which diet is an important consideration: all chronic gastrointestinal disorders, such as gallbladder stones, ulcerative colitis, enteritis, and diverticulitis; a variety of hereditary disorders such as phenylketonuria and galactosemia; atherosclerosis, especially when it is associated with elevated blood levels of cholesterol or triglycerides or both; liver disease such as cirrhosis; many of the endocrine diseases; kidney stones; and sometimes certain neurological diseases such as epilepsy. Diet also plays a special role in convalescence from most illnesses and in post-surgical care. A modified fat diet and low fat diet are recommended for some diseases of the liver and gall-bladder. A minimal residue diet is recommended for some digestive troubles and before and after gastrointestinal surgery.

Diet and Individual Differences

Most discussions about food and eating tend to suggest that all normal people have identical gastrointestinal and metabolic systems. This is simply not true. There are many individual differences that explain why one man's meat is another man's poison. A person's intolerance for a given food may be caused by a disorder, such as an allergy or an ulcer, and it is possible that many of these intolerances will ultimately be related to enzyme deficiencies or some other biochemical factor.

More subtle are the negative physical reactions to particular foods as a result of psychological conditioning. In most such cases, the choice is between avoiding the food that causes the discomfort or eating it and suffering the consequences. Of course, compulsive overeating can also cause or contribute to discomfort. Practically no one can eat unlimited quantities of anything without having gastrointestinal discomfort or *dyspepsia.*

The establishment of so-called daily minimum food requirements suggests that every day's intake should be carefully balanced. Although this is beneficial, it is by no means necessary. Freedom from such regimentation can certainly be enjoyed during a holiday, or a trip to another country, or on a prolonged visit to relatives with casual food habits.

Sometimes a change in diet is dictated by a cold or an upset stomach or diarrhea. Liquids containing carbohydrates, such as tea with sugar and light soups, should be emphasized in treating a cold, while at the same time solid food intake should be somewhat reduced. In the case of an upset stomach or diarrhea, the discomfort may be eased by not eating or drinking anything at all for a whole day. This form of treatment may be helpful for an adult, but since children with diarrhea can become dehydrated in a day or so, professional advice is indicated when cutting down liquid intake.

Diet and Disease Prevention

More and more, medical specialists agree that diet can be helpful in preventing various diseases. Consensus has become general that a diet low in cholesterol and saturated fats can help prevent cardiovascular disease caused by atherosclerosis. Among the foods that reduce total cholesterol levels are rice bran and oat bran. Other sources of the soluble fiber that decreases blood cholesterol include peas, lentils, barley, and pectin fruits like apples, oranges, pears, and prunes. Also recommended are skin-less poultry and fish, lean meat, and low-fat dairy products.

Food-Borne Diseases

There are several ways in which food can be the *cause* of disease, most commonly when it becomes contaminated with a sufficient amount of harmful bacteria, bacterial toxin, viruses, or other poisonous substances. The gastrointestinal diseases typically accompanied by nausea, vomiting, diarrhea, or stomach cramps that are produced in this way are not, strictly speaking, caused by the foods themselves, and are therefore called food-borne diseases.

Most food-borne illnesses are caused by a toxin in food contaminated by staphylococcal or salmonella bacteria. In general, milk, milk prod-ucts, raw shellfish, and meats are the foods most apt to be contaminated. This is most likely to happen when such foods are left standing at room temperature for too long between the time they are prepared and the time they are eaten. However, food can also become contaminated at many different points in time and at various stages of processing. Standards enforced by federal and local government agencies provide protection for the consumer for foods bought for the home as well as for use in restaurants, although whether the protection is adequate is a matter of dispute.

Food Storage

Food is best protected from contamination when it is stored below 40 degrees Fahrenheit or heated to 145 degrees or more. Cold slows bacterial growth; cooking kills it. Bacteria present in food can double in number every 15 minutes at room temperature.

All food stored in the refrigerator should be covered except ripe fruits and vegetables. Leftover foods cannot be kept indefinitely, nor can frozen foods be stored beyond a certain length of time. Specific information about these time periods for individual items is available from the Agricultural Extension Service in each state.

Commercially processed foods sold in the United States are under government control and generally are safe. However, any food can spoil or become contaminated at any point in time, and the consumer should not buy or serve food whose container (package or can) has been broken, cracked, or appears unusual.

Food Additives

From time to time, concern is expressed about one or another food additive as a hazard to health. Most of these additives are put into foods during processing in order to increase their nutritional value, or to improve their chemical or physical characteristics, such as taste and color. Perhaps as many as 2,000 different substances are used in this way in the United States. Some are natural products such as vanilla, others are chemicals derived from other foods, and a few, like artificial sweeteners, are synthetic. Other additives are referred to as indirect, since they are residues in the food from some stage of growing, processing, or packaging. Although additives are controlled and approved by agencies such as the federal Food and Drug Administration, they continue to be a cause of concern to many people.

Pesticides

The pesticides and fertilizers used in growing fruits and vegetables and the additives given to livestock may pose additional health hazards to humans. The National Academy of Sciences, for example, in 1988 estimated the national risk of cancer from pesticide use alone at as many as 20,000 cases a year.

Although it is not known how much is too much, it only makes sense to try and eliminate as much of the risk as possible. This is fairly easy to do. First of all, eat a wide variety of foods to help minimize your exposure to any one pesticide. Eat what's in season and what's grown locally or domestically. (The right season and less transportation mean less chemicals to ripen and preserve food; food and animals from abroad are subject to different health standards that are hard to regulate and check.) Wash all meat and produce carefully; many toxins are easily removed with soap and water. Peel any fruit or vegetable with a wax coating. (Although it is generally advisable to retain as much of the skin of produce as possible for higher vitamin content, wax coatings hold in toxic residues.) Trim produce.

You may also want to go further in reducing your chances of consumption of added toxins by buying organically grown and raised produce and meat. These foods are not widely available in all areas of the country, and they often cost quite a bit more than foods raised with chemicals, but many people not only feel safer eating these foods, but find them tastier as well. Home gardening without the use of chemical fertilizers and pesticides is another healthful option. Be sure to wash and trim carefully all organic or home-grown vegetables, however, to guard against ingestion of naturally occurring toxins such as fungus.

Psychological Aspects of Food and Meals

Food and meals play an important role in emotional well-being and interpersonal relationships as well as in physical health and appearance.

During Infancy

The infant whose needs are attended to by a loving family develops a general sense of trust and security. The major contribution to his emotional contentment is probably made at mealtimes, and perhaps in a special way if he is breast-fed.

For most infants, food comes to be identified with love, pleasure, protection, and the satisfaction of basic needs. If there is an atmosphere of tension accompanying his feeding times, his digestion can be impaired in such a way as to cause vomiting, fretting, or signs of colic. If the tension and the baby's reaction to it—and inevitably the mother's increasing tension as a consequence—become a chronic condition, the result may be a failure to gain weight normally, and in extreme cases, some degree of mental retardation. Throughout life, good nutrition depends not only on eating properly balanced meals that satisfy the body's physiological requirements, but also on a reasonable degree of contentment and relaxation while eating.

Everybody develops individual emotional reactions and attitudes about food and its role as a result of conditioning during the years of infancy and childhood. These attitudes relate not only to food itself and to mealtimes in general, but also to other aspects of eating, including the muscle activities of sucking, chewing, and swallowing.

If food symbolized contentment during the early years, it probably will have the same role later on. If it was associated with conflict, then it may be associated throughout life with strife and neurotic eating patterns.

During Childhood

For the preschool child, mealtimes should provide the occasion for the development of interpersonal relationships, because they are a daily opportunity for both verbal and nonverbal self-expression. The child who eats with enthusiasm and obvious enjoyment is conveying one message; the one who dawdles, picks at food, and challenges his mother with every mouthful is conveying quite a different one.

Meals can become either positive or negative experiences depending in large part on how the adults in the family set the stage. Communication can be encouraged by relaxed conversation and a reasonably leisurely schedule. It can be discouraged by watching television or reading while eating, by not eating together, or by eating and running.

Reasonably firm attitudes about eating a variety of foods in proper quantities at proper times and avoiding excessive catering to individual whims can also help in the development of wholesome eating patterns.

Those who select and prepare the food can transmit special messages of love and affection by serving favorite dishes, by setting the table attractively, and by creating an atmosphere of grace and good humor. Or they can show displeasure and generate hostility by complaining about all the work involved in feeding everyone, or by constant criticism of table manners, or by bringing up touchy subjects likely to cause arguments at the table.

Diet Fads

There are many fads and fallacies about losing weight. Everyone wants an easy solution; cosmetic and food product manufacturers know this and develop products that play to this desire. Thus we have pills that are supposed to burn fat while we sleep; machines that are supposed to give us a "workout" while we're lying down by electrically stimulating our muscles; plastic suits that we wear while exercising that are supposed to produce dramatic weight loss; and special creams and body scrubbers that are supposed to take away unsightly cellulite.

The truth is that a pill will not burn calories for you, a machine will not do your exercise for you, a plastic suit will only make you lose water, not fat, and the idea that there is a special kind of fat called cellulite is a myth.

Cellulite, in fact, is fat, plain and simple; there are no special varieties. Much of the body's fat is stored directly beneath the skin where there is also a sheath of connective tissue, which tends to compartmentalize the fat cells. The more fat the more this tissue is stretched and the more the fat bulges around and through it, producing cellulite's characteristic dimpled effect. Women tend to have thinner skin and less flexible connective tissue, making them more "prone" to cellulite than men. There is no point in spending money on special creams or brushes; you cannot scrub away excess fat. You have to reduce your intake and burn it through exercise.

Similarly, most diet programs that consist of pills, powders, or foolish eating habits are ineffective and usually harmful. Many of them are addictive and those who benefit from the diet programs often gain back the weight lost once they return to their "normal" eating habits.

One drug often used in diet pills is phenylpropanolamine hydrochloride (PPA). PPA is a decongestant, but it also acts as a stimulant and an appetite suppressant. Its side effects include dry mouth, nausea, insomnia, increased heart rate, and increased blood pressure. When PPA is used at the same time as certain other drugs, the elevation of blood pressure can be dramatic, increasing the risk of stroke. PPA can also aggravate glaucoma and kidney disease.

Benzocaine, an ingredient in diet products such as gums and candies, is a local anesthetic that numbs taste receptors, which may briefly suppress the urge to eat. Benzocaine, however, can cause potentially fatal allergic reactions in some individuals.

Although there is no substitute for regular exercise and eating health-

Fat Content of Some Common Foods

Food	Percentage of calories from fat
Brazil nuts	92
Pecans	90
Avocado	83
Almonds	81
Peanuts	79
Pistachio nuts	77
Sunflower seed kernels, roasted	76
Cheese, American processed	76
Cheese, Cheddar	71
Salami, cooked	71
Mozzarella, whole-milk	68
Ricotta, whole-milk	67
Cheese, Swiss	67
Pork, ground, cooked	64
Mozzarella, part-skim	63
Ground beef, lean, broiled	62
Pot roast, braised	62
Egg	59
Ground beef, extra lean, broiled	58
Ricotta, part-skim	52
Granola	51
Cheese, Swiss, reduced-fat	51
Milk, whole, 3.3% fat	48
Croissant	47
Yogurt, plain, whole-milk	45
Sockeye salmon, baked or broiled	44
Chicken, roasted, dark meat, without skin	41
Milk, low-fat, 2% fat	37
Pork loin, tenderloin, roasted	31
Chicken drumstick, without skin	31
Chicken, roasted, light meat, without skin	28
Milk, low-fat, 1% fat	26
Yogurt, plain, low-fat	25
Halibut, baked or broiled	23
Turkey leg, without skin	20
Chicken breast, without skin	19
Oatmeal, instant	17
Hamburger or hot dog bun	15
Whole wheat bread	13
Cottage cheese, 1% fat	11
Shrimp, steamed, poached, or broiled	11
Corn	10
Milk, skim	<10
Egg noodles	8
Kidney beans, dry	8
Rice, brown	8
English muffin	7
Garbanzo beans (chickpeas), canned, solids and liquid	6
Bagel, plain	5
Spaghetti or macaroni	5
Rice, white	<4
Fruits	0
Green, leafy vegetables	0

Note: The U.S. Government recommends that no more than 30 percent of daily calories come from fat.

fully, obesity, which increases the risk of serious health problems, may be managed with the help of physician-prescribed appetite suppressants. These drugs, such as sibutramine (brand name Meridia), may be used for a short time to achieve a loss of ten percent of body weight, an amount thought to reduce health risks. They are not a substitute for long-term behavioral changes in diet and exercise.

Anybody interested in losing a substantial amount of weight should consult with his or her physician. The physician will know of a nutritionist who can provide a healthy program for weight reduction.

Weight loss involves a complete change in one's lifestyle. The solution includes eating balanced meals, reducing the intake of fat, increasing proportionately the consumption of carbohydrates, and exercising three or four times a week. It is a slow process that does not offer the quick yet temporary loss offered by over-the-counter diet programs. Rather, it is a permanent commitment to a healthy way of life. Only then, can a person maintain an optimal weight.

28

Mental and Emotional Disorders

The ability to adapt is central to being emotionally fit, healthy, and mature. An emotionally fit person is one who can adapt to changing circumstances with constructive reactions and who can enjoy living, loving others, and working productively. In everyone's life there are bound to be experiences that are anxious or deeply disturbing, such as the sadness of losing a loved one or the disappointment of failure. The emotionally fit person is stable enough not to be overwhelmed by the anxiety, grief, or guilt that such experiences frequently produce. His sense of his own worth is not lost easily by a setback in life; rather, he can learn from his own mistakes.

Communication and Tolerance

Even the most unpleasant experiences can add to one's understanding of life. Emerging from a crisis with new wisdom can give a sense of pride and mastery. The emotionally fit person can listen attentively to the opinions of others, yet if his decision differs from that being urged by friends and relatives, he will abide by it and can stand alone if necessary, without guilt and anger at those who disagree.

Communicating well with others is an important part of emotional fitness. Sharing experiences, both good and bad, is one of the joys of living. Although the capacity to enjoy is often increased by such sharing, independence is also essential, for one person's pleasure may leave others indifferent. It is just as important to appreciate and respect the individuality of others as it is to value our own individual preferences, as long as these are reasonable and do not give pain to others.

Ways of Expressing Disagreement

Communication should be kept open at all times. Anger toward those who disagree may be an immediate response, but it should not lead to cutting off communication, as it so frequently does, particularly between husbands and wives, parents and children.

Emotional maturity enables us to disagree with what another says, feels, or does, yet make the distinction between that person and how we feel about his thoughts and actions. To tell someone, "I don't like what you are doing," is more likely to keep the lines of communication open than telling him "I don't like you." This is particularly important between parents and children.

It is unfortunately common for parents to launch personal attacks when children do something that displeases them. The child, or any person to whom this is done, then feels unworthy or rejected, which often makes him angry and defiant. Revenge becomes uppermost, and communication is lost; each party feels misunderstood and lonely, perhaps even wounded, and is not likely to want to reopen communication. The joy in a human relationship is gone, and one's pleasure in living is by that much diminished.

Function of Guilt

The same principles used in dealing with others can be applied to ourselves. Everyone makes mistakes, has angry or even murderous thoughts that can produce excessive guilt. Sometimes there is a realistic reason for feeling guilty, which should be a spur to take corrective action. Differentiate clearly between thoughts, feelings, and actions. Only actions need cause guilt. In the privacy of one's own mind, anything may be thought as long as it is not acted out; an emotionally fit person can accept this difference.

Understanding Mental and Emotional Disorders

As recently as 200 years ago it was believed that the emotionally ill were evil, possessed by the devil. Their illness was punished rather than treated. The strange and sometimes bizarre actions of the mentally ill were feared and misunderstood.

Beginning in the late 1800's, Sigmund Freud made significant steps toward understanding mental functions. Since then, a number of physicians, psychologists, and scholars have made major contributions to the area of mental health.

Today, mental disorders are viewed and evaluated in the same way as physical diseases. Many are treatable using techniques similar to those used for physical diseases.

Mental Retardation

According to the American Association on Mental Retardation (AAMR) and the Diagnostic and Statistical Manual of Mental Disorders, 4th edition (DSM-IV), the diagnosis of mental retardation is appropriate when intellectual functioning is significantly below average, adaptive skills are limited, and the onset of the retardation occurs before the age of 18.

The term "mental retardation," while still valid diagnostically, is no longer the favored term in common usage. Instead the term "developmental disability" is widely used to refer to both mental retardation and to any other condition that results from a congenital abnormality, trauma, disease or deprivation that interrupts or delays normal growth and development.

The most common identifiable form of mental retardation is Down Syndrome. Physical characteristics include slanting eyes, slightly protruding lips and tongue, small hands and feet, and a short trunk. Compared to the general population, individuals with Down Syndrome are more likely to have congenital cardiac abnormalities, digestive tract problems, and cervical vertebrae problems. They are also more likely to develop upper respiratory infections, leukemia, or

Alzheimer's Disease.

Other causes of mental retardation include hydrocephalus, an accumulation of fluid within the skull that destroys brain tissue; fragile X syndrome, a chromosomal abnormality resulting in moderate to severe retardation; phenylketonuria (PKU), the inability of a child's body to metabolize a certain kind of protein substance; Tay Sachs disease, an inherited disease that causes the progressive destruction of the central nervous system. Individuals with Tay Sachs disease appear to develop normally until about six months of age, when progressive deterioration of the infant's mental and motor skills begins. Most children who have the disease die from it before they are five years of age. Mental retardation from PKU can be prevented if the metabolic deficiency is detected within a few days after birth and treated with a special diet.

If a mother becomes infected with Rubella (German Measles) during her pregnancy, there is a chance her infant will be born with disabilities, including mental retardation. If a woman consumes alcohol during her pregnancy, there is a chance that her child will be born with Fetal Alcohol Syndrome (FAS). Characteristics of

FAS include mental and growth retardation, poor motor coordination, learning disabilities, and hyperactivity.

Early Intervention

An early intervention program is a very important part of the developmentally disabled child's life. It is an organized program of services necessary to prevent and/or minimize the effects of disability on young children with special needs. Programs are offered for children up to the age of 5 and may include speech, occupational and physical therapy, and medical care. Sometimes, early intervention programming is all that a child needs, and thereafter they enter regular schooling with little or no need for further intervention.

Effects on the Family

When a member of a family is diagnosed with a developmental disability, the entire family is affected. Depending upon the extent of the disability, the family members usually must rearrange their lives based upon the needs of the developmentally disabled child. Families must choose between trying to care for the child at home, or finding suitable placement in the community. They must arrange for any medical care and therapy their child might need. They must also manage the financial obligations that result from their child's needs, which can be considerable.

There are many organizations devoted to providing services and support to individuals with developmental disabilities and their families. The ARC of the United States has many state and local chapters, and can provide families with information regarding the services available in their community. To find the ARC chapter nearest to you, contact the national ARC office.

The ARC of the United States
500 East Border Street, Suite 300
Arlington, TX 76010
800-433-5255

Mental Illness

Most people occasionally experience spells of anxiety, blue moods, or temper tantrums, but unless the psychological suffering they endure or inflict upon others begins to interfere with their job or marriage, they seldom seek professional guidance. There is no exacting scientific standard for determining when an eccentric pattern of behavior becomes a mental illness. Norms vary from culture to culture and within each culture. Norms also change from generation to generation.

Just how can a determination be made as to who is mentally ill? No temperature reading, no acute pain, no abnormal growth can be looked for as evidence of a serious problem. Yet there are warning signs, and among the common ones are these:

- Anxiety that is severe, prolonged, and unrelated to any identifiable reason or cause
- Depression, especially when it is followed by withdrawal from loved ones, from friends, or from the usual occupations or hobbies that ordinarily afford one pleasure
- Loss of confidence in oneself
- Undue pessimism
- A feeling of constant helplessness
- Uncalled for or unexplainable mood changes.
- Rudeness or aggression that is without apparent cause or which is occasioned by some trivial incident
- An unreasonable demand for perfectionism, not only in oneself but in one's loved ones, friends, business associates, and even from things or situations

- Habitual underachievement, especially if one is adequately equipped to do the work one is called upon to perform
- The inability to accept responsibility, often manifested by a recurrent loss of employment
- Phobias
- Unreasonable feelings of persecution
- Self-destructive acts
- Sexual deviation
- A sudden and dramatic change in sleeping habits
- Physical ailments and complaints for which there are no organic causes

If one or more of these warning signs occur frequently or in severe form, a mental illness may be present, and professional help should be sought to evaluate the underlying problem.

Types of Mental Illness

The following discussion of classifications and types of mental illnesses is based on criteria compiled by the American Psychiatric Association in the *Diagnostic and Statistical Manual of Mental Disorders.*

Anxiety Disorders

Anxiety disorders are the most common emotional disorders. They are characterized by chronic feelings of uneasiness. The symptoms of an anxiety disorder are more persistent and intense than the typical feelings of nervousness or anxiety everyone feels at various times. In addition, the symptoms typically occur for no clear reason and do not go away.

There are several types of anxiety orders. Symptoms of these disorders range from a mild, chronic sense of worry, to an overwhelming emotional condition, accompanied by such physical reactions as muscle tension, racing heart, nausea, and an increase in perspiration and blood pressure.

Panic Disorder

A person with *panic disorder* has recurrent attacks of intense apprehension, fear, or terror. Panic attacks may occur unexpectedly and seemingly without reason. This unpredictability tends to further intensify the feelings of fearfulness and terror.

Agoraphobia

A person with an anxiety of any place or situation from which a quick departure would be difficult or embarrassing may suffer from *agoraphobia*. The anxiety of agoraphobia is so severe that it can result in the outright avoidance of certain places or situations.

Agoraphobia and panic disorder often occur together. People suffering from both have a fear of being in a place or situation in which they would not be able to get help if they had a panic attack.

Specific Phobias

A person with a *specific phobia* has an extreme or excessive fear of an object or situation that, under general conditions, is not harmful. The phobia often leads to avoidance of the object or situation altogether. People with specific phobias tend to realize that their reactions are irrational, but still are unable to overcome their fear without professional intervention. Common specific phobias include a fear of heights (acrophobia), a fear of flying (aerophobia), a fear of spiders (arachnophobia), a fear of confined spaces (claustrophobia), a fear of blood (hemophobia), and a fear of strangers (xenophobia).

Social Phobia

Also called *social anxiety disorder*, a *social phobia* is the fear of behaving in a way that could lead to public embarrassment or ridicule in specific social situations. A person with this phobia often avoids the problematic social situation altogether. Common social phobias include a fear of public speaking, a fear of using public restrooms, and a fear of meeting new people.

Obsessive-Compulsive Disorder

A person with *obsessive-compulsive disorder* experiences recurrent obsessions and recurrent compulsions. Obsessions are frequently occurring thoughts that usually reflect exaggerated anxiety or fears that have no foundation in reality. Although people with obsessions realize that their thoughts are irrational, this realization is not enough to alleviate their anxiety. Instead, they engage in repetitive rituals, or compulsions, to get rid of the obsessive thoughts and thereby reduce their anxiety. Compulsive behaviors can sometimes take up more than an hour a day, and can interfere with normal daily activities and social relationships.

Common obsessions, and the compulsions which result from them, include: a preoccupation with dirt or germs, resulting in repeated hand washing and the performing of excessive housekeeping chores; second-guessing previous actions, resulting in constant checking and rechecking to satisfy doubts; a need to have items in a very specific arrangement, resulting in strict regimens to ensure order and consistency.

Post-Traumatic Stress Disorder

Post-traumatic stress disorder is characterized by the repeated experiencing or "reliving" of a traumatic event, accompanied by extreme emotional, mental, and physical distress when exposed to situations reminiscent of the trauma. People with post-traumatic stress disorder repeatedly experience their ordeal through recurrent nightmares, memories of the event, and vivid flashbacks, which may make the person feel as if they were reliving the original event. Typical events which can result in post-traumatic stress disorder include: military combat, natural disasters, violent crime, and childhood abuse.

Acute Stress Disorder

Similar to post-traumatic stress disorder, *acute stress disorder* differs from it in duration. Whereas post-traumatic stress disorder lasts more than a month, acute stress disorder lasts a month or less; it occurs within a month after exposure to a traumatic event.

Generalized Anxiety Disorder

Generalized anxiety disorder is characterized by chronic and overwhelming anxiety that lasts for at least six months. People with this disorder experience such persistent worry and tension that it interferes with their daily lives. Symptoms of generalized anxiety disorder include: excessive concerns (about health, family, career, or finances) even when there is no apparent reason for such concern, inability to relax, tremors, insomnia, irritability, difficulty concentrating, fatigue, and headaches.

Substance-Induced Anxiety Disorder

In a *substance-induced anxiety disorder*, symptoms of anxiety are present because of drug abuse, the use of medication, or exposure to a toxin.

Mood Disorders

The predominant feature of these disorders is a serious disturbance in mood. Mood disorders can be caused by biological factors, drug abuse, use of medication, toxic substances, or various medical conditions—including thyroid disorders and Parkinson's disease. Some people have a genetic predisposition to developing mood disorders. The development and intensity of a mood disorder can also be affected by the personality of the individual. There are two types of mood disorders: *depressive* and *bipolar*.

Depressive Disorders

In a *major depressive disorder*, a person has strong feelings of depression for at least two weeks. The depression may have melancholic features—that is, there may be a loss of interest or pleasure in virtually all activities.

In a *dysthymic disorder*, a depressed mood exists for at least 2 years. This disorder is characterized by a moderate, lingering depression, in contrast to the more intense depression characteristic of a major depressive disorder.

Other symptoms of depressive disorders include periods of prolonged sadness, changes in appetite and sleep patterns, anger, anxiety, loss of energy, feelings of worthlessness, and recurring thoughts of death or suicide.

Bipolar Disorders

There are several variations of *bipolar disorders,* formerly known as *manic-depression*. These disorders are characterized by episodes of deep depression alternating with periods of extreme elation, or manic behavior. Examples of manic behavior include the need for less sleep without feeling tired, an increase in mental and physical activity, and exaggerated enthusiasm and feelings of self-worth. A person with a bipolar disorder might take unnecessary chances and engage in risky behavior.

Schizophrenia and Other Psychotic Disorders

The defining features of these disorders are psychotic symptoms, which include a loss of contact with reality, a disorganized thought process, hallucinations, and delusions.

A disorganized thought process is reflected by a person's actions and speech. The person may behave in a bizarre manner and not be able to give a coherent explanation for his or her actions. The person's speech will not make much sense to the average person.

Hallucinations are sensations that do not result from a "real" or external stimulus, although the person experiencing the hallucination might believe otherwise. They can occur with any of the five senses, but the most common are auditory hallucinations, particularly those of hearing voices.

Delusions are erroneous beliefs that usually involve a misinterpretation of experiences. One example of a delusion is the belief of being under surveillance by the police, although in actuality no surveillance is being made. A more extreme example of a delusion is the belief of certain people that their thoughts are under the control of or are being taken away by unknown entities. *Persecutory delusions*—delusions of being harassed, spied on, or tormented—are the most common type.

Schizophrenia

Schizophrenia is one of the most debilitating and puzzling mental illnesses. Symptoms may include not only psychotic symptoms—disorganized thought process, hallucinations, and delusions—but also withdrawal, social isolation, lack of emotional expression, and a decrease in normal thinking and speaking activity. Schizophrenia varies in severity from person to person, and, in a given individual, from one time to another.

Most mental health professionals agree that schizophrenia is a biological illness, and that it probably occurs in individuals with a genetic susceptibility to the illness who have been exposed to other factors. These factors include such prenatal problems as exposure to influenza or lack of nutrition while the individual was growing in the mother's womb. For someone with schizophrenia, stressful social and family interactions may affect the progression of the disease, but are they not the origin.

Contrary to popular belief, a schizophrenic does not have a "split personality." This notion probably developed from the fact that episodes of the illness may be separated by periods of normal behavior.

There are several types of schizophrenia, with behavior ranging from excitement and aggressiveness to withdrawal and immobility.

People with *paranoid schizophrenia* have strong feelings of persecution. They typically feel that someone (or a group of people) is plotting to harm or kill them.

People with *disorganized schizophrenia,* historically known as *hebephrenic schizophrenia*, experience such strong speech and behavior disorganization that their ability to perform daily activities is disrupted.

In *catatonic schizophrenia,* a person is usually in a state of extreme withdrawal and immobility. This may alternate with occasional periods of extreme agitation or excitement.

People with *residual schizophrenia* exhibit the absence of normal behaviors. For example, they may withdraw, lack emotional expression, isolate themselves from society, and experience a decrease in thinking and speaking activity.

In *undifferentiated schizophrenia,* a person exhibits a variety of schizophrenic symptoms, but none of them is dominant.

Psychotic Disorders

Other disorders included in the category of Schizophrenia and Psychotic Disorders follow, along with some defining features of each disorder.

Both *brief psychotic disorder* and *schizophreniform disorder* have the same symptoms as schizophrenia, but the symptoms do not last long enough to warrant a diagnosis of schizophrenia. In brief psychotic disorder, the symptoms last more than a day, but less than one month. In schizophreniform disorder, the symptoms last from one to six months.

In *schizoaffective disorder,* a person displays symptoms of a mood disorder—either bipolar or depressive—in addition to psychotic symptoms.

In a *delusional disorder,* a person experiences one or more delusions based on situations that could conceivably be happening to the person, but for which there is no evidence. The delusions must persist for at least one month in order to be classified as a delusional disorder.

In a *shared psychotic disorder,* a person is influenced by someone else who already has a similar delusion.

In a *substance-induced psychotic disorder,* the psychotic symptoms present are the result of drug abuse, the use of medication, or exposure to a toxin.

Personality Disorders

These disorders are characterized by a persistent pattern of noticeably unusual behavior and ways of thinking.

A *paranoid personality disorder* is characterized by a pattern of suspicion and distrust. A person with this disorder will misconstrue other people's intentions as being malicious.

A *schizoid personality disorder* is characterized by a pattern of disinterest in social relationships. A person with this disorder may be fearful of close interaction with others. They also have a limited range of emotional expression.

People with *schizotypal personality disorder* are socially and emotionally distant. Their thinking process is odd and distorted, and these oddities are evident through their speech and behavior.

An *antisocial personality disorder* is characterized by a pattern of disregarding and violating the rights of others. People with this disorder typically do not feel remorse or guilt after inflicting harm upon others. This disorder usually develops in adolescence and often continues into adulthood, although the severity of the disorder can diminish as a person ages.

A *borderline personality disorder* is characterized by a pattern of instability in relationships. A person with this disorder also displays symptoms of impulsiveness and irritability.

In *histrionic personalty disorder,* there is a pattern of attention-seeking behavior and excessive displays of emotion. A person with this disorder may easily fall under the influence of others in an effort to be the center of attention.

A *narcissistic personality disorder* is characterized by an exaggerated sense of self-importance. A person with this disorder requires excessive admiration and lacks empathy for others.

An *avoidant personality disorder* is characterized by feelings of inadequacy. A person with this disorder will avoid activities that require significant interpersonal interaction, and tends to be hypersensitive to negative evaluation.

A *dependent personality disorder* is characterized by an excessive need to be taken care of. A person with this disorder has a pattern of submissive and clinging behavior.

An *obsessive-compulsive personality disorder* is characterized by a preoccupation with orderliness, perfectionism, and control. A person with this disorder will appear inflexible and stubborn to others.

Dissociative Disorders

In these disorders, there is a disruption in consciousness, memory, identity, or perception. The disruption may occur suddenly, or it may gradually develop. It can also take the form of a brief affliction or a chronic condition.

A person with *dissociative amnesia* is unable to recall relevant personal information. The "forgotten" information is usually disturbing to the individual, and of a traumatic nature. For example, a person who attempts to commit suicide might not later remember anything at all regarding the incident.

A *dissociative fugue* is characterized by a sudden loss of personal identity and of the memory of one's past life. This is accompanied by the tendency to suddenly wander far from one's home or place of work. In some cases, the individual also assumes a new identity. The disorder can last from a couple of hours to several months. A dissociative fugue is usually brought on by traumatic events or an over-whelming accumulation of tension and stress. It is a rare disorder.

Dissociative identity disorder, formerly called *multiple personality disorder,* refers to the presence of two or more distinct personalities, each of which dominate an individual's behavior at different times. This disorder is also characterized by gaps in the individual's memory that vary, depending on which personality is currently dominant. For example, a weaker personality may not remember what happens during the times that a stronger personality is dominating the individual's behavior.

Depersonalization disorder is characterized by persistent feelings of detachment from one's own body or thoughts. The feelings of depersonalization can be severe and occur often enough that one's life is disrupted, and treatment is needed. In many cases, though, the sense of depersonalization is brief and minimal, and treatment is not needed.

Factitious Disorder

This disorder is characterized by physical or psychological symptoms that are deliberately produced or feigned in order to appear sick. People with this disorder might inflict harm upon themselves, exaggerate an existing medical complaint, or completely fabricate a new and false medical problem, for the sole purpose of appearing ill.

Somatoform Disorders

In these disorders, a person has physical symptoms of a physical disease, but does not have the disease. The physical symptoms are caused by psychological factors and are not intentionally produced by the individual. Examples of physical symptoms common in somatoform disorders include blindness, paralysis, respiratory distress, and heart problems.

A person with a *somatization disorder* has recurrent and multiple physical complaints and symptoms for which there is no known medical cause. There is evidence, or a strong presumption, that the symptoms are related to psychological reasons. Symptoms vary from person to person and also depend upon their underlying emotional conflict.

A person with a *conversion disorder* experiences emotional distress that is "converted" into physical symptoms. The physical symptoms have no biological cause, and are not a part of a somatization disorder. A person who witnesses a terrifying event and then develops blindness would be an extreme example of this disorder.

Hypochondriasis is the preoccupation with the fear of acquiring or the belief of having a serious disease. A person reaches this conclusion by overreacting to normal bodily functions and minor abnormalities. People with hypochondriasis will persist in their fears and beliefs despite medical tests and exams that prove that they do not have a serious disease.

A person with *body dysmorphic disorder* is preoccupied with an imagined or insignificant defect in one's own appearance.

Sexual and Gender Identity Disorders

These disorders involve sexual performance, sexual deviance, and concepts of appropriate gender roles. They include the categories of sexual dysfunctions, paraphilias, and gender identity disorders.

Sexual dysfunctions refer to changes in personal sexual desires and activities that the individual finds unfulfilling, or inadequate. Examples of sexual dysfuntions include pain during sexual activity and complications with sexual arousal and desire.

Persistent and intense sexual urges or behaviors that involve unusual objects or situations are called *paraphilias*. Examples of paraphilias include exhibitionism (exposing one's self), voyeurism (observing sexual activity), sadism (inflicting pain or humiliation), and masochism (receiving pain or humiliation).

A *gender identity disorder* is characterized by intense, persistent feelings of discomfort or inappropriateness with one's own gender, in addition to a strong identification with the opposite gender. People with gender identity disorders may engage in cross-dressing, hormone treatment, or surgery to acquire the physical appearance of the opposite sex.

Other Disorders

Several other types of disorders are discussed elsewhere in this encyclopedia. These disorders include:

Eating Disorders. See Chapter 3, *The Teens,* subtitles Anorexia Nervosa, and Bulimia.

Disorders Usually First Diagnosed in Infancy, Childhood, or Adolescence. See Chapter 2, *The First Dozen Years,* subtitles Autism, Brain Damage, Developmental Disability, Dyslexia, Hyperactivity, Learning Disability, Mental Illness, Mental Retar-dation, Pica, Speech Impediments, and Stuttering. Chapter 28, *Mental and Emotional Disorders,* subtitle Mental Retardation.

Sleep Disorders. See Chapter 2, *The First Dozen Years,* subtitles Dreams and Nightmares, Sleepwalking. Chapter 37, *Encyclopedic Guide to the Body, Health and Medicine,* subtitles Narcolepsy, Sleep, Sleep Apnea, Snoring. Chapter 5, *The Middle Years,* subtitle Rest and Sleep.

Treatment of Emotional Problems and Mental Disorders

W hen should help be sought for an emotional problem? Sometimes individuals themselves realize that they need help and seek it without urging. They may have symptoms such as anxiety, depression, or troublesome thoughts that they cannot put out of their mind. But many others who need help do not know it or do not want to know that they need it. They usually have symptoms that disturb others rather than themselves, such as irritability, impulsive behavior, or excessive use of drugs or alcohol that interferes with their family relationships and work responsibilities.

Other people in need of psychological guidance are those who have a physical disease that is based on psychological factors. They react to stress internally rather than externally. Instead of displaying anger, they feel it inside. We are all familiar with headaches or heartburn caused by tension.

The symptoms of many mental disorders seem only to be exaggerations of feelings and behavior found in "normal" people. At what point should help be sought for a problem? Generally, help should be sought when the problem begins to significantly and negatively impact the individual's life.

In all of the above situations, the individual's enjoyment of life is curtailed. He has no feeling of control over what he does and little or no tolerance for himself and others. Such an existence is completely unnecessary today, with the many agencies and specialists, capable of effectively treating these problems.

Mental Health Professionals

Who can help those with emotional problems? Confusion about the different professions in the mental health field is understandable. To add to the muddle, self-appointed counselors without professional training and experience have set themselves up in this field, so it is necessary to know whom to consult to obtain the best help possible. Every mental health professional you consult should be licensed, accredited, or associated with recognized groups of their peers.

Psychiatrists

Psychiatrists are medical doctors; that is, they have graduated from a medical school, served internships and afterwards residencies specializing in emotional disorders. They are specialists in the same way that a surgeon or an eye doctor is a specialist. Most are members of the American Psychiatric Association. They are experienced in treating medical illnesses, having done so for many years before being certified as specialists in emotional disorders.

The American Psychiatric Association, 1400 K St., N.W., Washington, D.C. 20005, can supply the names of members. The American Board of Psychiatry and Neurology, 500 Lake-Cook Road, Suite 335, Deerfield, IL 60015, examines and certifies psychiatrists who pass its tests. If a family physician is consulted about an emotional problem, he will often refer the patient to a psychiatrist, just as he would to any other specialist.

Psychologists

Psychologists have at least a master's degree in psychology; most psychologists have a doctoral degree. Like a psychiatrist, a psychologist can help you cope with many of life's problems. Unlike a psychiatrist, though, a psychologist is not a medical doctor and cannot prescribe medicine.

The American Psychological Association (APA), 750 First Street, NE, Washington, DC 20002, is the world's largest association of psychologists. They operate a telephone referral service. To find a psychologist in your area, call (800) 964-2000.

Psychotherapists

Psychotherapy is the general term for any treatment that tries to effect a cure by psychological rather than physical means. A psychotherapist may be a psychiatrist, or he may be a psychologist, or may have no training at all. Anyone can set up an office and call himself a psychotherapist, psychoanalyst, marriage counselor, family therapist, or anything else he desires. It is up to the patient to check on the training and background of a therapist. Any reputable therapist should be pleased to tell patients his credentials and qualifications for helping them.

Social Workers

Social workers are another group of trained persons who may also counsel those with emotional problems. They may work either with individuals, families, or groups after meeting the educational requirements for the profession, which include a bachelor's degree and two years of professional training leading to a master's degree in social work.

Types of Therapy

Emotional problems and mental illnesses can be treated in a variety of ways, including psychotherapy, medication, or physical treatments. Psychotherapy, or "talking therapy," is an effective and commonly prescribed method of treatment for mild to moderate cases of emotional and mental disorders. In more severe cases, psychotherapy is used in combination with medication or physical treatments.

Psychotherapy

As noted above, psychotherapy applies to various forms of treatment that employ psychological methods designed to help people understand themselves. With this knowledge, or insight, a person learns how to handle life—with all its relationships and conflicts—in a happier and more socially responsible manner.

The best known form of psychotherapy is *psychoanalysis,* developed by Freud but modified by many others, which seeks to lift to the level of awareness the individual's repressed subconscious feelings. The information about subconscious conflicts is explored and interpreted to explain the causes of the individual's emotional upsets.

Another form of psychotherapy is *behavior therapy,* treatment based on the belief that many types of behavior are learned. Instead of probing an individual's unconscious, as in psychoanalysis, a behavior therapist focuses on the individual's observable behavior and tries to help the individual control it. In a method called *operant conditioning,* behavior is controlled using a *reinforcer,* anything that increases the likelihood that a particular behavior will be repeated. Praise or gifts given for good behavior are common examples of reinforcers.

Cognitive therapy is another form of psychotherapy. Unlike behavior therapy, cognitive therapy is based on changing thoughts. Cognitive therapy involves helping people change the patterns of thinking responsible for their emotional distress. The change is made by monitoring negative or distorted thoughts, then correcting or replacing them with positive thoughts.

Group therapy is a form of psychotherapy treatment in which a group of people, usually ten or fewer, discuss their mental and emotional problems. The group is under the guidance of a psychiatrist or clinical psychologist. By talking to one another about mutual problems and by interacting with one another emotionally under skillful guidance, people are often helped more quickly than when treated individually.

Psychodrama is a therapeutic technique in which an individual or members of a group create and act out situations based on their personal conflicts.

Play therapy is a type of treatment for young children who can more easily act out their problems through play activity, as opposed to discussing them. Play therapy may be a form of individual psychotherapy or group therapy. In both instances, the therapist observes the play activity.

Family problems can be treated with *family therapy.* Family members are sometimes able to discuss their problems of relating to each other within the context of a group better than they can on an individual basis with a therapist.

Medication

In the last half of the 20th century, the study of the relationship between biochemical processes of the brain and mental illness resulted in the development of psychiatric medication. Many people with mental illnesses have greatly benefitted from the use of these medications. However, many psychiatric drugs have side effects, some of which are severe, so close medical supervision is necessary while taking the drugs. With proper monitoring, psychiatric drugs can be a part of a safe, therapeutic approach to alleviating the negative effects of mental illness.

Depression is believed to be caused by low levels of *neurotransmitters*, chemicals of the nervous system. *Antidepressant drugs*, used to relieve the symptoms of depression, work by increasing the level of neurotransmit-

ters present in the brain.

Antipsychotic drugs, sometimes called major tranquilizers, are used to relieve delusions, hallucinations and other psychotic symptoms. Antipsychotic drugs work by blocking the neurotransmitter *dopamine* from completing its function in the brain.

Antianxiety drugs, sometimes called sedatives or minor tranquilizers, are used to relieve anxiety or tension. By suppressing the brain chemistry responsible for anxiety, these drugs provide a sense of relaxation. They may also act as a muscle relaxant, and alleviate mild insomnia.

Mood stabilizers, like lithium, are used to treat bipolar depression. It is not known how lithium alleviates the symptoms of bipolar disorder, but it is effective. The blood level of lithium must be monitored carefully. If the level is too low, the medication will not be effective in stabilizing the person's mood, and if the level is too high, adverse side effects may result.

Physical Treatment

Electroconvulsive therapy (ECT) is a form of therapy in which regulated electric shocks are delivered to the brain to induce seizures. It is an effective treatment for severe depression, often providing relief much more quickly than psychiatric medication. Although psychiatric medication and psychotherapy are used much more frequently as treatments for depression, ECT is generally used in life-threatening situations or other circumstances where immediate relief from depression is needed.

Psychosurgery is another form of physical treatment. It involves physically altering the structure of the brain in an attempt to alleviate severe mental illness. Psychosurgery was widely used in 1950's. The use of psychosurgery has greatly diminished with increased knowledge of psychiatric illness and with the development of psychiatric drugs. Current pyschosurgery methods involve only microscopic alterations to the brain, and are only used in extreme cases of mental illness with a definite biological cause.

Options Available for the Mentally Ill

The last two decades have seen a number of changes in the facilities for treatment of mental disorders in the United States. The great majority of severely ill mental patients used to be cared for in county or state mental hospitals, many of which were crowded and able to offer custodial care but very little in the way of therapeutic programs. The picture has changed, however, and the extent and quality of care in these hospitals is expanding and improving. Also, other facilities now offer treatment for mental illnesses, including general hospitals, private psychiatric hospitals, mental heath clinics, and various social agencies.

Results of Treatment

There will always be things in life that are disappointing or otherwise upsetting. No treatment can eliminate such problems. After successful treatment, however, one should be better able to handle these stresses with flexible and constructive responses and to see individual difficulties in relation to the problems of others.

To feel emotionally fit is to have a capacity for enjoying life, working well, and loving others. Fear, shame, and guilt about undergoing needed treatment should not prevent anyone from reaching that potential.

29

Substance Abuse

"**D**rug-Related Deaths up 59%." "Driving-and-Drinking Accident Claims 5 Lives." "Teen Drug Abuse—The News Is Bad."

The headlines tell a story with a moral, or lesson. The lesson is that the United States has a major health and social problem. Once called by a number of names, including *alcoholism, drug addiction,* and *drug abuse,* the problem today goes by the designation *substance abuse.* In this usage, the phrase applies to all forms of addiction or abuse, whether the substance is alcohol or such vegetation-derived drugs as marijuana, cocaine, and heroin.

In a broad sense, substances include any material aside from food that can be imbibed, injected, or taken into the body in any way and that changes or affects the body or mind. This definition covers aspirin, many medications, tobacco, and a broad range of other substances. But *substance abuse* refers to unhealthy or excessive use of any material, alcohol, or addictive drugs at an individual's discretion and not according to a physician's prescription.

The dimensions of the substance-abuse problem are almost incalculable. Americans in 1986 spent an estimated $110 billion on addictive drugs alone. At least 40 percent of all Americans between the ages of 18 and 25 had experimented with one or more illegal substances. As one authority wrote,

Not only the poor, the uneducated, the deprived, or the shadow types are being destroyed. We're dealing with the privileged, the successful, the professional.

Alcohol Abuse

Alcohol abuse is not unique to the United States or to the twentieth century. Alcoholic beverages, and their use or abuse, have an ancient history.

Long before humans began to keep records of any kind, these beverages were valued as food, medicine, and ceremonial drinks. When people today have a beer with dinner, or toast newlyweds with champagne, or share wine at a religious ritual or festival, they are continuing traditions that have deep roots in the past.

The consumption of alcoholic beverages has always been a fact of life. So has, in a sense, alcohol abuse. The immigrants who came to the United States brought their ethnic ceremonies and drinking habits with them. The frontiersmen who moved continually west found liquor to be a source of release and comfort. Inevitably, alcohol use and abuse occurred.

Most drinkers have been, and are, able to control what they are doing and are none the worse for the habit. However, of the estimated 100 million drinkers in the United States, about 10 million have some kind of problem with alcohol: they are *alcohol abusers.* The 10 million alcoholics cost the economy some $60 billion annually. Drunken drivers are implicated in about half of the nearly 50,000 traffic deaths occurring yearly.

Scientists have come to believe that habitual alcohol abuse is a disease and should be treated as such. In 1956, the American Medical Association officially termed alcoholism an illness and a medical responsibility.

Kinds of Alcohol

The alcohol in beverages is chemically known as *ethyl alcohol.* It is often called *grain alcohol.* It is produced by the natural process of *fermentation:* When certain foods such as honey, fruits, grains, or their juices remain in a warm place, airborne yeast organisms begin to change the sugars and starches in these foods into alcohol. Ethyl alcohol is in itself a food in the sense that its caloric content produces energy in the body, but it contains practically no essential nutriments.

Methyl alcohol, also called *wood alcohol,* because it is obtained by the dry distillation of maple, birch, and beech, is useful as a fuel and solvent. It is poisonous if taken internally and can cause blindness and death. Other members of the same family of chemicals, such as *isopropyl alcohol,* are also used as rubbing alcohols—as cooling agents and skin disinfectants—and are also poisonous if taken internally.

Present-Day Drinking Trends

On a per capita basis, Americans drink twice as much wine and beer as they did a century ago, and half as much distilled spirits. Where the drinking takes place has also changed. There is less hard drinking in saloons and more social drinking at home and in clubs. The acceptance of drinking in mixed company has made it more a part of social situations than it used to be.

Here are some facts about the current consumption of alcoholic beverages in the United States:

- Drinking is more common among men than among women, but the gap is closing.

- It is more common among people who are under 40.

- It is more common among the well-to-do than among the poor.

- Beyond the age of 45, the number of drinkers steadily declines.

Teenagers and Alcohol

One fact emerges clearly and consistently from all the surveys of teenage drinking in all parts of the country: the drinking behavior of parents is more related to what children do about drinking than any other factor. It is more influential than children's friends, their neighborhoods, their religion, their social or economic status, or their local laws.

Statistics on teenage (and adult) drinking vary from one ethnic group or one part of the country to another. But overall, the statistics show that about two-thirds of all Americans 18 and older consume alcoholic beverages. Some three-quarters of all students in the tenth to twelfth grade range also drink.

In general, drinking is an activity that is associated with growing up. For boys, it represents manhood; for girls, sophistication.

Kinds of Alcoholic Beverages

The way any alcoholic drink affects the body depends chiefly on how much alcohol it contains. The portion of alcohol can range from less than 1/20th of the total volume, in the case of beer, to more than one-half in the case of rum. As a general rule, distilled drinks have a higher alcohol content than fermented ones.

The five basic types of beverages are beers, table wines, dessert or cocktail wines, cordials and liqueurs, and distilled spirits such as brandy and whisky. The labels of beers and wines usually indicate the percentage of alcohol by volume. The labels of distilled spirits indicate *proof.*

Proof

The proof number is twice the percentage of alcohol by volume. Thus a rye whisky that is 90-proof contains 45 percent alcohol, 80-proof bourbon is 40 percent alcohol, and so on. The word *proof* used in this way comes from an old English test to determine the strength of distilled spirits. If gunpowder soaked with whisky would still ignite when lighted, that fact was "proof" that the whisky contained the right amount of alcohol. The amount, approximately 57 percent, is still the standard in Canada and Great Britain.

How Alcohol Affects the Body

The overall effects of alcohol on the body and on behavior vary a great deal depending on many factors. One factor should be noted at once: if the blood reaching the brain contains a certain percentage of alcohol, there are marked changes in reaction. As the percentage increases, the functioning of the brain and central nervous system is increasingly affected. As the alcohol is gradually metabolized and eliminated, the process reverses itself.

If at any given time the blood contains a concentration of about 3/100 of one percent (0.03 percent), no effects are observable. This amount will make its way into the bloodstream after you have had a highball or cocktail made with one and one-half ounces of whisky, or two small glasses of table wine, or two bottles of beer. It takes about two hours for this amount of alcohol to leave the body completely.

Twice that number of drinks produces twice the concentration of alcohol in the bloodstream (0.06 percent) with an accompanying feeling of warmth and relaxation.

If the concentration of alcohol in the bloodstream reaches 0.1 percent—when one part of every thousand parts of blood is pure alcohol—the person is legally drunk in most states. The motor areas of the brain are affected; there is a noticeable lack of coordination in standing or walking. If the percentage goes up to 0.15 percent, the physical signs of intoxication are obvious, and they are accompanied by an impairment of mental faculties as well.

A concentration of as much as 0.4 percent can cause a coma. At the level of 0.5 to 0.7 percent there may be paralysis of the brain centers that control the activities of the lungs and heart, a condition that can be fatal.

Alcohol affects the brain and nervous system in this way because it is a depressant and an anesthetic.

How Alcohol Moves through the Body

Although it is negligible as nourishment, alcohol is an energy-producing food like sugar. Unlike most foods, however, it is quickly absorbed into the bloodstream through the stomach and small intestine without first having to undergo complicated digestive processes. It is then carried to the liver, where most of it is converted into heat and energy. From the liver, the remainder is carried by the blood-stream to the heart and pumped to the lungs. Some is expelled in the breath and some is eventually eliminated in sweat and urine. From the lungs, the alcohol is circulated to the brain.

People who use good judgment when drinking rarely, if ever, get drunk. The safe and pleasurable use of alcoholic beverages depends on the drinker's weight and his or her physical condition and emotional state. Other factors include the following:

1. *The Concentration of Alcohol in the Beverage* The higher the alcohol content in terms of total volume, the faster it is absorbed. Three ounces of straight whisky—two shot glasses—contain the same amount of alcohol as 48 ounces (or four cans) of beer.

2. *Sipping or Gulping* Two shots of straight whisky can be downed in seconds or, more normally, in a few minutes. The same amount diluted in two highballs can be sipped through an entire evening. In the latter case, the body has a chance to get rid of much of the alcohol.

3. *Additional Components of the Drink* The carbohydrates in beer and wine slow down the absorption of alcohol in the blood. Vodka mixed with orange juice travels much more slowly than a vodka martini.

4. *Food in the Stomach* The alcohol concentration in two cocktails consumed at the peak of the hunger before dinner can have a nasty effect. Several glasses of wine with a meal or a brandy sipped after dinner get to thebloodstream much more slowly and at a lower concentration. The sensible drinker doesn't drink on an empty stomach.

The Hangover

The discomfort that sometimes sets in the morning after excessive drinking is known as a hangover. It is caused by the disruptive effect of too much alcohol on the central nervous system. The symptoms of nausea, headache, dry mouth, diarrhea, fatigue, dizziness, heartburn, and a feeling of apprehension are usually most acute several hours after drinking and not while there is still any appreciable amount of alcohol in the system.

Although many people believe that "mixing" drinks, such as switching from whisky drinks to wine, is the main cause of hangovers, a hangover can just as easily be induced by too much of one type of drink or by pure alcohol. Nor is it always the result of

drinking too much because emotional stress or allergy may well be contributing factors.

Some aspects of a hangover may be caused by substances called *congeners*. These are the natural products of fermentation found in small amounts in all alcoholic beverages, among them tannic acid and fusel oil. Some congeners have toxic properties that produce nausea by irritating certain nerve centers.

In spite of accumulated lore about hangover remedies, there is no certain cure for the symptoms. A throbbing head and aching joints can sometimes be relieved by aspirin and bed rest. Stomach irritation can be eased by bland foods such as skim milk, cooked cereal, or a poached egg. Persons seeking relief may also try analgesics such as aspirin or acetaminophen for the headache, antacids if the problem is upset stomach, or over-the-counter medications for the diarrhea.

Alcohol and General Health

It is known that alcohol has harmful effects when consumed in large quantities, but studies in the 1990s showed that alcohol may provide some health benefits. Moderate consumption—no more than one drink a day for women or two for men—has been associated with a lower risk of heart disease in some individuals. Some people, however, should not drink at all; for example, children and adolescents, people who cannot control their consumption, women who are pregnant or trying to become pregnant, and anyone taking medication. No one should drink before driving. The adverse effects of alcohol are detailed below.

Tissue Impairment

Habitual drinking of straight whisky can irritate the membranes that line the mouth and throat. The hoarse voice of some heavy drinkers is the result of a thickening of vocal cord tissue. As for the effect on the stomach, alcohol doesn't cause ulcers, but it does aggravate them.

There is no evidence to support the belief that port wine or any other alcoholic beverage taken in moderation will cause gout. Studies have shown that as many as 60 percent of all patients with this disease had never drunk any wine at all.

Brain Damage

Alcohol abuse continued over many years has been found to contribute to cognitive defects. These may, in turn, indicate brain impairment. Researchers do not know what the defects represent—whether greater susceptibility to the problems of aging or an actual, alcohol-caused "premature aging" effect. Whatever the case, long-term chronic alcohol abuse leads to more rapid aging of the brain. Neuropsychologically, the alcoholic's brain resembles that of an older nonalcoholic.

Long-term abuse can have many other effects. These include withdrawal symptoms beginning 12 to 48 hours after a person stops drinking, sometimes followed by *delirium tremens* (DTs), which brings hallucinations and can be fatal; the Werner-Korsakoff syndrome, a type of beriberi characterized by a lack of the B vitamins; alcoholic peripheral neuropathy, involving damage to the nerve tissue outside the brain and spinal cord; and liver damage, including alcoholic hepatitis and cirrhosis. In the latter the liver becomes hard and yellowed.

Alcohol and Immunity to Infection

Moderate drinkers who maintain proper health habits are no more likely to catch viral or bacterial diseases than nondrinkers. But heavy drinkers, who often suffer from malnutrition, have conspicuously lower resistance to infection. Even well-nourished heavy drinkers have a generally lower immunity to infection than normal. When the blood-alcohol level is 0.15 percent or higher, the alcohol appears to weaken the disease-fighting white blood cells.

Alcohol and Stroke

Studies have shown that heavy drinkers face nearly three times the teetotaler's risk of hemorrhagic stroke. Light drinkers face twice the risk. About one stroke in four occurring in the United States is hemorrhagic, but these strokes are more likely to be fatal than those caused by blood clots.

Alcohol and Life Expectancy

It is difficult to isolate drinking in itself as a factor in longevity. One study reported the shortest life span for heavy drinkers, a somewhat longer one for those who don't drink at all, and the longest for moderate drinkers. But other factors, such as general health and heredity, play important roles.

Alcohol and Sex Activity

Alcohol in sufficient quantity depresses the part of the brain that controls inhibitions. This liberating effect has led some people to believe that alcohol is an aphrodisiac, in men. This is a conclusion that is far from the truth. At the same time that alcohol increases the sexual appetite, it reduces the ability to perform.

Alcohol as an Irritant

Many otherwise healthy people cannot tolerate alcoholic beverages of any kind, or of a particular kind, without getting sick. In some cases, the negative reaction may be psychological in origin—connected with a disastrous experience with drunkenness in the early years or with an early hatred for a drinker in the family. Some people can drink one type of beverage but not another because of a particular congener, or because of an allergy to a specific grain or fruit. People suffering from such diseases as peptic ulcers, kidney and liver infections, and epilepsy should never drink any alcoholic beverages unless allowed to do so by a physician.

Uses and Hazards

At practically all times and in many parts of the world today, alcoholic beverages of various kinds have been and are still used for medicinal purposes. This should not be taken to mean that Aunt Sally is right about the curative powers of her elderberry wine, or that grandpa knows best when he says brandy is the best cure for hiccups. Today an American physician may recommend a particular alcoholic beverage as a tranquilizer, a sleep-inducer, or an appetite stimulant.

Use of Alcohol with Other Drugs

Alcoholic beverages should be avoided by anyone taking barbiturates or other sedatives. See "Drug Use and Abuse" later in this chapter for a discussion of barbiturates.

Alcohol and Driving

For many people, coordination, alertness, and general driving skills are impaired at blood-alcohol levels below the legal limit (0.1 percent). There are some people who become dangerous drivers after only one drink. Attempts are constantly being made, but so far with less than perfect success, to educate the public about the very real dangers of drunken driving.

Possible Causes of Alcohol Abuse

A popular myth holds that alcohol causes alcohol abuse. It doesn't—any more than sugar causes diabetes. Various theories have been evolved to explain what does cause alcohol abuse.

Physiological Causes

Although several physiological factors seem to be involved in the progression of alcohol abuse, no single one can be pinpointed as the cause of the disease. Among the theories that have come under investigation are the following: abnormal sugar metabolism, disorders of the endocrine glands, and dietary deficiencies.

Psychological Causes

Recent studies have pointed to a possible relationship between personality and alcohol abuse. Researchers indicate that one definable segment of the alcoholic population has the character disorder known as *antisocial personality*. Once called a *sociopath,* the person with an antisocial personality is usually charming in a social sense, manipulative, impulsive and rebellious, and egocentric. An estimated 25 percent of the alcoholic population falls in this category; in the general population the prevalence of antisocial personalities is about 3 percent.

Sociological Factors

Practically all studies of alcohol abuse in the United States indicate that ethnic groups vary dramatically in their rates of problem drinkers. A great deal of attention has therefore been focused on *learned attitudes* toward alcoholic beverages and how they are used or abused. Generally, in the low-incidence groups attitudes toward drinking are clearly defined and understood by all the members of the group. Drunkenness is consistently frowned upon. In the high-incidence groups, researchers have found extensive conflict over alcohol. The basic rules aren't clearly defined, and there are no clear-cut standards for acceptable and unacceptable drinking behavior.

Genetic Factors

Research into the genetics of alcohol abuse has led to a theory of "familial abuse." The theory holds that the person with a close relative who is alcoholic is at far greater risk of succumbing to the disease than are others without such connections. Familial abuse or "familial alcoholism" characterizes as many as three in four of all abusers. Therapy has thus begun to focus on the families of alcohol abusers—particularly young sons—as the ones most susceptible to the disease.

Recognizing the Danger Signals of Problem Drinking

The chronic alcohol abuser shows physical symptoms that a physician can recognize. Among them are hand tremors, deterioration of eye functions, reduced bladder control, liver disorders, anemia, memory lapses, and others. But there are many other symptoms that family members and friends can observe, among them these:

- Alcohol use as a way of handling problems or escaping from them

- Increased use of alcohol with repeated occasions of unintended intoxication

- Sneaking drinks or gulping them rapidly in quick succession

- Irritation, hostility, and lying when the subject of alcohol abuse is mentioned

- A noticeable deterioration in appearance, health, and social behavior

- Persistent drinking in spite of such symptoms as headaches, loss of appetite, sleeplessness, and stomach trouble

Treatment

Methods of treating alcohol abuse fall generally into three categories. Choice of any one form of treatment depends on the particular needs of a client, including the degree of dependency. The three categories include the hospital, the intermediate, and the outpatient settings. Other approaches to treatment may be geared to individual or group needs.

The family physician can in most cases provide guidance on what kind of treatment would most benefit a particular patient. The alcohol abuser may be referred first to a toxicologist for an interview and recommendations on treatment. A review of the patient's history is a typical first step in treatment. Family involvement during therapy may be critically important. More than 4,200 centers offer treatment programs; of these, many are nonprofit clinics while others are units owned by for-profit health care chains. Many centers and clinics specialize in team approaches to therapy.

The Hospital Setting

Whether undertaken voluntarily or involuntarily (for example, by court order) the treatment formats offered in a hospital can be individualized. Where some patients adjust best to inpatient care, others prefer partial hospitalization. In the latter case the patient is allowed to go home or to work at appropriate times, otherwise living in the hospital. In a hospital detoxification program, one designed to end physical addiction, the patient has a variable period, usually two weeks to a month, during which he or she undergoes a programmed regimen of activities. These may range from exercise classes to medications to bed rest and regulated diets.

The Intermediate Setting

The intermediate settings usually include at least halfway houses, quarterway houses, and residential care sites. The first of these offer not only living quarters but also job counseling, psychotherapy, and other services. In quarterway houses, the patient receives more attention in the form of counseling and psychotherapy. Residential care centers usually offer little beyond living quarters.

The Outpatient Setting

Again in the outpatient setting the patient has a range of treatment choices. Among them typically are individual counseling sessions held by a paraprofessional; individual therapy sessions with a professional who may have an advanced degree in social work, psychology, medicine, or a related specialty; and group therapy sessions supervised by either a paraprofessional or a professional.

Chemical Treatments

Some treatment programs utilize medications to help patients to "shake the habit." Tranquilizers may be used to reduce tensions and prepare the patient for a follow-up stage. In a program of *aversion therapy* a substance called emetine may be prescribed. Taken before an alcoholic drink, emetine causes nausea. The treatment should be undertaken only under medical supervision.

Where to Find Help

Volunteer organizations of various kinds offer the alcohol abuser and his or her family a wide range of services and programs. The best known is Alcoholics Anonymous (AA), which is supported by contributions from members. AA utilizes a group-support approach to treatment. Most larger communities have AA chapters as well as Al-Anon and Alateen units for family members, relatives, and friends of abusers. Alateen works with young people between 12 and 20 years of age. Counseling and referrals may be obtained from a local Alcoholic Treatment Center.

Information may also be obtained from the following national headquarters of organizations established to help alcohol abusers:

Alcoholics Anonymous World
   Services
475 Riverside Drive
New York, NY 10163

National Association for Children
   of Alcoholics
11426 Rockville Pike, Suite 100
Rockville, MD 20852
(888) 554-2627

Al-Anon Family Group
   Headquarters
1600 Corporate Landing Parkway
Virginia Beach, VA 23454-5617
(888) 425-2526

National Council on Alcoholism
   and Drug Dependence
12 W. 21 Street
New York, NY 10010
(800) 622-2255

Drug Abuse

Like alcohol abuse, drug abuse can wreck lives and break up families. But to many experts the problem of drug abuse is far more serious than alcohol abuse. The trade in addictive, harmful drugs is not only unlawful; it has grown year by year, to the point where many believe it is out of control. Since the mid-1980's the U.S. government has spent approximately one and half billion dollars a year to combat illegal drug importation, calling on units of the military to join the campaign. Nevertheless, the amount of illegal drugs seized and the amount estimated to elude detection increase each year.

The forms that drug abuse takes, and the numbers of drugs, are numerous and increasing. Many authorities believe we should examine our whole American society for the "pill-happy" context in which drug abuse occurs. Dr. Joel Fort, former consultant on drug abuse to the World Health Organization, called America

> "a drug-prone nation. . . . The average 'straight' adult consumes three to five mind-altering drugs a day, beginning with the stimulant caffeine in coffee, tea, and Coca Cola, going on to include alcohol and nicotine, often a tranquilizer, not uncommonly a sleeping pill at night and sometimes an amphetamine the next morning."

The social effects of drug abuse rank among the most alarming of all the symptoms of what has been called the drug crisis. By estimate, drugs are involved in one-third to one-half of all crimes committed in the United States in a typical year. In a single recent year, medical treatments for drug abusers cost the nation more than $2 billion. The costs of abuse to families, communities, and to abusers themselves cannot be calculated.

Making the problem of control of drug abuse unbelievably complex is the fact that literally thousands of drugs and drug combinations have basic roles in medical treatments. Legal and illicit uses may, because of the close connections, become confused. Physicians' instructions regarding use of such legal drugs as sleeping pills may be ignored or neglected. Legitimately prescribed drugs may, in some cases, unintentionally lead to abuse or dependency.

Other facts make it difficult to control drug abuse. More and more, for example, abusers are turning to multiple substance abuse. Cocaine "sniffers" may take alcohol in one form or another to soften the uncomfortable and even painful effects of cocaine withdrawal. Physicians report that "polydrug" abuse leads to progressive worsening of such medical symptoms as stomach ailments and liver problems.

Designer drugs add another complicating factor. Made in clandestine chemical laboratories, these drugs are created by altering the existing molecular structure of other drugs, such as cocaine, heroin, amphetamines, and many other controlled substances. The chemical composition of a designer drug is enough like that of the banned or controlled drug it imitates that it produces similar effects, but it is different enough to be a new drug. The federal Drug Enforcement Administration must then take steps to declare the new drug illegal. Far more powerful than the basic drugs they imitate, the designer forms have been implicated in hundreds of deaths.

A designer drug called Ecstasy is an imitation methamphetamine (speed). It contains the industrial chemical MPTP, a suspected causative element in cases of Parkinson's disease. A number of Ecstasy abusers also had classic Parkinson's symptoms: rigidity, tremors in the arms, legs, and even the head, and slow or difficult movement. Thus new research has focused on MPTP as a possible clue to the degenerative brain processes that lead to Parkinson's.

Over-the-Counter Drugs

Americans consume over-the-counter (OTC) drugs in enormous quantities. Purchasable without a physician's prescription, these drugs have limited but real potential for abuse. They range from headache remedies to cold nostrums and from acne ointments to vitamins. In general, good practice is to use OTC drugs as seldom as possible, for short-term, minor illnesses. Medicines of proven effectiveness should be used exclusively: taking an aspirin for a headache is a good example. The U.S. Public Health Service offers these guidelines:

• Self-prescribed drugs should never be used continuously for long periods of time. . . . A physician is required for abdominal pain that is severe or recurs periodically; pains anywhere, if severe, disabling, persistent, or recurring; headache, if unusually severe or prolonged

more than one day; a prolonged cold with fever or cough; earache; unexplained loss of weight; unexplained and unusual symptoms; *malaise* lasting more than a week or two. . . .

The Food and Drug Administration (FDA), a branch of the U.S. Public Health Service, is responsible for establishing the safety and usefulness of all drugs marketed in the United States, both OTC and prescription. You can be assured that OTC drugs are safe provided you take them in strict accordance with the label instructions. These indicate the appropriate dosages, among other things, and carry warnings against prolonged or improper use, such as "discontinue if pain persists," or "do not take if abdominal pain is present." This labeling information is regulated by the FDA.

Drug Classifications

In addition to alcohol, the drugs of potential abuse fall into six categories: stimulants, depressants, and narcotic preparations, all of which can have legitimate medical uses; hallucinogens; cannabinoids such as marijuana; and inhalants (or volatile inhalants) such as aerosol sprays, glues, and fuels. See the accompanying table:

Drug abuse can lead to at least three kinds of addiction or dependency. *Physical addiction* results in unpleasant withdrawal symptoms, including, nausea, headache, or cold

Major Drug Classification	
Type	**Examples**
Stimulants	Amphetamines Cocaine derivatives
Depressants	Valium Seconal
Narcotics (opioids)	Morphine Codeine
Hallucinogens	LSD Mescaline Psilocybin

Marijuana	Marijuana
(cannabinoids)	Hashish
Inhalants	Gasoline
	Amyl nitrate

sweats when the abuser does not take the drug. Sudden withdrawal from some physically addictive drugs can cause heart failure. *Psychological addiction,* more subtle, is a stage at which the abuser believes he or she cannot cope without the drug. In *functional addiction,* the abuser grows dependent on such drugs as decongestant nasal sprays to remain free of an annoying physical condition.

Definitions of Dependence and Addiction

Dependence and addiction is used to describe the compulsive and uncontrollable use of a substance. The use continues despite negative effects on health, lifestyle, work, or other aspects of one's life. Lack of the substance leads to craving, physical or psychological discomfort, and, at times, an overwhelming desire to obtain more of the substance to alleviate the negative sensations experienced from withdrawal.

Psychological dependence or addiction occurs when the user feels he or she cannot manage without the drug. This can occur for several reasons, with several types of drugs. The condition can be mild or can be extraordinarily severe.

Psychological addiction to painkillers — and this can include ibuprofen (Motrin), aspirin, and acetaminophen (Tylenol) — occurs when the user feels that pain may be too great without regular medication. As pain occurs without use, it fulfills the user's expectations. The pain may be real or may be psychosomatic (triggered by psychological expectations of pain), but it reassures the user that the drug is needed and does good. The problem is that with many types of drug, the effectiveness decreases as use increases.

Psychological addiction can accompany physical addiction, and it is usually difficult to distinguish where psychological needs leave off and physical needs begin. Many addictions are a combination of psychological and physical.

Physical dependence or addiction occurs when the body has developed a physical need for the drug. Physical dependence is usually recognized when the user stops taking the drug. Withdrawal symptoms occur when the body is denied the chemicals to which it has become habituated. Withdrawal symptoms can include dizziness, anxiety, restless sleep, dull ache, acute pain, heart tremors, seizures and convulsions, and heart attack. Sudden withdrawal from some physically addictive drugs can kill the user. Many of the street drugs, such as cocaine and heroin, and many of the prescription drugs, such as Xanax and codeine, can produce severe symptoms if withdrawal is sudden from quantities that were abusive.

Tolerance is the term used for the effect that occurs when the quantity of drug is progressively increased to achieve the desired result. For some chemicals, the body becomes habituated to one quantity and the dosage must be increased to maintain the same level of relief or pleasure experienced from the drug. Increased tolerance for some drugs is what frequently leads to levels that are physically addictive.

Three Classes of Prescription Drugs

Among the drugs that may be prescribed for you are some that have a tremendous potential for abuse. They include *stimulants,* such as amphetamines; *depressants,* such as sleeping pills; and *narcotic* painkillers, including morphine and codeine. When abused (that is, when taken in any way other than according to a physician's strict instructions) these drugs constitute a substantial part of America's burgeoning national drug problem.

Stimulant Drugs

The legitimate use of stimulant drugs and their great capacity for abuse stem from the same property: their ability to speed up the processes of the central nervous system. Physicians may prescribe amphetamines primarily to curb the appetites of patients who are dieting or to counteract mild depression. More rarely, they use stimulant drugs to treat *narcolepsy,* a disease in which the patient is subject to irresistible bouts of sleep, and to counteract the drowsiness caused by sedatives. Amphetamines and an amphetamine-like drug (Ritalin) may be used to treat some hyperactive children who are extremely excitable and easily distracted. For reasons that are imperfectly understood, the drug calms these children instead of stimulating them.

Amphetamines

The major forms of the amphetamines are: amphetamine (Benzedrine), the more powerful dextroamphetamine (Dexedrine), and methamphetamine (Methedrine, Desoxyn). The street name for these drugs is "speed."

The consumption of amphetamines is reportedly far greater than the prescription books indicate. Some 10 billion tablets are produced in the United States annually, enough for 50 doses for every man, woman, and child. Of this amount, probably half is diverted into illicit channels. Underground laboratories manufacture even more.

Abusers of amphetamines include students cramming for exams, housewives trying to get through the day without collapsing from exhaustion, and the businessman who has tossed and turned all night in a strange hotel bedroom and needs to be alert for a conference the next morning.

Used judiciously, amphetamines can improve performance, both mental and physical, over moderate periods of time. In effect, they delay the deterioration in performance that fatigue normally produces. Required to carry out routine duties under difficult circumstances and for extended periods, some astronauts have used amphetamines under long-range medical supervision.

Amphetamines give some persons feelings of self-confidence, well-being, alertness, and an increased ability to concentrate and perform. Others may experience an increase in tension ranging from the uncomfort-

able to an agonizing pitch of anxiety. High doses may produce dry mouth, sweating, palpitations, and raised blood pressure. Because amphetamines only defer the effects of fatigue, the letdown can be dangerous, especially for such users as long-distance truck drivers. In addition, the feelings of self-confidence about improved performance may be highly deceptive. Some college students who have crammed for exams while on speed have turned in blank examination books, or written a whole essay on one dense line.

Amphetamine abusers quickly develop a tolerance to the drug. They may have continually to increase dosages, and may undergo different kinds of drug experiences. Psychological dependence can build rapidly.

Amphetamine-like Stimulants

Several drugs that are chemically unrelated to the amphetamines produce very similar effects on the body. They are, also, equally amenable to abuse.

Among them are methylphenidate (Ritalin) and phenmetrazine (Preludin). The latter has been commonly used as a diet pill.

Cocaine

Ranked as powerful stimulants to the central nervous system, cocaine and its derivatives have become the trendy drugs of the late 20th century. An alkaloid found in the leaves of the coca bush, *Erythroxylon coca,* cocaine in its crystalline form is a white powder that looks like moth flakes. Cocaine can be sniffed, smoked, or taken intravenously. Abusers of cocaine may or may not develop a tolerance for the drug. But some evi-

dence indicates that the same dose repeated frequently will not produce similar effects over a period of time.

Very little street-purchased cocaine is pure. Usually, the drug is mixed, or cut, with other drugs or with substances that resemble it, such as talcum powder or sugar.

Physical dependence on cocaine is rare. Psychological dependence is much more common. When physical dependence occurs, the withdrawal symptoms may include hunger, irritability, extreme fatigue, depression, and restless sleep. With psychological dependence, abusers come to need the feeling of euphoria induced by cocaine. When a dose wears off, the abuser may go into a period of deep depression.

The use of cocaine as a legal anesthetic need not lead to addiction. It has been used particularly in surgical operations on the mouth, eyes, and throat because it can constrict blood vessels and because it is rapidly absorbed by the mucous membranes.

Cocaine's effects as a stimulant last only a short time. Generally, the effects depend on the size of the dose. A small dose may produce sensations of euphoria and illusions of increased strength and sensory awareness. A large dose may magnify these effects. The abuser may engage in irrational behavior, and may experience such physical side effects as sweating, dilation of the pupils, and rapid heartbeat.

In extreme cases abusers may have hallucinations and feelings of paranoia and depression. They may imagine that insects are crawling over their skins (formication) and may have chest pains. Injections by needle may produce skin abscesses. Both heavy and light users may develop runny noses, eczema around the nostrils, and deterioration of the nasal cartilage. The latter occurs because cocaine is usually "snorted" into the nostrils through a straw or a roll of paper, or from a spoon.

Death results, occasionally, from overdoses of cocaine, with respiratory arrest as a prime cause. The abuser may also have high fever, heart rhythm disturbances, or convulsions.

Crack Cocaine

By a simple process dealers in cocaine can convert cocaine in white powder form, cocaine hydrochloride, into cocaine alkaloid, called *freebase*. The process involves mixing powdered cocaine with baking soda and water to form a paste. Once the concoction hardens, it looks like lumpy, off-white granulated sugar. Unlike powdered cocaine, the drug in this form, called *crack* or *rock,* can be smoked, eliminating the need for needles.

However made, crack is a purified cocaine base that is usually smoked in a special pipe with wire screens, or sprinkled on a tobacco or marijuana cigarette. The drug produces a high that may start in eight seconds and last two minutes. By contrast, snorted cocaine takes effect after about five minutes.

Crack produces a very intense euphoria along with other physical symptoms. Because the drug in this form is far more potent than powdered cocaine, the heartbeat speeds up and the abuser's blood pressure may rise. Heart-lung problems may follow, and seizures can occur. Death may ensue. Because of the variations in the strength and purity of crack, and because of the variability of a body's response, death can occur on the first use or the thousandth. Abuse of crack may lead to physical addiction in weeks, with the victim needing continually larger doses to achieve a high.

Depressant Drugs

Making up a second class of medically useful drugs that are also widely abused, the depressants act as sedatives on the central nervous system (CNS). They may also act as hypnotic, or sleep-inducing, agents.

The depressants include mainly the barbiturates, which are both sedative and hypnotic, and the tranquilizers, which can calm without producing sleep. Though they are available as main or secondary constituents of more than 80 brand name preparations, the barbiturates are readily abused.

Tranquilizers act selectively on the brain and the central nervous system. Divided into major and minor tranquilizers, these drugs are similar to barbiturates in many ways, including their sedative or calming effect. The major tranquilizers, called *neuroleptics* because they are useful in the treatment of mental disorders, are *haloperidol* and *chlorpromazine*. These drugs lead to virtually no addiction or dependence even in long-term therapy.

The minor tranquilizers, among them *meprobamate* (Miltown), *chlordiazepoxide* (Librium), and *diazepam* (Valium), are, by contrast, highly addictive. Abusers take such drugs to achieve euphoric states as well as to offset the effects of alcohol, amphetamines, and other drugs.

Barbiturates

Barbiturates have many legitimate uses. For example, they may be prescribed to overcome insomnia, reduce high blood pressure, alleviate anxiety, treat mental disorders, and sedate patients both before and after surgery. Barbiturates may help to bring epileptic and other convulsions under control.

Barbiturates are metabolized, or broken down chemically, by the liver. They are then eliminated by the kidneys at different speeds depending on their types: slow- or long-acting, intermediate and short-acting, or ultra-short-acting. The first of these, primarily phenobarbital and barbital, take effect on the brain in one to two hours and last for six to 24 hours. The intermediate and short-acting barbiturates, including secobarbital and pentobarbital, take effect in 20 to 45 minutes and last five to six hours. The best known of the ultra-short-acting drugs, sodium pentothal or thiopental, can produce unconsciousness in a few minutes. Used mostly in hospitals as an anesthetic, pentothal is also injected by dentists to produce instant unconsciousness.

Abuse

Barbiturate abusers usually select the ultra-short-acting form of the drug because of the rapid action. Abusers as a group generally fall into four categories, with some overlap.

The "silent abuser" takes sleeping pills at first to get some sleep, probably with a physician's prescription. Progressively, the drug helps the abuser to deal with tension and anxiety. Indulging at home, he or she finds the barbiturates producing an alcohol-like high, with slurred speech, confusion, poor judgment and coordination, and sometimes wild emotional swings. Eventually the abuser is obtaining the drug through illicit channels. Some may end up spending most of their time in bed.

A second group, taking barbiturates for stimulation, has already developed a high tolerance that makes drug stimulation possible. Some other abusers find that the drug releases inhibitions.

Made up mostly of young people who are experimenting with various drugs, a third group uses barbiturates to "come down" from an amphetamine high. Members of this group may find themselves in a vicious cycle of stimulation and sedation. To obtain both effects at once, some abusers take the barbiturate-amphetamine combination in the same swallow—a so-called "set-up."

A fourth group, abusers of heroin and other narcotics, uses barbiturates as a substitute when drugs of choice are not available. They may also combine barbiturates with heroin to prolong its effect. In one hospital surveyed, 23 percent of the narcotics users said they were also dependent on barbiturates.

Effects and Dangers

Barbiturate abuse is generally considered to be far more dangerous than narcotic abuse. Every year brings some 3,000 deaths from barbiturate overdose, accidental or intentional. For such reasons many physicians believe barbiturates are the most dangerous of all drugs. Chronic abuse can lead to psychological dependence and increased tolerance, followed often by physical dependence of a particularly anguishing kind.

Abrupt withdrawal from barbiturates can be much more dangerous than withdrawal from heroin. Within a day the abuser withdrawing from bar- biturates may experience headaches, muscle twitches, anxiety, weakness, nausea, and blood pressure drops. If the abuser stands up suddenly he or she may faint. Delirium and convulsions may come later. The latter can be fatal. Thus the withdrawal must always be undertaken under medical supervision. Even with supervision, a withdrawal from barbiturates may take two months.

Abuse of barbiturates presents other dangers. Unintentional overdosing frequently occurs when a person takes a regular dose to get to sleep and then remains awake or awakens soon afterward; tired and confused, the person may take another or repeated doses. Death may result. Mixing barbiturates and alcohol can produce the same outcome.

Other Barbiturate-Type Drugs

Some depressants are chemically unrelated to the barbiturates but have similar effects. These include *glutethimide*, *ethchlorvynol* (Placidyl), and *methyprylon* (Noludar). These too lead to tolerance when abused and sometimes to psychological and physical dependence.

Tranquilizers

The minor tranquilizers are manufactured as capsules and tablets in many sizes, shapes, and colors. They may also be purchased in liquid form for injection. Used legitimately to treat emotional tension and as muscle relaxants, these tranquilizers have high abuse potential because they produce both psychological and physical dependence. Tolerance develops with prolonged abuse.

Miltown, Librium, and Valium produce effects similar to those of barbiturates. But the minor tranquilizers act more slowly and have longer duration. Once considered completely harmless, these drugs came into such vogue that in the 1970s the federal government intervened. Both Valium and Librium as well as some other drugs were placed under federal control. From 1975 on anyone requiring a prescription for these drugs was limited to five prescription refills within a six-month period following the initial prescription. If more of the medication was required after that, a new prescription had to be written.

Withdrawal from the minor tranquilizers can be as dangerous and painful as withdrawal from barbiturates. Combining the tranquilizing drugs with others, including alcohol, is a highly dangerous form of abuse. Each drug reinforces the effects of the other. The result may be greater than the combined effects of the different drugs.

Narcotics (Opiates)

Narcotics are drugs that relieve pain and induce sleep by depressing the central nervous system. Under U.S. law, narcotics are addictive drugs that produce rapid and severe physical and psychological dependence; that category includes opium and such opium derivatives as heroin, morphine, and codeine. The narcotics, or *opioids,* also include the so-called synthetic opiates, among them *meperidine* and *methadone.*

Varieties of abused drugs

Name	Form	Drug
amphetamine methamphetamine	capsule, pill, liquid, powder, tablet, lozenge; swallowed	stimulant
barbiturate	sleeping pills, capsules, tablets; swallowed; injected	depressant, sedative
cocaine	white powder; sniffed, smoked, injected	stimulant, local anesthetic
hashish	resin; smoked	relaxant, euphoriant, hallucinogen (in large or strong doses)
heroin	powder; injected, or sniffed	narcotic
inhalants (for example, gasoline, paint, glue, aerosols, amyl nitrite)	aerosols, volatile substances, solvents; sniffed	
LSD (d-lysergic acid diethylamide)	tablet, capsule, liquid; swallowed	hallucinogen (psychedelic)
marijuana, marihuana	dried leaves; smoked	relaxant, euphoriant, hallucinogen (in large or strong doses)
mescaline	tablet, capsule; swallowed	hallucinogen
PCP	powder; smoked, swallowed	anesthetic (used only with animals)

Opium

The seedpods of the opium poppy, *Papaver somniferum,* produce a gummy resin that has narcotic effects when eaten or smoked. Opium has been used in many lands and many cultures since prehistoric times. It was used medicinally in ancient Egypt. But not until recently did its addictive properties become known. Of the more than two dozen active compounds, or *alkaloids,* that can be isolated from opium, the two most important are morphine and codeine.

Morphine

Morphine, named after Morpheus, the Roman god of dreams, is the chemical substance in opium that gives it sedative and analgesic properties. Isolated initially in the early 1800s, morphine was later synthesized in pure form. On the illicit drug market it appears usually as a white powder.

Morphine can relieve almost any kind of pain, particularly dull, continuous pain. It may also relieve the fear and anxiety that go with such suffering. In addition to drowsiness, euphoria, and impairment of mental and physical performance, morphine may have adverse effects including nausea, vomiting, and sweating. Intravenous injections of the drug may produce an orgasmic high sensation beginning in the upper abdomen and spreading throughout the body.

Taken in overdose, morphine can lead to respiratory depression that is sometimes severe enough to cause coma and death. Morphine is highly addictive and is used only short-term in hospitals because longer exposure easily leads to problems. Naloxone (Narcan) may be administered intravenously as an antidote for morphine overdose.

Codeine

Taking its name from the Greek word *kodeia,* meaning poppyhead, codeine is a mild pain-reliever that can be produced from gum opium or through conversion from morphine. The effects of codeine peak in 30 to 60 minutes; they disappear in three to four hours. Codeine is milder than either morphine or heroin in analgesic effect, and is the most effective cough medicine available. All forms can induce addiction problems with regular use.

Heroin

Originally thought to be nonaddictive, heroin was for a time used as a cure for opium and morphine addiction. It was then found to be more addictive than either of those drugs. It was prohibited in the United States in 1924 and became a staple on the drug black market. Heroin is several times as powerful as morphine.

All of the opiates, including heroin, produce feelings of well-being or euphoria. They also lead to dulled senses and to reduction or elimination of normal fears, tensions, and anxiety. The drug also produces sleepiness and lethargy; *nodding* is one of the characteristic symptoms of abuse. Possible side effects include nausea, flushing, constipation, slowed respiration rates, retention of urine, and, eventually, malnutrition resulting from loss of appetite. When first injecting heroin, nausea and vomiting can occur almost immediately.

The heroin abuser rapidly develops tolerance to the drug. Continually larger doses are then required to produce the same degree of euphoria. Used chronically, heroin leads to both psychological and physical dependence. The former is far more important, and is more difficult to break.

Caught in a cycle involving desperate efforts to obtain enough money, often by criminal means, and getting high, the heroin abuser is not necessarily driven by the search for escape. He or she may want, equally, to avoid withdrawal symptoms. For the chronic abuser these symptoms can be difficult and painful, and may include anxiety, sweating, muscle aches, vomiting, and diarrhea.

Heroin sold on the streets is cut with quinine, milk sugar, or baking soda. It may be cut several times before reaching the abuser. A bag may contain only 1 to 5 percent heroin. If the addict unknowingly buys a dose containing 30 percent or more pure heroin, the higher concentration can spell grave illness or death.

Because heroin can be taken in different ways, the drug's narcotic effects are variable. Sniffing is the mildest form of abuse, followed by skin-popping or subcutaneous injection anywhere on the body, and mainlining, injection directly into a vein, usually the large vein inside the elbow. Abscesses at the preferred site of injection are common, and the vein may become inflamed.

Heroin use does not necessarily lead to dependence. Many persons have experimented with the drug without becoming addicted. Others "joy-pop"—use the drug on weekends, usually for recreational purposes or "kicks."

Little agreement exists regarding treatments for heroin abuse. A promising yet controversial method is the substitution of controlled doses of *methadone* for heroin. Methadone is a synthetic opiate that does not produce the euphoria of heroin. The substitution can help the abuser to lead a normal life, but he or she may still be addicted—to methadone.

Other forms of treatment utilize group psychotherapy, often in live-in communities modeled after the West Coast's *Synanon*. Some experts believe that only multiple-approach treatment formats, combining chemical treatment, psychiatry, user communities, and rehabilitation, can be effective. But the five-year cure rate for heroin abusers is low—only about one-third of that for alcoholics.

Synthetic Opiates

Prescription pain-relievers such as Demerol, Dilaudid, Pantopon, and other synthetic opiates can become addicting if used indiscriminately. They occasionally appear on the illicit drug market. With the increased availability of methadone in treatment clinics, methadone itself is used illicitly, often in combination with alcohol or other drugs, and especially when heroin is in short supply.

The Hallucinogens: LSD and Others

LSD (lysergic acid diethylamide) is one of a class of drugs legally classed as *hallucinogens*—agents that cause the user to experience hallucinations, illusions, and distorted perceptions. Others include *mescaline, psilocybin* and *psilocin, PCP, DMT* (dimethyltryptamine), and *DOM* or *STP*.

A colorless, tasteless, odorless compound, LSD is a semisynthetic acid of immense potency. A single effective dose requires, on the average, only 100 millionths of a gram. A quantity of LSD equivalent to two aspirin tablets would furnish 6,500 such doses. When sold on the street, LSD is generally mixed with colored substances. It may be manufactured in capsule, tablet, or liquid form.

History of LSD

With names such as *California sunshine, acid, purple haze,* and others, LSD reached a peak of popularity in the 1960s. Today it cannot be made legally except for use in certain supervised experiments. Physicians may use it to treat alcoholism and some mental disease, but without uniformly convincing results. It may be sold illegally in sugar cubes, candy, cookies, on the surfaces of beads, even in the mucilage of stamps and envelopes. One dose may produce a 4- to 18-hour *trip,* a hallucinogenic experience.

In the 1960s this trip made LSD the drug of choice for many substance abusers. Among those who claimed that LSD and other psychedelic drugs were consciousness-expanding were well-known public figures. The drugs, in brief, were supposed to enhance the user's appreciation of everything in the environment, to increase creativity, open the gates of awareness to mind-bending mystical or religious experiences, and perhaps to bring about profound changes, hopefully for the better, in the user's personality.

While some users reported such results, various studies suggested that the improvements were illusory. Members of some groups nonetheless felt that it was "in" to be an *acidhead,* an LSD user. One authority estimates that less than 1 percent of the total population have experimented with LSD. Partly because knowledge of dangers in LSD use has become common, the drug has passed the peak of its popularity even though it can still be obtained illegally.

Addictive Aspects

Abuse of LSD is difficult; the drug produces such a spectacular high that daily ingestion is virtually out of the question. Thus LSD use does not lead to physical dependence. But the heavy user can develop a tolerance for the drug very quickly. The tolerance disappears after a few days of abstinence.

Effects

Taking LSD, the individual is usually prepared for minor physical discomforts: a rise in temperature, pulse, and blood pressure; the sensation of hair standing on end; and some nausea, dizziness, and headache. The trip begins about an hour after the drug is first taken. Vision is affected the most profoundly. Colors become more intense and more beautiful; those in a painting may seem to merge and stream. Flat objects become three-dimensional.

The LSD user's reactions are closely related to his or her expectations. Thus one trip may be mind-expanding, filled with brilliant sights and sensations as well as euphoric feelings of oneness with the universe. Another trip may bring anxiety, panic, fear, and depression verging on despair. The latter experience can be terrifying; some bad trips have ended in psychiatric wards, with the tripper suffering from a severe mental disorder, a *psychosis*. An individual's body image may be distorted; in the LSD-induced vision he or she may have no head, for example. Such psychotic episodes, or breaks, may clear up within a day or two. Others can last for months or years.

Some trips have ended in tragedy. Convinced that they could fly or float through the air, some trippers have walked through high windows to their deaths. Others have walked in front of trains or cars.

In effect, no one can predict what psychological changes LSD use will produce. One reason is that no one really knows how LSD works inside the body to affect the mind. What is known is that the drug moves quickly to the brain and throughout the body, acting on both the central and autonomic nervous systems. But all traces of the drug disappear from the brain in some 20 minutes. The effects, as noted, last many more hours.

As with all drugs, LSD should not be ingested by persons who have psychotic tendencies or who are unstable. A disquieting side effect, usually occurring after chronic or heavy use, appears in the flashback, a reexperiencing of the effects of the drug weeks or months after a trip. One theory holds that flashbacks are induced by stress or fatigue, or by resort to other drugs, but the theory remains a theory.

Studies have reported some statistical findings. One research project found that the children of LSD users are 18 times more likely to have birth defects than the children of nonusers. Some research also suggests that the drug may have toxic effects on some cells of the human body. An unproved, and possibly unprovable, theory indicates that there may be a link between LSD use and breaks in chromosomes that could conceivably lead to leukemia or to birth defects in users' children.

Other Hallucinogens

Many other substances, both natural and synthetic, are used as hallucinogens. Most of them produce effects similar to those of LSD, but are far less potent.

Mescaline

Mescaline is the active ingredient of *peyote,* a Mexican cactus that has been used by American Indians for centuries to achieve mystical states in religious ceremonies. Users consume cactus "buttons" either ground up or whole. Mescaline itself may be obtained as a powder or a liquid. It can also be synthesized in a laboratory.

Psilocybin and Psilocin

Psilocybin and psilocin are the active hallucinogenic ingredients in the Aztec mushroom *Psilocybe mexicana.* The mushroom grows in southern Mexico and has been eaten raw by the natives since about 1500 B.C. Both derivatives can be made in the laboratory.

PCP (Phencyclidine Hydrochloride)

First developed in 1959 as an anesthetic, PCP in its pure form is a white crystalline powder that is readily soluble in water or alcohol. It appears on the drug black market as tablets, capsules, and colored powders. Abusers snort, smoke, or eat PCP. They can also inject the drug, but do not usually do so. PCP appears as an adulterant in many drug mixtures—in mescaline, psilocybin, or LSD, for example. PCP reportedly has as many or more undesirable effects as positive ones, among them forgetfulness, loss of behavior control, feelings of depersonalization, paranoid episodes, hallucinations, and suicidal impulses.

DMT (Dimethyltryptamine)

Called the "businessman's high" because its effects may last only 40 to 50 minutes, DMT is similar in structure to psilocin. DMT can be smoked or injected; in either case the effect is a powerful wave of exhilaration. An ingredient of various plants native to South America, DMT has long been used by Indian tribes in the form of intoxicating drinks or snuff, often very dangerous. In the United States, DMT is synthesized from tryptamine in the laboratory.

DOM or STP

DOM or STP is a synthetic compound originally developed by the Dow Chemical Company for possible use in the treatment of mental disorders. The drug was never released. Manufactured illicitly, it was allegedly given the name STP for Serenity, Tranquillity, Peace. The drug is powerful, it produces vivid hallucinations, and it seems to last as long as LSD. It is also extremely poisonous, and can bring on fever, blurred vision, difficulty in swallowing, and occasionally death from convulsions. In some cases abusers suffer from manic psychoses lasting for days.

Marijuana (Cannabinoids)

Marijuana, or *marihuana,* is a Mexican-Spanish word originally used to refer to a poor grade of tobacco. Later it came to mean a smoking preparation made from the Indian hemp plant (*Cannabis sativa*). A tall, weedy plant related to the fig tree and the hop, cannabis grows freely in many parts of the world and in a variety of grades depending on climate and method of cultivation. The different grades produce drugs of varying strengths. Some 300 million people around the world obtain drug preparations of one kind or another from cannabis.

Drugs are obtained almost exclusively from the female hemp plants. The male plants produce the fiber for hemp. When the female plants are ripe, late in the summer, their top leaves and especially the clusters of flowers at their tops develop a minty, sticky, golden-yellow resin, which eventually blackens. This resin contains the highest concentrations of THC (tetrahydrocannabinol), the group of substances containing the active principles of the drug. The pure resin of carefully cultivated plants is the most potent form of cannabis. It is available in cakes, called *charas* in India, and as a brown powder called hashish in the Middle East.

An estimated 15,000 tons of marijuana are illegally smuggled into the United States annually. But cannabis cultivation has become a major underground business inside the United States. Most illegal shipments of the drug come from Colombia, Jamaica, and Mexico.

Abuse Potential

Marijuana has puzzling aspects. Scientists have not succeeded in establishing exactly what substances in the cannabis plant produce drug effects, or how. THC is, of course, believed to be the most important active element, but chemists believe it is not the only one.

Beyond that, marijuana seems to be in a special class as a drug. It is classed as a hallucinogen, but is less potent than the true hallucinogens. It is not a narcotic, and it resembles both stimulants and depressants in some of its effects. Its use does not lead to physical dependence, nor does the user or abuser develop tolerance. Some users, in fact, find that with regular use they need less marijuana to achieve the desired high.

Users do acquire a slight to moderate psychological dependence—less, in some experts' opinions, than do regular users of alcohol or tobacco. Thus much of the theorizing about marijuana is conjecture despite the fact that millions of persons use it regularly or occasionally.

Effects

Experimenters and newcomers to marijuana smoking may experience little at the beginning. A sense of panic may accompany early exposure to the drug. More serious reactions have been reported, however, including *toxic-psychosis* (psychosis caused by a toxic agent) with accompanying confusion and disorientation. But such reports are rare. Experimenters using large doses of marijuana, hashish, or THC have induced what they termed hallucinations and psychotic reactions.

The experienced smoker may feel halfway between elation and sleepiness. He or she may have some altered perceptions of sound or color, for example, and a greatly slowed-down sense of time. It is usually possible to control the extent of the high by stopping when a given point is reached. The smoker often experiences mild headache or nausea.

Medical Evidence

Research and medical use of marijuana have led to some relatively tentative findings. Some evidence indicates, for example, that the drug may produce genetic damage. More definitely, marijuana has been found to be effective for reducing the pressure of fluids in the eyes of patients suffering from glaucoma. In a 1976 case, the Food and Drug Administration (FDA) approved the use of marijuana for such treatment.

In 1985 the FDA licensed a small drug firm to manufacture THC for use in combating the nausea associated with cancer chemotherapy. Other studies indicated that the drug may also be useful in the treatment of such other diseases as multiple sclerosis.

The debate over full legalization of marijuana promises to continue. Few argue that all penalties for major suppliers should be dropped, at least as long as marijuana remains illegal. But many persons see a contradiction in sending a young person to prison for smoking a marijuana cigarette while his or her parents can drink three martinis every evening.

Inhalants

The inhalants as a class include solvents used in cleaning compounds, aerosol sprays, fuels, and glues. Abusers of these substances sniff or inhale the fumes for recreational and mind-altering purposes. But the substances, primarily chemical compounds, were never meant for human consumption. With some exceptions, they are available commercially and thus have appeal for persons who cannot afford or cannot obtain the more conventional drugs.

Strictly speaking, tobacco, cocaine, and marijuana could be considered inhalants. But the term more commonly refers to three categories of products: solvents, aerosols, and anesthetics. Among the solvents are commercial items such as gasoline, transmission fluid, paint thinner, and airplane cement. The aerosol products include shoeshine compounds, insecticides, spray paints, and hair spray. The type of inhalant used appears to vary according to geographic location, the ethnic backgrounds of abusers, and availability.

Anesthetics comprise a special group of inhalants. Some of them, including nitrous oxide, ether, and chloroform, were used recreationally before medical applications were found for them. Because they are not widely available, they are not abused as much as solvents and aerosols.

Abuse Patterns

Young teenagers are primary inhalant abusers. But some groups or classes of adults, such as prisoners in institutions, also use inhalants. Reasons for abuse vary; among teenagers they range from hostility and lack of affection to peer pressure. Adults, say authorities, are attracted by the ready availability of many inhalants. Alcoholics may resort to inhalants while trying to forestall the symptoms of withdrawal from alcohol.

Effects

Among the active chemicals in many inhalants are toluene, naphtha, carbon tetrachloride, acetone, and others. The fumes from these chemicals enter the bloodstream quickly. They are then distributed to the brain and liver. Entering the central nervous system, the fumes depress such body functions as respiration and heartbeat. It is possible for even first time users to be killed by "huffing."

Classed as depressants, inhalants are sometimes referred to as "deliriants." The reason is that they can produce illusions, hallucinations, and mental disturbances. These effects usually result in cases of overdose; in moderate doses, the abuser feels sedated, has changed perceptions and impaired judgment, and may experience fright or even panic. Depending on the dosage, the abuser may also feel intoxicated, and may have lowered inhibitions along with feelings of restlessness, uncoordination, confusion, and disorientation.

Prolonged abuse can lead to nausea, muscular weakness, fatigue, and weight loss. Other effects of such abuse can be extensive damage to the kidneys, bone marrow, liver, and brain. Inhalants have been implicated in some forms of cancer. A high can last from a few minutes to an hour or more. Repeated dosing can produce physical and psychological dependence.

In the 1960s the many deaths resulting from glue-sniffing made inhalant abuse a matter of nationwide concern. Studies reported later that about two-thirds of these deaths came about because the abusers, usually children, put plastic bags over their heads to intensify the effect and suffocated.

In recent years, inhalant abuse has become a serious problem. It is the fourth most commonly abused substance among eighth graders and is abused nearly as frequently as marijuana. Still, 9 out of 10 parents believe their children have never abused inhalants.

Where to Find Help

Substance abuse has many disturbing aspects aside from the physical, psychological, and social damage that it can cause. With addictive medicines, the progression from a *therapeutic* dose—the amount prescribed by a physician—to a *toxic* dose may seem, to some persons, natural and even inevitable. Ingestion or injection of a *lethal* dose may follow as an unintended consequence.

Other factors are causes for concern. The proliferation of illicit street drugs, the rapidity with which dependence or addiction can develop, and the costs and complexity of treatment or detoxification programs all add to the dangers inherent in abuse as a spreading phenomenon. Researchers are discovering weapons that may help in some cases to make treatment more effective: *naloxone* (Narcan), for example, can be given intravenously to reduce the toxic effects of narcotics. But too often a drug has done irreversible harm in a human system before help arrives.

American society has begun to mobilize resources to aid those who need information, assistance, or counsel, for themselves or others, in cases of substance abuse. A National Partnership to Prevent Drug and Alcohol Abuse has established a network of community groups to inform teenagers about narcotics and their potentially disastrous effects. Since 1997 it has been possible for parents to test their children's urine for traces of drugs with kits available over the counter at pharmacies.

Those seeking further information or help may call a toll-free number 800-COCAINE, where counselors are linked to a network of treatment centers and hospitals throughout the country. The addresses and telephone numbers of four national groups are:

Cocaine Anonymous World
　Services (CAWS)
P.O. Box 2000
Los Angeles, CA 90049-8000
(310) 559-5833

National Family Partnership (NFP)
11159-B South Towne Square
St. Louis, MO 63123
(314) 845-1933

National Parent Resource Institute
　for Drug Education (PRIDE)
3610 DeKalb Technology Parkway
Suite 105
Atlanta, GA 30340
(770) 458-9900

Narcotics Anonymous
P.O. Box 9999
Van Nuys, CA 91409
(818) 700-0700

30

The Environment and Health

How pure is the soil in which our food grows? How clean is the air we breathe or the water we drink? How healthy are the animals that provide substantial portions of our diets?

The Environmental Protection Agency (EPA) monitors, among other things, the level of pollutants in drinking water, the disposal of toxic wastes, the threat of radiation from nuclear power plants and the seepage of poisonous chemicals.

Harmful ingredients in the environment may be the result of pollution, accidental or intentional. Some enter the environment as a result of deliberate planning. Asbestos, for example, a mineral fiber that will not burn, was used widely to insulate and fireproof buildings. The EPA banned the use of asbestos in construction in the 1970s, after researchers proved the fiber caused diseases and several forms of cancer.

Major health hazards fall in four categories: Air, water and noise pollution and food contamination. Other hazards include toxic wastes, nuclear radiation, and work-place dangers.

Air Pollution

Air pollutants can damage health in a number of ways. Even where little scientific proof links these pollutants to specific maladies, much statistical or circumstantial evidence suggests that air pollution can lead to various forms of respiratory disease. Some cases of air pollution outside the workplace and exclusive of nuclear radiation hazards have been documented.

Sulfur Dioxide

Sulfur dioxide enters the air from many sources. In the main, however, it is spewed into the atmosphere when heavy fuel oil and coal are burned to provide heat, generate electricity, and provide industrial power. Large cities are especially vulnerable because of their concentrations of heavy industry.

Sulfur dioxide apparently irritates the lungs and leads to a reduction of the lungs' oxygen-handling capacity. Persons who are particularly susceptible to carbon and sulfur dioxide-filled smogs are those suffering from bronchial asthma, chronic bronchitis, and emphysema. The respiratory systems of such persons are already defective. In emphysema, for example, the elasticity of the air sacs in the lungs has progressively broken down, usually after prolonged infection or repeated bronchial irritation. Cigarette smoking can produce such irritation; the sulfur dioxide only worsens the situation.

Lead

Substantial evidence indicates that lead in the air can cause neurological harm and impair body chemistry and bone growth. Most airborne lead comes from combustion of solid waste, coal, and oils; emissions from iron and steel production and lead smelters; and tobacco smoke. Children are most immediately affected because they have fewer natural defenses against toxic absorption than adults. But adults too may feel the effects of such absorption. They may, for example, feel tired, cramped, or confused.

Because their bodies absorb and metabolize substances rapidly, children may have rates of lead absorption four times as high as those of adults. Workers in some industries, including the ceramic, glass, and lead industries, are also at risk. One study showed that 44 percent of the lead workers in two U.S. smelters suffered from clinical poisoning.

Specific effects of lead poisoning range across a broad spectrum. The formation of red blood cells may be inhibited even by low-level exposure to lead in the air. At higher levels, lead may cause anemia. In children, bone cell growth may be stunted; in pregnant women, lead may prevent the normal development of the fetal skeleton. But lead affects the brain primarily, in some cases interfering with motor skills, auditory development, memory, and the nervous system. Children with higher levels of lead absorption have been found to have serious learning disabilities. Fortunately, lead levels may fluctuate, and the lead in blood and soft tissue may pass out of the human system four to six weeks after exposure ends. But lead remains in bone for periods lasting as long as three decades.

Other Fuel Contaminants

Auto exhausts are major sources of air pollutants. Exhaust emissions may include nitrogen oxides, carbon monoxide, hydrocarbons, and soot. The latter is made up of visible particles of carbon suspended in the air.

Nitrogen oxides irritate the eyes and the respiratory tract. When nitrogen oxide and hydrocarbons mix in sunlight, they form other noxious substances in the typical photochemical smog that has a yellowish cast. The new ingredients include *ozone,* a poisonous form of oxygen, and peroxyacetyl nitrate (PAN), which is intensely irritating to the eyes. Los Angeles was the first city to experience these smogs; they now occur in many other cities as well.

Worst of all, auto exhaust hydrocarbons include varieties that are possible *carcinogens,* causes of cancer in susceptible individuals.

Acid Rain

While so-called *acid rain* has not been found to harm humans directly, scientists say it has begun to damage the natural food chain in certain regions. As industrial smokestacks emit pollutants, including sulfur and nitrogen oxides, these rise into the upper atmosphere. Mixed with water vapor and other substances, the airborne chemicals are changed by sunlight, becoming tiny acid droplets. The droplets fall to earth as rain or snow, raising the acid content of freshwater lakes and damaging trees and other plants. Under conditions of extreme acidity, fish populations have disappeared. Where the food web is disrupted, aquatic animals, algae, and bacteria may dwindle in number. The effects of acid rain on crops and trees are less apparent but are thought to be harmful.

To some extent, acid rain is a geographic phenomenon in North America. Factories in the midwestern industrial belt throw off most of the pollutants, which are then carried east and north. Southeastern Canada and the northeastern and eastern regions of the United States are the areas primarily affected.

Indoor Air Pollution

Reports of illness associated with office and other nonresidential buildings have given rise to what has been termed the "sick building syndrome." The causes of this syndrome, or complex of symptoms, have not been completely and precisely explained. Among the possible explanations are the following:

- Building ventilation has been reduced to conserve energy, with the result that ventilation is simply inadequate

- Indoor air has become contaminated by emissions from the building fabric and associated systems, furnishings, office equipment, or maintenance materials

- Entrainment or cross contamination has taken place, with contaminants generated in a different part of the building or in a separate building drawn in by an air-handling system

- Bioeffluents, or volatile human substances, spread throughout a building, polluting the air with pyruvic acid, lactic acid, acetaldehyde, butyric acid, carbon dioxide, and other body effluents

- Combustion byproducts from smoking tobacco have produced substances, smoke included, that contaminate indoor air

- Microorganisms or airborne particles from molds, dust mites, and other sources cause such illnesses as Legionnaires Disease

A common tendency has been to identify a public building's heating, ventilating, and air conditioning (HVAC) system as the cause of indoor air pollution. But that conclusion may be premature and overly nonspecific. The symptoms described by persons affected by the sick building syndrome should be studied closely. At least four separate illnesses have been isolated according to their symptoms and causes. Hypersensitivity Pneumonitis and Humidifier Fever usually produce such symptoms as coughing, wheezing, chest tightness, muscular aches, chills, headache, fever, and fatigue. While these conditions are rarely fatal, Legionnaires Disease, produced by the bacterium *Legionella pneumonophilae,* is notable because of its 15 to 20 percent mortality rate. Both Legionnaires Disease and the relatively less serious Pontiac Fever are identified by their pneumonia-like symptoms.

Carbon Monoxide

Carbon monoxide poisoning is one of the most common dangers of modern living. A colorless, odorless and tasteless gas produced whenever organic, or carbon-containing, substances burn, carbon monoxide can be lethal in poorly-ventilated spaces. The gas rapidly combines with hemoglobin to replace oxygen in the blood. The heart and the brain are most vulnerable, since they rely heavily on oxygen to function properly, and symptoms generally mimic those associated with impaired heart or brain functions: shortness of breath, nausea, headache, fatigue, weakness, dizziness, irritability, and reduced ability to concentrate. During winter is when most deaths attributed to carbon-monoxide poisoning occur, primarily due to clogged furnace exhaust systems and doors and windows too tightly sealed against the cold. Other common sources are tobacco smoke, motor vehicle exhaust, house fires, wood-burning stoves and fireplaces, factory machines with gas-powered engines, charcoal-burning barbecues, kerosene heaters and water heaters that run on gas or oil. Improvements in ventilation systems and public warnings to consumers have lowered the number of carbon monoxide deaths in recent years. In addition, most hardware stores sell carbon monoxide detection devices that sound an alarm when unsafe levels of carbon monoxide are reached. Many cities now require all homeowners and landlords to install them.

Secondhand Smoke

While it has long been established that cigarettes are harmful to smokers, only in the last two decades has research begun to establish the risks of cigarette smoke to nonsmokers, those who passively inhale "secondhand" smoke. In 1986, the Surgeon General's Report examined the smoke inhaled directly by smokers and the smoke passively inhaled by nearby nonsmokers, concluding that the chemical composition of both types of smoke was similar enough to warrant further study and to issue a preliminary warning about the potential dangers. Since then, a heated debate has raged. While some research has linked passive smoking to an increased risk of diseases, including lung cancer, other research indicates a negligible effect. Despite the frequent contradictions in data, public opinion has sided with nonsmokers who fear potential harm from environ-mental tobacco smoke. Fewer and fewer public places even allow smoking and many places, including New York City, Boston, and the state of California, have legislatively declared most public spaces to be smoke-free environments.

The only exception to the debate on the risks of passive smoking are very young children exposed to passive smoke. Studies have proven that pregnant women who smoke not only increase their risk of miscarriage and stillbirth, but also risk delivering infants with low birthweight who, as a result, are highly susceptible to health and development problems. Infants and toddlers of smoking parents have an increased incidence of bronchitis and pneumonia and are much more likely to be hospitalized for respiratory infections than children of nonsmoking parents.

Household Chemicals

Depending on its location, structural characteristics, and other factors, the typical home may have as many as 350 or more organic chemical pollutants in its interior air. Household chemical products like spray paints, insecticides, and furniture polish disperse tiny (and toxic) droplets into the air, adding the propellant to the chemicals in the basic product. Among the hazard-producing chemicals, some solvents in particular are known or suspected carcinogens. One of the worst is methylene chloride, found in paint sprays and paint strippers and in some hair sprays and insecticides. Product labels may identify methylene chloride as a "chlorinated solution" or as "aromatic hydrocarbons."

Radon

After cigarette smoking, say scientists, the second leading cause of lung cancer may be radon gas. Considered by many to be the most dangerous of all indoor air pollutants, radon, a naturally occurring radioactive gas, diffuses out of the ground into houses that happen to be built above subsurface sources.

Invading homes, according to the U.S. Environmental Protection Agency, radon causes between 5,000 and 20,000 lung cancer deaths annually. The gas breaks down into unstable elements called "radon daughters"; these become attached to particles of dust or other matter floating in the air. If breathed in, the radon daughters lodge in the linings of the lungs. Radioactive decay takes place almost at once, with the daughters emitting alpha particles that damage the adjacent lung cells, sometimes causing cancer.

Private homes can be tested for radon and, if hazardous levels are found, can be equipped with ventilation or other equipment to remove the health threat. A charcoal-based detector is available. Finally, many firms can conduct home radon checks for a fee.

Water Pollution

To an increasing extent, water pollution has prevented or limited use of many once-valuable sources of water. This progressive deterioration of the nation's water supply has resulted from years of abuse in which natural lakes and waterways were inundated with quantities of raw sewage, waste products of industrial plants and slaughterhouses, petroleum residues, poisonous herbicides and insecticides, and so on. But the pollutants generally fall into two categories: materials that change with time and contact with water, and materials that remain unchanged in form. Organic materials in sewage and such industrial wastes as pulp and paper effluents belong in the first group; inorganic salts like sodium sulfate and such inert inorganic materials as pesticides represent the second.

Communities generate thousands of tons of municipal sewage daily. Industries, the greatest users of water, utilize more than half of all the water consumed in the United States for raw material, heating and cooling processes, and transporting, sorting, and washing operations. Agriculture, the second largest user, requires millions of gallons of water for irrigation and drainage; for spraying orchards and crops, often with insecticides, fungicides, or herbicides; for removal of animal and other organic wastes; and for manufacturing operations such as meat packing and canning.

Chemical Contamination

The continuing proliferation of chemicals, many of them toxic, suggests the dimensions of the problems relating to water pollution. One estimate by the EPA's Office of Toxic Substances indicated that more than

70,000 chemicals are manufactured or processed commercially in the United States. About 1,000 new chemical compounds are added annually. Literally hundreds of these compounds find their ways into the nation's water supply, some in potentially dangerous concentrations.

How directly and to what degree chemical contaminants contribute to America's health bill cannot be gauged with accuracy. But the roles of these contaminants as carcinogens is widely accepted. Federal health officials have estimated that environmental carcinogens, including those in water, account for 55 to 60 percent of all U.S. cancer cases annually. Some estimates run much higher.

Heavy Metals

A study by the U.S. Geological Survey reported that small amounts of seven toxic metals were present in many of the nation's lakes and streams, with dangerous concentrations occurring occasionally. The metals are mercury, arsenic, cadmium, chromium, cobalt, lead, and zinc. Aside from being generally poisonous, some of these metals are implicated in specific health problems. Cadmium, as one example, has been linked to hypertension caused by kidney malfunction. Some other substances represent special situations.

Mercury

Because mercury is heavier than water, experts thought for years that it could be dumped into lakes, the oceans, and waterways. In theory, the mercury would lie harmlessly on the bottom. In reality, bacteria can convert some of the metallic part of the element into water-soluble form. The new compound enters the food chain and ends up in fish. When dangerous levels of this form of mercury were found in some waters and in food fish, warnings were issued regarding canned tuna and swordfish.

The government later announced that 97 percent of the tuna on the market was safe to eat. But lakes and rivers across the country were closed to commercial and sport fishing.

An extremely toxic substance, mercury can, even in small concentrations, produce blindness, paralysis, and brain damage. The U.S. Food and Drug Administration has established the safe limit of mercury in food at half a part per million—about the equivalent of a thimbleful in an Olympic-sized swimming pool.

PCBs

Among the chief water pollutants today are the *polychlorinated biphenyls* (PCBs), highly toxic chemicals used industrially in carbonless copying paper and as an additive in lubricants, paints, printing inks, coatings, waxes, and many other products. PCBs, which are *biodegradable* (capable of decomposing) only over a period of years, have been found in unusually large quantities in waterways downstream from manufacturing plants. The EPA banned the direct discharge of PCBs into any U.S. waterway in 1977 after tests showed that fish in some rivers, like the Hudson, had levels of PCBs far higher than the permissible levels.

No one knows what the long-term effects of ingesting small quantities of PCBs will be. But the chemical is a suspected carcinogen. PCB's have also caused severe skin and eye irritations and have been implicated in reproductive disorders, kidney damage, and liver ailments. Researchers believe that the millions of pounds of PCBs in the nation's water or in landfills will take many years to dissipate.

Sludge

Sewage treatment plants around the country also face the major health challenge of disposing of the sludge, or solid matter, that is removed from sewage in the treatment process. Sludge contains not only human wastes but the residues of petroleum products, detergents, toxic heavy metals such as cadmium, lead, and zinc, and many other contaminants. Disposal methods range from dumping on land to burning and to composting for use as fertilizer. But environmental experts maintain that the use of sludge as fertilizer constitutes a health hazard; and major food processors will not accept food grown with sludge as fertilizer. In refusing such food, the companies are following guidelines set by the National Food Processors Association, which has expressed concern for farm workers' health and for the health of the consumer.

The sludge comes from an estimated 6.8 billion gallons of sewage flushed daily into America's sewers. The sewage itself contains microorganisms that can endanger health. You may be risking gastrointestinal upsets if you swim at a beach that is posted with a sign proclaiming "polluted water." Scientists warn that the fish caught in sewage-polluted coastal waters and harbors may not only be cancerous, they may also be carcinogenic. A number of states including Michigan and New York have restricted or banned sales of tainted fish such as naturally grown carp, catfish, and striped bass.

Oil Spills

With the increasing reliance on supertankers to carry industrial and heating oil from abroad, the danger of major water-polluting oil spills in coastal areas has grown substantially. Several of these huge ships have gone aground and broken apart under heavy pounding by sea waves. Their cargoes have spilled into the oceans, where currents usually carry them many miles before they float ashore or sink to the ocean floor. The oil reaching land fouls beaches and kills water birds. Similar accidents on inland waterways have polluted rivers and lakes, killing fish and spoiling recreational areas.

Noise Pollution

"Pollution" refers generally to the various forms of physical pollution by liquids, gases, or solids. Few persons realize that we are all threatened by a pollutant so common that it tends to be overlooked: noise.

Noise assails us nearly everywhere. It fills homes with loud music or the dog's barking or the grinding of the washing machine and the workplace with the chatter of drill presses and the roar of huge engines. Neither city dwellers nor country people can live noise-free today; none of us can escape car and truck horns, motorcycles that belch sound, and the noisy throb of machinery.

Effects of Sound on the Eardrum

Noise is not just annoying; it is potentially dangerous, both physically and mentally. It has been described as "a slow agent of death." A form of energy, sound or noise is caused by anything that vibrates, that moves back and forth. Our ears receive the effects of this vibrating motion from a distance, great or small, via sound waves. These waves are successive series of regions of compressed air and partial vacuums, or areas of high and low air pressure. Sound can also travel through liquids and solids. We *hear* sound because our eardrums are moved back and forth by the changes in air pressure. The eardrum, or *tympanic membrane,* may perceive a sound that moves it only one billionth of a centimeter—the threshold of hearing. If the intensity of sound pressure becomes too great, we experience pain, and the eardrum or the delicate structures inside the ear may be damaged.

The intensity of sounds is often measured in units called *decibels,* or *db.* These units are logarithmic, that is, 10 db is ten times as powerful as 1 db, 20 db is 100 times as powerful, 30 db is 1,000 times as powerful, and so on. On this scale, 0 db is at the threshold of hearing; rustling leaves, 20 db; a quiet office, about 50 db; conversation, 60 db; heavy traffic, 90 db; a pneumatic jackhammer six feet away, 100 db; a jet aircraft 500 feet overhead, 115 db; a Saturn rocket's takeoff, 180 db.

For most people, the pain threshold is about 120 db; deafening ear damage can result at 150 db. But damage of various kinds can come from much lower exposures. Temporary hearing impairment can result from sounds over the 85 db now found in modern kitchens with all appliances going. If the ears do not get a chance to recover, the impairment will become permanent.

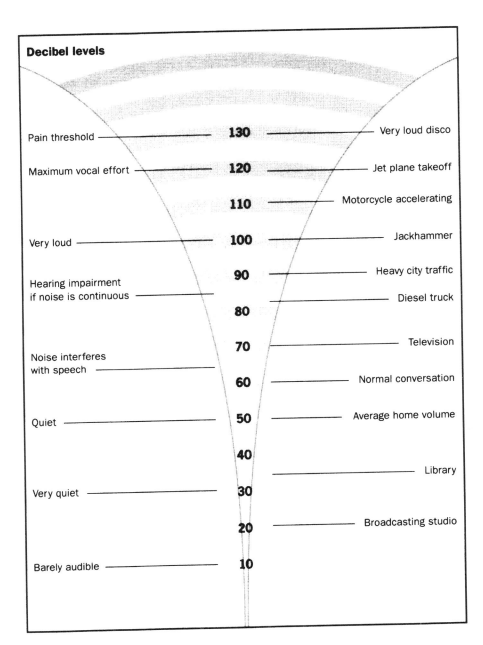

Decibel levels

Pain threshold	130	Very loud disco
Maximum vocal effort	120	Jet plane takeoff
	110	Motorcycle accelerating
Very loud	100	Jackhammer
	90	Heavy city traffic
Hearing impairment if noise is continuous		Diesel truck
	80	
	70	Television
Noise interferes with speech	60	Normal conversation
Quiet	50	Average home volume
	40	
		Library
Very quiet	30	
	20	Broadcasting studio
Barely audible	10	

Damage to the Inner Ear

Although very loud noise can damage the eardrum, most physiological damage from noise occurs in the snail-shaped, liquid-filled *cochlea,* or inner ear. Sound transmitted to the cochlea produces waves in the liquid, which in turn move delicate and minute structures called hair cells or *cilia* in that part of the cochlea known as the organ of Corti. The motion of the cilia is transformed into electrical impulses that conduct the sensation of sound to the brain.

The cilia can easily be fatigued by noise, causing a temporary loss of hearing, or a shift in the threshold of hearing. If they are not given a chance to recuperate, they will be permanently damaged, and irreversible hearing loss will result. There are some 23,000 cilia in the average cochlea; different sets of cilia respond to different frequency bands. The cilia responding to sound frequencies of 4,000 to 6,000 cps (cycles per second) are especially vulnerable to damage. The region of 85 to 95 db is generally regarded as the beginning of dangerous sound intensities. In general, the louder the noise, the longer it lasts, the higher it is, and the purer in frequency, the more dangerous it is. Thus, jet engines and powerful sirens are particularly hazardous.

Noise and Stress

The EPA has estimated that some 20 million Americans live or work at noise levels that could cause hearing losses; about 18 million have experienced at least some hearing loss because of noise exposure. But sound, or noise, can lead to physical and psychological problems ranging from irritability to migraine headaches. Linked with many such problems is stress, which has been found to cause high blood pressure, insomnia, ulcers, digestive disorders, alcoholism, anxiety, and many other ills.

Excessive noise has been implicated in such problems as adrenaline flow, elevated heart rates, and blood pressure. All are associated with heart disease. Noise can also affect children in special ways. For example, researchers believe it can retard language development and impair reading ability. Pregnant women exposed to excessive noise may show symptoms of stress and may pass on the harmful effects to their unborn babies. Studies in several countries have shown that the newborns of women living near airport runways experience a higher than normal incidence of birth defects.

Noise-related stress has a definite effect on mental well-being. No one knows exactly how, but noise can produce irritability, tension, and nervous strain. More seriously, British medical authorities have reported a significantly higher incidence of mental illness among people exposed constantly to aircraft noise.

Workplace Noise

Workplace noise presents special problems. Persons working in such industries as construction, mining, steel, lumber, and textiles are almost universally exposed to loud noises. Certain operations in other industries expose workers to high decibel levels. Overexposure takes place when employees work eight hours a day at sites with noise levels exceeding 90 decibels. Such standards, established by the government's Occupational

Safety and Health Administration (OSHA), provide also that overexposure occurs where workers are subjected to higher decibel levels for shorter periods.

Workplace noise can lead to problems similar to those produced by overexposure elsewhere. But many workers have little choice as regards the places where they work. For their parts, companies may have limited options insofar as noise control or abatement is concerned. Changing the gears of a machine or building an enclosure around it may not always be feasible.

Some professional musicians find it difficult or impossible to avoid excessive noise on the job. Rock music artists, for example, spend hours at a stretch in enclosed places that magnify sound that is already greatly amplified. Such persons may be at serious risk of incurring hearing losses.

Food Hazards

Contaminants found in water often make their way into food products in the cooking and packaging processes, so that many of the comments on water pollution apply here. Some dilute water pollutants become highly concentrated as they pass up the food chain and end in fish or other foods for man. Mercury was cited earlier as one example. Contamination of food with harmful microorganisms is an everpresent concern wherever standards of cleanliness and sanitation are low.

Additives

Food entails a whole new set of problems because of the thousands of new ingredients that have been added to it, directly and indirectly, in recent years. These substances include many that have been deemed necessary because of the revolution in food technology: the rise of packaged convenience foods of all kinds. Labels on today's convenience foods list preservatives, nutrients, flavors, colors, and processing agents. The trouble with food additives is that we have had little time to learn about their long-term effects on the body. The Food and Drug Administration does set standards in this area; but in the opinion of many experts, these safeguards are inadequate.

What do the additives do and what are they? What kinds of health hazards do they present? The principal kinds are explained below.

Nutrients

Some additives are simply vitamins and minerals that increase the nutritional value of food. Iodine is added to salt as a goiter preventative; vitamins A and D go into fortified milk. The vitamin and mineral additives are generally beneficial.

Preservatives

Preservatives do what the name implies: they protect against spoilage from molds, yeasts, or bacteria, or prevent oxidation. In the first category are such substances as salt, sugar, vinegar, and—among the controversial additives—sodium nitrate, sodium nitrite, and the sulfiting agents. Where some of these substances guard against illnesses like salmonella and *Clostridium botulinum,* or botulism, a deadly form of food poisoning, the controversial types may cause serious illnesses and even cancers. For example, nitrates and nitrites can combine with the amines in protein to become nitrosamines, powerful carcinogens.

The antioxidants include lecithin from soybeans, ascorbic acid (vitamin C), and *butylated hydroxytoluene* (BHT) and *butylated hydroxyanisole* (BHA). The latter two have been studied because they appear to protect against stomach cancer and liver damage.

Flavors

Of the more than 1,500 different flavors used in food, some are natural and some synthetic. Among the natural flavors are cinnamon, vanilla, and citrus oils. The synthetics, some of which, like vanillin, have exactly the same chemical compositions as their originals, include monosodium glutamate (MSG), hydrolyzed vegetable protein, and maltol. MSG in particular has become controversial because it can cause "Chinese restaurant syndrome," with temporary headaches, dizziness, and other unpleasant symptoms.

Colors

As a group, the color additives are the most controversial. But they range from beta carotene, a yellow coloring that is used in carrots and sweet potatoes and is beneficial, to a number of coal tar dyes. The FDA has banned as unsafe more than a dozen of the latter in recent years. Others are readily available and are widely used in cereals, baked goods, ice cream, and beverages.

Processing Agents

Many useful processing agents, including yeast and baking soda, are standard kitchen items. They help to control stability, moisture, texture, and other food qualities and characteristics.

Chemical Residues

Some toxic substances found in food appear in the natural environment. An example: the trace amounts of arsenic in cow's milk. Other poisons are introduced into the environment by humans. These, including fungicides, herbicides, and pesticides, have aroused deep concern among environmentalists and a growing number of private physicians.

American farmers use more than 350 approved agricultural chemicals, including about one billion pounds of insecticides annually. Because of such heavy use, about 52 percent of the average American's diet contains one or more kinds of chemical residues. Measured often in parts-per-billion, these can collect in human bodies.

Permanent damage can result, according to researchers. Among the compounds are not only weed- and bug-killers like parathion but also growth-enhancers like daminozide.

Researchers warn of other problems with contaminated food. The use of antibiotics in livestock feed, for example, promotes the development of bacteria that resist antibiotics. As one result, humans who eat beef or pork that is improperly cooked may acquire infections that resist penicillin or tetracycline.

Irradiated Foods

Consumer groups have urged further study and cautious use of irradiation as a means of preserving many foods. At least 30 countries have approved radiation exposure to retard spoilage and aging; but concerns remain. They focus particularly on the nutritional losses thay may occur if foods are exposed to more than one kind of preservative, on the effects of radiation exposure on workers handling irradiated foods, and on environmental hazards that could emerge in the transport, storage, and handling of radioactive food-processing wastes.

The possible long-term effects of irradiation have led to other concerns. Radiation kills the salmonella microorganism, but may not affect more virulent and dangerous bacteria such as those responsible for botulism and may, over time, strengthen those other organisms. Irradiation might even produce dangerous mutations of some bacteria. Researchers point out further that meat can become contaminated after irradiation, indicating that other preservatives might have to be used.

Other Hazards

Toxic Wastes

Various estimates place the number of toxic-waste disposal sites in the United States at 14,000 to 20,000. Poisonous substances left over from industrial processes are buried or simply dumped at these sites, many

of which present serious health hazards. Primarily, according to scientists, the open dumps, landfills, bulk storage containers, and surface impoundments at the thousands of sites spill toxic chemicals into the surrounding soil and through it into groundwater systems. Noxious fumes and even flames burst from some sites at unpredictable moments. The wastes include a huge variety of substances, among them chlorinated solvents, aromatic hydrocarbons, pesticides, trace metals, and PCBs.

The locations of many waste disposal sites remain unknown, often, until a health or environmental problem is detected. Thus the health threats posed by waste dumps may lie dormant for years and may surface only after a container has rusted through or seepage has brought poisonous slush into contact with drinking-water sources.

Waste chemicals can enter the body through skin contact and inhalation as well as ingestion. But the latter is the most common method. Where dosage is substantial, ingestion usually leads to toxic effects on the liver and kidneys. Other parts of the body may be affected as well. Skin contact may produce lesions while inhalation can have direct respiratory effects.

Improved methods of disposing of toxic wastes have combined with public awareness and governmental action to build hopes of reduced waste problems in the future. In the meantime, as environmentalists contend, the thousands of existing toxic-waste sites pose continuing health hazards.

Nuclear Radiation

Among the most dangerous of all pollutants is nuclear or "ionizing" radiation. Made up of particles of energy, this radiation can attack the atoms that form the body's cells, causing both short- and long-term damage. Human tissues like skin, bone-marrow, and intestinal cells, all of which reproduce rapidly, feel the impact of radiation most intensely. But different isotopes in ionizing radiation concentrate in different body tissues, sometimes causing cancer or genetic mutations many years after exposure. Of the most common radioactive elements in radiation from a nuclear power plant, barium resembles calcium and therefore concentrates in the bones while iodine 131 concentrates in the thyroid.

Completely invisible, radiation reaches the earth from various natural and manmade sources. Some comes from the sun and outer space; larger amounts are given off by radioactive materials, including waste from nuclear power plants, the fallout from nuclear weapons explosions, and various electronic devices. The numbers of such devices are increasing steadily; among them are lasers, X-ray machines, TV sets, and microwave ovens.

The damage done to the human body as a result of exposure to radiation varies with the intensity of the "dose" and the isotopes involved. A dose of radiation above 1,000 rem, a unit of measurement, is always fatal. Smaller doses, with exposure over an extended period of time, may also be fatal. Victims can protect themselves to a limited degree if given time. For example, they can guard against thyroid cancer by taking potassium iodide. Ingested in pill form, the medication loads the thyroid gland with iodine, thus "blocking" the iodine 131 isotope and preventing its concentration in the thyroid.

In a simple operation physicians can transplant marrow into persons exposed to the barium isotope, and thus reduce the possibility of bone-marrow syndrome. This illness cripples the body's immune system. But donor marrow must match that of the victim, and the relatives of a victim are those most likely to supply marrow that is a genetic match. If the relatives have also been exposed to radiation, no donors may qualify.

Workplace Dangers

Air and noise pollution are, as noted, common in certain industries. The materials and machines used in manufacturing processes are the usual causes of such pollution. Many controls have been mandated by the federal Occupational Safety and Health Administration, but researchers have reported that some industries are experiencing increased health hazards, largely because of the materials they use.

High-tech microelectronics plants are especially threatened. According to scientists, many such plants use toxic chemicals that have been linked to reproductive disorders in both men and women. Among the high-tech hazards usually cited are glycol ethers, widely used as a solvent by manufacturers of printed circuit boards; arsenic, an element in the manufacture of some semiconductor chips; and lead, used in soldering and other operations. Some semiconductor plants are also employing radiofrequency radiation in potentially dangerous amounts to etch and clean silicon wafers.

Musculoskeletal Disorders

Carpal tunnel syndrome and other neurological and musculoskeletal disorders frequently occur in the workplace and are usually the result of a repetitive motion or series of movements which strain or damage nerves and muscles. Poor posture, uncomfortable or poorly-designed chairs and equipment, and lengthy periods of the same repetitive motion exposes the nerves and muscles of the body, often the hands and arms, to agonizing pain. In most cases, behavior modification, exercises, surgeries, and specially-designed furniture or equipment can completely eradicate pain and incidence of these disorders. A physician should be consulted for individualized diagnosis and treatment.

31

Health Insurance

ealth insurance has two basic purposes. It provides for reimbursement to families or individuals for health care costs. It may also guarantee replacement income when a person is unable to work because of sickness or injury. Reimbursement insurance can cover virtually all types of expenses connected with hospital care, medical treatment, and related services. Disability insurance usually calls for periodic payments to make up for lost income.

From another perspective, health insurance offers protection to both groups and individuals. The groups may be company workforces that have *group insurance* as a benefit. Individuals can buy insurance from as many as 1,800 commercial insurance companies offering a huge variety of plans.

Some insurers are general insurance companies. Others are hospital and medical service plans such as Blue Cross and Blue Shield, group medical prepayment plans such as health maintenance organizations (HMOs), and others.

What Health Insurance Is and Does

"Health insurance" means a number of things. It may be called "accident and health insurance" or "disability insurance." Various types of policies have other names. The different descriptions indicate that the policies vary as regards the types of expenses covered. While some policies cover hospital expenses only, others may cover virtually all kinds of medical expenses.

Two Types of Coverage

In general, private health insurance coverage is one of two kinds: *group* and *individual.* Employers, unions, and other kinds of organizations typically provide group insurance as an employee or membership benefit. An individual can buy individual insurance whether or not he or she is covered under a group policy. But a good group policy usually covers all the major health problems or contingencies that a person could face under normal circumstances.

Group insurance has a number of specific advantages over individual coverage, among them the following:

- Because a number of people can be included under a single contract, with consequent savings to the insurer in sales, administrative, and claims costs, the insurer can charge less per individual covered.

- In most cases the company, union, or organization holding the group contract pays part or all of the individual premiums.

- With group insurance the health of the individual insured person is usually not a major factor in determining eligibility. The insurance company is more interested in the average age and overall health status of the group. The health of individuals may become a selection factor, however, where small groups, 10 or fewer persons, are involved.

- Unless an individual leaves a job or gives up a membership, his or her group coverage cannot be canceled. Termination of the group plan itself would, of course, terminate coverage.

Despite such advantages, individual and family policies fulfill at least two fundamental needs. First, they provide coverage for persons who are not members of an insured group. Such policies may also cover those who cannot, for whatever reason, obtain group coverage. Second, the individual or family policy can provide supplementary coverage where a group plan does not meet all basic health insurance needs.

Group and individual plans differ in basic ways. Where a group policy establishes the level of benefits for all group members, the individual policy can more easily be tailored to specific requirements. With the individual policy, too, each person or family is enrolled separately. The cost of individual insurance is usually substantially higher because the insurer considers the age, health status of the insured, and other factors when setting premium rates.

Principles of Health Insurance

Private or commercial health insurance programs function according to some key principles. Primarily, these programs are based on the theory that a relatively small, regular payment, the premium, can protect the insured against what might be a sizable loss.

A companion principle holds that the insured must pay the expenses of operating an insurance system. These expenses include the costs of maintaining offices, investigating claims, and otherwise administering the system as well as paying benefits.

Two other principles underlie the operation of most health insurance programs:

- The *large-loss principle,* which holds that the insured should try to obtain protection only against those costs or losses that he or she could not bear financially. Under this principle the contract may exclude from reimbursement some specific kinds of costs. Most such policies contain a "deductible"

clause specifying that the insured must pay a certain amount of initial costs.

Major medical insurance plans probably exemplify best the large-loss, or large-risk, principle. These policies nearly always provide for a deductible. The higher the deductible, as a rule, the lower the premium.

- The *first-dollar principle,* under which the policy pays the full cost of all covered hospital and medical expenses. Policies of this kind have no deductible clauses.

Advocates of first-dollar policies stress the need for preventive health care. The policy in theory encourages the insured to see a physician and obtain treatment before a health problem becomes worse or even unmanageable.

Kinds of Insurance Plans

Voluntary or private health insurance plans offer protection against a broad range of hospital and medical expenses. Some policies offer protection against a single illness such as

cancer while others insure individuals, families, or groups against nearly all medical contingencies. Some of the many kinds of coverage are as follows:

Hospital

Blue Cross plans and most other commercial plans provide room benefits at a specified rate per day. Usually, they also cover miscellaneous hospital services, including drugs, operating

room, and laboratory services up to a given cost level. Some commercial plans and most Blue Cross plans cover all costs in a semiprivate, or shared, room.

Surgical

Typically, health insurance policies

cover the costs of surgery according

to a schedule that establishes specified amounts for listed procedures. The insurance contract sets a payment of so many dollars for an appendectomy or a tonsillectomy, for example, with that payment going toward coverage of the surgeon's bill. In the case of Blue Shield, certain surgeons perform surgical operations for low-income subscribers for no additional charge.

Regular Medical

This is a form of insurance that provides coverage of physicians' fees in cases that do not involve surgery. The medical care may be provided in the home, in a hospital, or in a physician's office. A regular medical policy may also cover diagnostic X-ray and other laboratory expenses.

Major Medical

As noted, major medical policies usually provide for deductibles. After an insured has reached a specified hospital-medical expense level, the insurer will also pay, for example, 80 percent of all remaining expenses to a set maximum. The maximum may be $1 million or more. Some policies offer unlimited coverage. In some cases the policy sets a maximum, perhaps $5,000, $10,000, or $25,000, for a given illness in a one- or three-year period. Where an insurance company and the insured pay percentages of all costs beyond a deductible, the policy is said to be a form of "coinsurance."

Comprehensive or Comprehensive Major Medical

This kind of health policy combines hospital, major medical, and surgical coverage in one contract. Generally, little or no deductible applies to hospital and surgical charges. But the major medical coverage ordinarily comes with a deductible.

Dental

Basic or comprehensive protection, covering the costs of hospital care, surgery, and physicians' services, may also include dental insurance. A basic plan may establish a set of allowances for each procedure to an annual maximum of, for example, $500 or $1,000. A comprehensive policy would cover, typically, 80 percent of all dental expenses above a specified minimum.

Special Perils

While frowned upon by many insurance experts, "special perils" plans continue to appear. They cover such specific health hazards as cancer, polio, and vision problems.

Auto and Travel

Many insurance companies offer auto and travel policies that cover insured persons in the event of injury or death in an accident. Such policies may provide protection against almost any travel accident in various kinds of vehicles.

Income

Insurance against loss of income gives the insured person a flow of cash if, because of illness or disability, he or she cannot work. A commercial policy that limits coverage to accidental disability usually costs much less than broader coverage, or it provides for greater benefits. Accidental disability payments, usually monthly, may continue for life. Payments for disability resulting from illness are commonly limited to 6, 12, or more months depending on the terms of the contract.

Many policies provide only for *hospital income insurance*. Such insurance pays a stipulated cash payment for every day of hospitalization. Insurance companies offer these policies to individuals only, not to groups.

Basic Protection

Of the various kinds of comprehensive health insurance, the so-called "basic protection" plan ranks among the most common. Basic protection offers coverage for the costs of hospital care and services and physicians' services.

Most basic protection policies specify that hospital room and board benefits will be paid in one of two ways. One kind of policy provides for reimbursement for actual room and board charges up to a set daily maximum. Another kind offers a service type of benefit equaling the hospital's established semiprivate room and board rates. If the insured occupies a private room, he or she pays the additional room charge.

Surgical-Expense Insurance

Basic policies that provide hospital expense coverage generally offer surgical-expense benefits as well. That means coverage may extend to operations and postoperative, inpatient physicians' visits. The policy then becomes a "hospital-and-surgical-expense" or "hospital-surgical" plan.

Surgical-expense insurance normally pays benefits whether illness or accident makes the surgery necessary. Coverage may include benefits for anesthetics. A schedule of surgical procedures and specified maximum benefits for each may be part of such a policy. Physicians' fees may be covered to a "reasonable and customary" level for the particular city or region. In this case the policy would not contain a surgical schedule.

Physician's-Expense Insurance

The counterpart of the surgical-expense policy is the physician's-expense plan. This policy offers benefits to help cover the costs of nonsurgical physicians' services in a hospital, home, or office. The terms of the policy usually provide for maximum payments for specified services. The latter may include diagnostic X-ray and other laboratory expenses.

Policy Provisions

Purchasing health insurance calls for close attention to the provisions of any given policy. Little standardization exists among the hundreds of types of policies, a factor that makes the buyer's task a difficult one. In four areas in particular the buyer should scrutinize closely the "fine print" in an individual policy.

Provisions Relating to Other Policies

Many policies include clauses that limit or prohibit payments where the policyholder has other insurance covering the same loss or expense. In this way insurers protect themselves against overpayments for specific losses. A typical clause of this kind reduces benefits payments to the policy's prorated share of the insured person's actual expenses.

Cancellation and Renewal

All health policies contain cancellation and renewal provisions. One type, the most favorable to the policyholder, specifies that the insurer cannot cancel or refuse to renew the policy before the insured turns 65. The same clause may state that the premium cannot be increased. Because it provides guaranteed coverage, this kind of policy is usually the most expensive.

Many policies contain a widely used modification of the no-cancel, guaranteed renewal clause. This alternative provides that the company must continue the coverage until the insured reaches 65, but that the premium can be increased for entire groups of insured persons. In a third variation, some policies permit the insurer to cancel or refuse to renew the coverage at anytime by giving written notice to the policyholder. This kind of policy is the least advantageous to the insured.

"Good-Health" Discounts

Increasingly, the disability, hospital, or medical policy provides for discounts for persons in good health. For example, the policy may specify that the applicant be a nonsmoker who exercises three to five times a week and does not have a high-risk job or hobby. Race-car driving would fall in the latter category.

Discounts of 5 to 15 percent have

been available to nonsmokers since the 1960s. New discount arrangements broaden the range of qualifying factors and increase the discount levels. The new trend takes as a model the life insurance plan that may offer discounts of up to 50 percent if the applicant observes basic rules of health and safety. These include, in addition to those named, adhering to a nutritious diet, using seat belts while riding in a car, and avoiding excess salt in diet.

Meeting Special Needs

Some health insurance policies are designed to meet special needs. They tend to provide coverage for individuals with long-term medical problems or chronic health conditions who represent above-average risks for insurers. Special policies may totally exclude coverage for the specified health problem while providing all other standard benefits, or they may impose a waiting period before beginning coverage of the problem. The section below provides more information regarding preexisting medical conditions.

Some insurance policies that were initially designed to meet special needs are now common to the point of being standard. For example, dental-expense coverage is now available through a majority of group and individual insurance plans. Many group policies also make provisions for the cost of eye care.

Making Insurance More Widely Available

From its inception, the health insurance industry has restricted a number of people from obtaining adequate, uninterrupted coverage. Such coverage was denied because of preexisting medical conditions, unemployment or a change in jobs, or a host of other reasons. From July 1997, however, the Kennedy-Kassebaum bill changes the law and effectively ends most of these exclusions.

Preexisting Medical Conditions

Preexisting conditions are physical or health problems which existed before a person's health policy was to take effect. Previously, insurers would not cover claims related to these conditions at all, or at least not for a certain period of time. Now, provided the medical problem has existed for 12 months or more, coverage cannot be denied. It is, however, important to note that people with preexisting conditions may still have to pay higher rates for individual health insurance policies. This is simply because they are above-average risks, and insurers might stand to lose money in paying their claims.

Unemployment and Job Changes

Because most health insurance is a job-related benefit, many people find their coverage terminates when they become unemployed. After July 1997, this can no longer happen, as long as individuals have had insurance for at least 12 months prior to losing their jobs. For those who become unemployed, their former employer's insurer must provide an individual health insurance policy. For those who change jobs, their new employer's insurer must accept them into the group health insurance policy. Individuals who previously did not have insurance, or who had it for fewer than 12 months before losing their jobs, still face being uninsured while unemployed.

Remaining Problems

Even with the improvements of Kennedy-Kassebaum, satisfactory health insurance is not universally available. The mentally ill may find their insurance policies inadequate because the laws regulating coverage of physical ailments do not extend to mental health problems. Additionally, those who depend upon their spouses for coverage in a group plan may find their insurance terminated upon divorce. Many states have enacted laws to provide continued coverage for a short period following the divorce, but as the federal government has not yet addressed this question, laws and policies vary widely.

"Medigap Insurance"

An estimated 95 percent of all Americans over 65 are protected by Medicare. Yet this government program covers only a portion of all possible physician and health expenses. To help bridge the gap between Medicare and the 100 percent coverage that most people want, private insurance companies have developed "medigap" policies.

The terms of these policies vary, but most simply expand existing Medicare coverages. Few offer even partial protection against hospital and medical costs that Medicare does not cover in full or at all. Areas not covered by many medigap policies include hearing tests and hearing aids, most dental care and vision care, and long-term care in-home or at a nursing facility. Clearly, policies with such exclusions still leave people vulnerable. Those trying to supplement their Medicare coverage must search out more complete policies, such as Blue Cross/Blue Shield's.

When considering a medigap policy, consumers are well-advised to first research the reputation of the insurer by calling the Better Business Bureau. Understanding all the terms of coverage before buying the policy will prevent unpleasant surprises later. Basing decisions on premium levels is rarely wise: rates can and do increase at all companies. Finally, older people should make sure they have both parts of Medicare coverage (medical insurance *and* hospitalization) before purchasing additional policies.

Five Innovative Plans

Pressures to cut the costs of medical care have given rise to basic changes in the methods of delivering such care in the United States. Most people no longer call their family physicians and, if so advised, go to the nearest hospital. Insurance plans and programs now offer both more choices and more restrictions. Five programs in particular are changing the face of health insurance.

Health Maintenance Organizations (HMOs)

Operating clinic-style facilities, HMOs require that their subscribers pay a set monthly premium. In return, the HMO provides full medical care. However, members have to select their physicians from a list provided by the HMO. If hospitalization is necessary, the subscriber goes to a hospital selected by the organization.

Charging premiums that are lower than those for equivalent insurance coverage, HMOs provide incentives to avoid unnecessary expenses or treatments. They generally encourage subscribers to make use of preventive care to stay healthy. Thus, most HMOs offer eye and hearing check-ups, as well as podiatric and dental services, at little or no cost beyond the monthly fee.

There are drawbacks for HMO subscribers. Most HMOs try to keep costs low by regimenting the length of hospital stays for specific health problems, i.e. two days for pneumonia, and disregard the individual circumstances of each patient. In some cases, HMO physicians under great pressure to minimize costs have failed to recommend expensive treatments even when they were the most promising options.

HMOs already account for a large share of the health care market. As they grow in number, new and better regulations will be developed to ensure a higher standard of care for subscribers. Many state and federal laws passed in recent years have already contributed to notable improvements in HMOs, and the future is similarly promising.

Preferred Provider Organizations (PPOs)

In the PPO, subscribers receive care at a discount if they go to physicians and hospitals recommended by the insurer. Generally, the insurance company underwriting the PPO allows employees in insured groups to go to a nonparticipating physician. But in such a case the costs of care rise considerably, sometimes to twice those charged by the listed physicians.

Under the PPO arrangement, physicians, hospitals, and insurers work together to keep down overall costs. A PPO hospital provides care for insured persons at reduced rates. In

exchange, the hospital enjoys increased utilization of its facilities.

Managed Care

Unlike the HMO and the PPO, a managed care program gives members the freedom to pick the physicians and hospitals they prefer. But severe cost-containment rules apply. The restrictions may include the following:

• Preadmission reviews of hospital stays by panels of physicians and nurses. A panel would have to agree in all cases, except for maternity care and emergencies, that hospitalization and the proposed care are necessary.

• Reviews during hospitalization to ensure that continued inpatient care is necessary.

• Mandatory second opinions before some operations to make certain a particular procedure is necessary.

• As in some newer group plans, surgery is performed on an outpatient basis where possible.

Companies adopting managed care plans may offer HMO and PPO plans as well. An eligible employee in such a firm then has a choice of program.

Hospital Chains

Competition among health care providers has led to still another approach to both cost control and hospital utilization. Some for-profit hospital chains have bought insurance companies to obtain insurance licenses, then provided health insurance programs that required the insured to use the chain's facilities.

A variation on the HMO and PPO systems, the hospital chain approach makes possible insurance costs that are 10 to 15 percent lower than those of traditional plans. Chain officials

contend that the lower charges are justified by more efficient hospital operation.

Insurance experts note characteristics of the hospital chains' programs that appear to justify caution on the part of the potential buyer. For example, the policies sold by the chains usually impose limits on lifetime benefits. Unlike the plans of such nonprofit groups as Blue Cross/Blue Shield, the chains' policies provide for the termination of certain benefits at specified ages.

Long-Term Care

Increasingly, major insurance companies have begun to devise policies that cover the costs of long-term care for the elderly, in-home or at a nurs-

ing care facility. The terms of these policies vary, and a number of them fall short of expectations. For example, rather than providing a live-in companion as soon as health begins to decline, many insurers will provide in-home care only after a stay in the hospital. Even individuals who have specific in-home care policies find that their insurers use their own stringent guidelines to determine if and when that care is needed.

Such specialized plans face a double financial difficulty. First, the insurance company needs to make a profit. Second, the costs of nursing home and in-home care ranging from $15,000 to $50,000 and more per year raises the possibility of enormous claims that could continue for many years. Some companies work through organizations like the American Association of Retired Persons (AARP). The memberships of such groups are usually large enough to reduce the premiums for the buyers and the risks of major claims for the insurers.

With long-term care policies in particular, it is important for people never to buy more insurance than they can afford, as they may never need to make a claim. They should also plan ahead as far as possible: purchasing coverage for the retirement years in advance of need tends to secure lower premiums and better benefits. And, as with all policies, individuals should understand all the terms of coverage and the exclusions before purchase.

32

Home Care of the Sick

Patients suffering from serious illnesses or from certain communicable diseases should be hospitalized. Home care facilities do not normally include the expensive and delicate medical equipment required for the complete care of these diseases.

If, however, the physician in charge of a case decides that his patient does not need hospitalization and that adequate home nursing care can be provided, the well-being of the patient can be greatly enhanced by his being cared for in the comfortable and familiar surroundings of his own home.

When the decision to treat a patient at home is made, it must be understood that the physician's orders regarding rest, exercise, diet, and medications have to be rigorously adhered to. Nursing responsibilities assigned to the patient and whoever else is tending to the patient's recovery should be carried out as conscientiously as they would be if the patient's care were entrusted to a team of medical professionals in a hospital environment.

The physician in charge of a case should, of course, be notified of any significant changes in the condition of the patient. The physician should be contacted if, for example, the patient complains of severe pain, pain of long duration, or pain that apparently is not directly related to an injury or surgical procedure. The location and characteristics of the pain should be noted, and the physician will want to know whether the pain is affected by changing the position of the patient or if it seems to be related to the intake of food or fluids.

In addition to being informed of such potentially dangerous developments, the physician should get daily or frequent reports on the patient's progress. The easiest and best way to see that this is done is to keep a written record of the following functions, symptoms, and conditions of the patient:

- Morning and evening body temperature, pulse rate, and respiration rate

- Bowel movements—frequency, consistency of stools, presence of blood

- Urination—amount, frequency, presence of burning sensation, color

- Vomiting or nausea

- The amount and kind of solid foods and liquids taken by the patient

- Hours of sleep

- Medications given (should be administered only on the instructions of the physician)

- Patient's general appearance (includes any unusual swelling, skin rash, or skin discoloration)

- General mental and psychological condition of the patient, such as signs of irritability or despondency

Checking the Pulse and Respiration

The pulse and respiration are usually checked in the morning and again in the evening; the physician may recommend other times as well.

Pulse

The home nurse should learn how to measure the pulse rate in beats per minute. A watch with a second hand or a nearby electric clock will help count the passage of time while the pulse beat is counted. The pulse can be felt on the inner side of the wrist, above the thumb; the pulse also can be checked at the temple, the throat, or at the ankle if for some reason the wrist is not conveniently accessible.

The patient should be resting quietly when the pulse is counted; if the patient has been physically active the pulse count probably will be higher than normal, suggesting a possible disorder when none actually exists. Temperature extremes, emotional upsets, and the digesting of a meal also can produce misleading pulse rates.

What is a normal pulse rate? The answer is hard to define in standard or average terms. For an adult male, a pulse rate of about 72 per minute is considered normal. The pulse of an adult woman might range around 80 per minute and still be normal. For children, a normal pulse might be one that is regularly well above 100 per minute. Also, a normal pulse may vary by a few beats per minute in either direction from the average for the individual. The home nurse with a bit of practice can determine whether a patient's pulse is signifi-cantly fast or slow, strong or weak, and report any important changes to the physician.

Respiration

The patient's respiration can be checked while his pulse is taken. By observing the rising and falling of the patient's chest, a close estimate of the rate of respiration can be made. An average for adults would be close to 16 per minute, with a variation of a few inhalations and exhalations in either direction. The rate of respira-tion, like the pulse rate, is higher in children.

Sometimes the respiration rate can be noted without making it obvious to the patient that there is concern about the information; many persons alter their natural breathing rate unconsciously if they know that function is being watched.

Body Temperature

A fever thermometer, available at any drugstore, is specially shaped to help the home nurse read any tiny change in the patient's temperature, such changes being measured in tenths of a degree. Instead of being round in cross-section like an ordinary thermometer, a fever thermometer is flat on one side and ridge-shaped on the other. The inner surface of the flat side is coated with a reflective material and the ridge-shaped side actually is a magnifying lens. Thus, to read a fever thermometer quickly and properly, one looks at the lens (ridged) side.

How To Take the Temperature

The usual ways of taking temperature are by mouth (oral) or by the rectum (rectal), and fever thermometers are specialized for these uses. The rectal thermometer has a more rounded bulb to protect the sensitive tissues in the anus. Normal body temperature taken orally is 98.6° F. or 37° C. for most people, but slight variations do occur in the normal range. When the temperature is taken rectally, a normal reading is about 1° F. higher—99.6° F. or about 37.5° C.—because rectal veins in the area elevate the temperature slightly.

Before a patient's temperature is taken, the thermometer should be carefully cleaned with soap and water, then wiped dry, or sterilized in alcohol or similar disinfectant. The thermometer should then be grasped firmly at the shaft and shaken briskly, bulb end downward to force the mercury down to a level of 95° F. or lower—or 35°

C. or lower if the thermometer is calibrated according to the Celsius temperature scale. See the chart *Body Temperature in Degrees* for comparative values of the Fahrenheit and Celsius scales.

If the temperature is taken orally, the thermometer should be moistened in clean fresh water and placed well under the tongue on one side. If the temperature is taken rectally, the thermometer should be dipped first in petroleum jelly and then inserted about one inch into the opening of the rectum. If an oral thermometer is used in the rectum, special care should be taken to make sure that the lubrication is adequate and that it is inserted gently to avoid irritating rectal tissues. Whichever method is used, the thermometer should be left in place for at least three minutes in

Body Temperature in Degrees		
Fahrenheit		**Celsius**
105.5		40.8
105		40.6
104.5		40.3
104		40
103.5		39.7
103		39.4
102.5		39.2
102		38.9
101.5		38.6
101		38.3
100.5		38.1
100		37.8
99.5		37.5
99		37.2
98.6	Normal	37.0
97.8	Range	36.6

order to get an accurate reading.

If circumstances preclude an oral or rectal temperature check, the patient's temperature may be taken under the arm; a normal reading in that area is about 97.6° F. or 36.5° C.

Above-Normal Temperature

If the patient's temperature hovers around one degree above his normal reading, the home nurse should note the fact and watch for other signs of a fever that would indicate the presence of an infection or some other bodily disorder. A mild fever immediately after surgery or during the course of an infectious disease may not be cause for alarm. Also, the normal body temperature of a mature woman may vary with hormonal changes during her menstrual cycle. But when oral temperatures rise above 100° F. the change should be regarded as a warning signal. A rise of as much as three degrees above normal, Fahrenheit, for a period of several hours or more, could be critical, and a physician should be notified immediately.

Sleep

Another item to be checked each day for the at-home medical records is the patient's sleeping habits. While there is no standard number of hours of sleep per day preferred for healthy individuals, a regular pattern of sleep is very important during recovery from disease or injury, and an obvious change from such a pattern can suggest tension, discomfort, or other problems. Typical daily sleep periods for most adults range from 7 to 9 hours, while children and infants may sleep as much as 12 to 20 hours per day and be considered normal; sleep in the form of naps should be included in total amounts per day.

Making the Patient Comfortable

A good deal of the patient's time at home will be devoted to sleep or rest, most or all of it in bed. The bed should give firm support to the body; if the mattress does not offer such support, place a thick sheet of plywood between the springs and mattress. Pillows can be placed under the head and shoulders of the patient to raise those parts of the body from time to time. When the patient is lying on his back, a small pillow can be slipped under the knees to provide support and comfort. A small pillow can also be placed under the small of the back if necessary. Additional pillows may be placed as needed between the ankles or under one foot or both feet.

If the pressure of bed clothing on the feet causes discomfort, a bridge made from a grocery carton or similar box can be placed over the feet but beneath the blankets. To help maintain muscle tone and circulation in the feet and legs, a firm barrier can be placed as needed at the foot of the bed so the patient can stretch his legs and push against the barrier while lying on his back.

Changing Position

Helping the patient change position in bed is an important home-nursing technique. Unless a definite effort is made to help the patient change positions at regular intervals, the sick person may tend to curl up into a sort of fetal position, with the hips and knees flexed and the spine curved. While this position may be preferred by the patient in order to increase body warmth or to relieve pain, the practice of staying in one position for longer periods of time can lead to loss of muscle tone and even deformities.

Moving or positioning the patient in bed should, of course, be done according to directions outlined by the doctor for the specific medical problem involved. Body movements should not aggravate any injury or other disorder by placing undue strain or stress on a body part or organ system that is in the healing stage. At the same time, the patient should be stimulated and encouraged to change positions frequently and to use as much of his own strength as possible.

If the patient is likely to need a very long period of bed rest, and the family can afford the modest expense, it may be wise to purchase or rent a hospital-type bed. The basic hospital bed is higher from the floor than ordinary beds, making the tasks of changing bed linens, taking temperatures, etc., easier for the home nurse. More sophisticated hospital beds have manual or electrical controls to raise the head and foot of the bed.

Helping the Patient Sit Up

The patient can be helped to a sitting position in bed by placing one arm, palm upward, under the patient's shoulder while the patient extends an arm around the nurse's back or shoulders. The nurse also may slip both hands, palms facing upward, under the patient's pillow, raising it along with the patient's head and shoulders. The same procedures can be used to help move a patient from one side of the bed to the other if the patient is unable to move himself.

When the patient has been raised to a sitting position, he should try to brace his arms behind him on the bed surface with elbows straightened. If the patient feels dizzy or faint as a result of the effort, he can be lowered to the back rest position again by simply reversing the procedure.

When the patient is able to support himself in a sitting position, he should be encouraged to dangle his legs over the side of the bed, and—when his strength permits—to move to a chair beside the bed and rest for a while in a seated position.

Bathing the Patient

A patient who is unable to leave the bed will require special help in bathing. When bath time comes, the nurse will need a large basin of warm water, soap, a washcloth, and several towels, large and small. A cotton blanket also should be used to replace the regular blanket during bathing, and pillows should be removed from the bed unless they are necessary at the time.

One large towel should be placed under the patient's head and another should be placed on top of the bath blanket, with part of the towel folded under the bath blanket. This preliminary procedure should help protect the bed area from moisture that may be spilled during the bathing procedure.

The bath should begin at the area of the eyes, using only clear water and brushing outward from the eyes. Soapy water can be applied to the rest of the face, as needed, with rinsing afterward. After the face, bathing and rinsing are continued over the chest and abdomen, the arms and hands, the legs and feet, and the back of the body from the neck downward to the buttocks. The external genitalia are washed last.

During the washing procedure, the nurse uses firm strokes to aid circulation and checks for signs of pressure areas or bed sores. Skin lotions or body powders may be applied, and a back rub given, after washing. The teeth may be brushed and the patient may want to use a mouthwash. After the personal hygiene routine is completed, a fresh pair of pajamas can be put on. If bed linen needs to be changed, the bathing period provides a good opportunity for that chore.

Changing the Bed Linen

Changing the bed linen while the patient is in bed can be a challenge for any home nurse. However, there are a few shortcuts that make the task much easier. First, remove all pillows, or all but one, as well as the top spread if one is used. Loosen the rest of the bedding materials on all sides and begin removing the sheets from the head of the bed, top sheet first. By letting the patient hold the top edge of the blanket, or by tucking the top edges under his shoulder, the blanket can remain in place while the top sheet is pulled down, under the blanket, to the foot of the bed. If the top sheet is to be used as the next bottom sheet, it can be folded and placed on the side with the top spread.

Next, the patient must be moved to one side of the bed and the bottom sheet gathered in a flat roll close to the patient. Then the clean bottom sheet is unfolded on the mattress cover and the edges, top, and bottom,

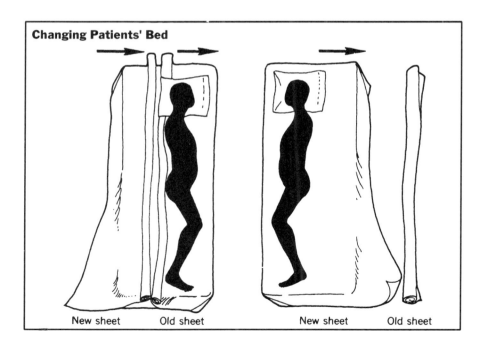

Changing Patients' Bed

New sheet   Old sheet   New sheet   Old sheet

tucked under the mattress. The rest of the clean sheet is spread over the empty side of the bed and pushed in a flat roll under the soiled sheet next to the patient's back.

The next step is to roll the patient from one side of the bed onto the clean sheet that has been spread on the other side. The soiled bottom sheets can be pulled out easily and the new bottom sheet spread and tucked in on the other side.

The new top sheet can be pulled up under the blanket, which has been used to cover the patient throughout the change of bed linens. Finally, the top spread and pillows can be replaced, after the pillow cases have been changed. A special effort should be made, meanwhile, to keep the mattress cover and bottom sheet of the patient's bed as flat and smooth as possible and to allow room for the feet to move while the sheets are firmly tucked in at the foot of the bed.

The home nurse should handle the soiled linens carefully if the patient is being treated for an infectious disease; they should never be held close to the face.

Bowel Movements and Urination

If the patient is expected to remain bedridden for a long period of time, the home nurse should acquire a bedpan and perhaps a urinal from a drugstore. A sheet of oilcloth, rubber, or plastic material should also be provided to protect the bed during bowel movements and urination.

If the patient is unable to sit up on a bedpan because of weakness, his body can be propped up with pillows. If he is capable of getting out of bed but is unable to walk to the bathroom, a commode can be placed near the bed and the patient can be helped from the bed to the commode and back. Another alternative is to use a wheelchair or any chair with casters to move the patient between the bedroom and bathroom.

Administering an Enema

Occasionally, a physician may recommend an enema to help the patient empty his bowels or to stimulate the peristaltic action associated with normal functioning of the intestinal tract.

Since enemas are seldom an emergency aspect of home nursing, there usually is time to purchase disposable enema units from a drugstore. The disposable enema contains about four or five ounces of prepared solution packaged in a plastic bag with a lubricated nozzle for injecting the fluid into the patient's rectum. The entire package can be thrown away after it has been used, thus eliminating the need to clean and store equipment. The alternative is to use a traditional enema bag filled with plain warm water or a prescribed formulation.

An enema is best administered while the patient is lying on his side with his knees drawn up toward his chest. When using the disposable enema unit, the home nurse simply squeezes the solution through the lubricated nozzle that has been inserted into the rectum. When using an enema bag, the home nurse should lubricate the nozzle before insertion.

After insertion of the nozzle, the enema bag should be held or suspended above the patient so that, upon the opening of the valve that controls the flow of the enema, the liquid will flow easily into the patient's rectum.

Feeding the Patient

It may be necessary at times for the home nurse to feed a patient unable to feed himself. An effort should be made to serve meals to the patient in an attractive and, when possible, colorful manner. The bedding should be protected with towels or plastic sheeting and the patient made as comfortable as possible with his head raised.

Liquids should be offered in a spoon filled about two-thirds full with any drops on the bottom of the spoon carefully wiped off. The spoon should be held so that the area between the tip and the side touch the patient's lower lip. Then the spoon is tilted toward the tip so the liquid will run into the patient's mouth. The process takes time, and much patience is required of the nurse. The patient may be slow to swallow and in no hurry to finish the meal.

If the patient can take liquids through a glass tube or plastic straw, the home nurse should see to it that the end of the tube inserted in the container of liquid is always below the surface of the fluid so that the patient will swallow as little air as possible.

A patient who can drink liquids from a spoon or tube may be able to drink from a cup. In making the step from tube or spoon to cup, the home nurse can help the patient by holding the cup by its handle and letting the patient guide the cup to his lips with his own hands.

The nurse should always make sure the patient is fully alert before trying to put food or liquid into his mouth; a semiconscious person may not be able to swallow. The nurse also should test the temperature of the food; cold foods should be served cold and warm foods should be served warm. But foods should never be too hot or too cold for the patient. Finally, the dishes, tubes, or other devices used to feed the patient should be carefully cleaned before storing them.

Ice Bags and Hot-Water Bottles

Ice bags and hot-water bottles frequently are used in home nursing to relieve pain and discomfort. The temperature of the water in a hot-water bottle or bag should be tested before it is placed near a patient's body. The maximum temperature of the water should be about 130° F., and preferably a few degrees cooler. The hot-water container should never be placed directly against the skin of a patient; it must be covered with soft material, such as a towel, to protect the patient against burns. A patient who is receiving pain-killing medications could suffer serious tissue damage from a hot-water bottle without feeling severe pain.

When ice is the preferred method of relieving pain, it can be applied in a rubber or plastic bag sealed to prevent leakage and covered with a soft cloth. Cold applications to very young and old persons should be handled cautiously and with medical consultation, particularly if ice packs are to be applied to large body areas for long periods of time; individuals at both age extremes can lack the normal physiological mechanisms for coping with the effects of cold temperatures.

Steam Inhalators

If the at-home patient suffers from a respiratory ailment that is relieved by steam inhalation, there are several devices to provide the relief he needs. One is the commercial electric inhalator that boils water to which a few drops of a volatile medication are added to provide a pleasantly moist and warm breathing environment. If a commercial inhalator is not available, a similar apparatus can be made by fashioning a cone from a sheet of newspaper and placing the wide end of the cone over the top and spout of a teapot containing freshly boiled water. The narrow end of the cone will direct the hot water vapor toward the face of the patient. If a medication is to be added, it can be applied to a ball of cotton placed in the cone; the steam or water vapor will pick up the medication as it passes through the cone.

If medicated vapor is intended for a small child or infant, the end of the cone can be directed into a canopy or tent made of blankets placed over a crib or the head of a bed. This arrangement should produce an effective respiratory environment for the child while keeping his body safely separated from the hot teakettle.

Still another method of providing steam inhalation for a patient requires only an old-fashioned washstand pitcher and bowl plus a grocery bag. An opening is cut in one corner of the bottom of the bag which is placed upside down over the pitcher filled with hot steaming water and, if needed, a medication. The patient simply breathes the hot moist air seeping through an opening in the bag. The pitcher of steaming water is placed in a bowl or basin as a safety precaution.

Improvising Sickroom Devices

With a bit of imagination, many sickroom devices can be contrived from items already around the house. A criblike bed railing can be arranged, for example, by lining up a series of ordinary kitchen chairs beside a bed; if necessary, they can be tied together to prevent a patient from falling out of bed. The bed itself can be raised to the level of a hospital bed by placing the bed legs on blocks built from scrap lumber. Cardboard boxes can be shaped with scissors and tape into bed rests, foot supports, bed tables, or other helpful bedside aids.

Plastic bags from the kitchen can be used to collect tissues and other materials that must be removed regularly from the sickroom. Smaller plastic bags may be attached to the side of the bed to hold comb, hairbrush, and other personal items.

Keeping Health Records

The family that keeps good records of past injuries and illnesses, as well as immunization information and notes on reactions to medications, has a head start in organizing the home care of a member who suddenly requires nursing. The file of family health records should include information about temperatures and pulse rates taken during periods of good health; such data can serve as benchmark readings for evaluating periods of illness. Also, if each member of the family can practice taking temperatures and counting pulse and respiration rates during periods of good health, the family will be better able to handle home nursing routines when the need arises.

Home Care Equipment Checklist

Following is a convenient checklist of basic supplies needed for home care of the sick:

1. Disinfectants for soaking clothing and utensils used by the sick. Not all disinfectants are equally effective for every purpose. For clothing and food utensils, corrosive or poisonous disinfectants are to be avoided. Antiseptics do not kill bacteria; they only retard their growth. Among the common disinfectants that can be used in the home are:

- Alcohol, 75 percent by weight, used for disinfecting instruments and cleaning the skin

- Lysol, for decontaminating clothing and utensils

- Soap with an antibacterial agent for scrubbing the hands

- Carbolic acid (phenol) for disinfecting instruments and utensils (it is corrosive, poisonous, and very effective if used in 5 percent solution)

- Cresol in 2.5 percent solution for disinfecting sputum and feces (less poisonous than phenol and can be obtained as an alkali solution in soap)

- Boric acid, a weak antiseptic eyewash

- Detergent creams, used to reduce skin bacteria

2. Disposable rubber gloves, to be used when handling patients with open wounds or contagious diseases, as well as for cleaning feces.

3. Paper napkins and tissues for cleaning nasal and oral discharges.

4. Rectal and oral thermometers. The former is used primarily for infants, while the latter is used for adults and older children. Thermometers should always be thoroughly disinfected after use by soaking in isopropyl alcohol, and they should be washed prior to reuse.

5. Eating and drinking utensils to be used only by the patient. Disposable utensils are preferable.

6. Urinal, bedpan, and sputum cup for patients who cannot go to the toilet. After use, they should be thoroughly disinfected with cresol and washed with liquid soap containing an antibacterial agent.

7. Personal toilet requisites: face cloths and towels, toilet soap, washbasin, toothbrush and toothpaste, comb, hairbrush, razor, and a water pitcher (if running water is not accessible to the patient).

8. Measuring glass graduated in teaspoon and tablespoon levels for liquid medication.

9. Plastic waste-disposal bags that can be closed and tied.

33

Health Care Delivery

A Changing Service

Unending change has characterized American health care in recent decades. The general practitioner in private practice, once the institutionalized symbol of medical care in the United States, has largely given way to specialists of many kinds. Where the general practitioner once sent a handwritten bill for services to the family home, he or she may now send a computerized invoice to an insurance company or a government agency. The "house call" has virtually disappeared.

Technology has taken over. Hospitals and other health care institutions may pay sums in seven figures for equipment that can save lives but that also demands to be used. A "technological imperative" requires that the new approach or instrument or drug at least be tried—experimented with, proven useful or useless, and made available to those who need it. In diagnosis and therapy in particular, physicians and other professionals are continually seeking the new and better.

Some seven million people work in the American health care system. Half a million of those are physicians. The facilities in which the system's personnel work range from rural clinics to high-technology urban medical centers. On balance, the consumer dealing with this system has many choices. Understanding those choices may make the difference between a beneficial experience and a frustrating search for help.

Health care reaches the American public at three broadly defined levels. The three are primary, secondary, and tertiary care.

Primary Care

Essentially, *primary care* refers to "first contact" care as provided in physicians' offices or hospitals. Such care may also be provided in emergency rooms and outpatient clinics. The individual can obtain primary care without referral by a physician, but referrals from this level of care are generally necessary to ensure that the patient will receive treatment at the next higher level. Among the types of services provided at the primary care level are health maintenance for infants and children, screening for infectious and communicable diseases, and treatment for minor injuries.

Secondary Care

At the *secondary care* level the patient usually comes under the care of a specialist, often in a community hospital or other, similar setting. Secondary level specialties include such well-known areas of medicine as obstetrics and gynecology, dermatology, otolaryngology, and cardiology. While physicians often refer their patients for secondary level care, many persons "refer themselves."

Tertiary Care

At the tertiary care level, the patient receives highly specialized, high-technology care and treatment. Complex programs and unusual procedures, among them open heart surgery, heart or kidney transplantation, and neurological surgery, are provided by physicians with extensive training and the advantages of sophisticated equipment for diagnosis and treatment. Often, care at this level is obtainable only if the patient enters a hospital with specialized facilities. Of the various tertiary care institutions, three key ones are hospitals specializing in a certain disease or a group of diseases, hospitals associated with medical schools, and large regional referral centers. Many such institutions would be expected to have diagnostic equipment for such procedures as cardiac catheterization, nuclear magnetic resonance testing, and CT scanning.

Importantly, the three levels of care overlap. The distinctions among them are not always clearly drawn or defined. For the patient, the most important factor may be the need for referrals at some levels and not at others.

Health Care Delivery Formats

The average American visits a physician five times a year. That statistic appears in a U.S. Public Health Service survey that also defines a visit as an encounter with a physician or other health professional under a physician's direction or supervision. The "encounter" can take place in the physician's office, in the patient's home, by telephone, or in some other ambulatory care setting. The physician initiates about half of the encounters, usually as part of follow-up care.

Office and Clinic Care

In the main, the patient sees his or her physician in an office or at a site reserved for group practice; in a hospital outpatient department; in an ambulatory surgical center; or in a freestanding surgical center.

Office-Based Practice

Most physicians practice on their own; even so, the solo practice is declining as a way of medical life. The solo practitioner survives in isolated or rural areas, but hardly at all elsewhere. For the physician, solo practice is both simpler because of the independence and freedom it guarantees and more complex because the service responsibility may continue 24 hours a day, seven days a week. For the patient, the main advantage of solo practice is both the closer relationship that can develop and less fragmented care.

Partnerships

Very common today is the partnership, an agreement between two or more physicians under which the participants share office space, staff, and equipment. The physicians retain their independence in the sense that they have their own practices, but they usually share patient responsibilities under given circumstances. A physician who has to be out of contact with the office may, for example, give a patient another partner's number so as to have continuous backup. Spreading the care responsibilities and reducing the workload, each physician may also have more time for each patient.

The patient may find major advantages in the partnership. He or she can become acquainted with the physician's partner and in this way obtain personalized care at all times. Backup support may be especially important in obstetrics, where deliveries may occur without warning, and in cardiology, where emergencies are equally unscheduled.

Groups

Where three or more physicians associate in an arrangement that is normally less formal than a partnership, it is termed a *group*. The physicians belonging to the group may practice in a single specialty or in diverse fields of medicine. An example of the latter would be a group of three doctors offering internist, obstetrics-gynecological, and pediatric services. In other ways the group shares the advantages and disadvantages of the typical partnership. Like the partnership, the group has one particular advantage, however: other physicians are available for consultation and education. The group format may also make possible relatively sophisticated laboratory and other facilities.

Health Maintenance Organizations

The health maintenance organization (HMO) ranks as a special kind of group practice, one that involves a fixed monthly or annual fee system rather than a fee-for-service arrangement. The fixed fee ensures that the HMO member will receive, at no additional charge, all necessary health services, including hospitalization and the care of specialists. Preventive medicine at no extra cost to the member is a feature of the HMO that has ensured reduced usage of hospital facilities.

Preferred Provider Organizations

Like the HMO, the preferred provider organization (PPO) is at least partly a response to rising health-care costs. Forming a PPO, a group of physicians contracts individually with an insurance company or employer to provide health services for fees that are usually lower than those prevailing in the community or area. The PPO does charge on a fee-for-service basis, but employees making use of the organization's medical services save money because they avoid the copayments of conventional insurance plans and the standard deductibles. Physicians belonging to the PPO have a stable pool of employed members whose health problems may be extremely diverse. For the employer or insurance company, a particular advantage is the ability to bargain for lower fees.

Three Alternative Systems

Obviously, office and clinic care takes many forms. Three alternatives that provide relatively minor, low-level services are the hospital outpatient department, the ambulatory surgical center, and the freestanding emergency center. Each plays a particular role in the health care delivery network.

Hospital Outpatient Departments

Outpatient departments once offered free services as a means of training medical students and residents or because physicians volunteered their services for such departments. Today, outpatient departments charge for their services while delivering health care that varies broadly as regards quality. One hospital in three has an outpatient department or a clinic for ambulatory care while nine of ten community hospitals offer outpatient care in their emergency departments.

Ambulatory Surgical Centers

Sometimes called surgicenters, the ambulatory surgical center may be attached to a hospital or be completely independent. In either case, the surgicenter may be an effective alternative in the traditional situation where a patient needs an abortion, a dilatation and curettage (D & C), hernia repair, or tissue biopsy. Because they perform lower-risk procedures, ambulatory surgical centers can keep costs down. Local anesthesia is the norm, and usually the patient goes home on the day of the operation.

Freestanding Emergency Centers

Sometimes called *urgicenters,* freestanding emergency centers resemble hospital emergency departments. But private, for-profit groups usually run them. Open from 12 to 24 hours daily, they operate on a drop-in basis, meeting a definite need where a hospital emergency room is far away or when all physicians' offices have shut down for the day. Typically, emergency centers treat sprains and bruises, cuts that require stitches, and upper respiratory infections. Charges for such services usually range from visits to physicians' offices on the low side to hospital emergency rooms on the high side.

Community Health Care Facilities

Providing more evidence of the complexity of the United States' health care delivery complex, community health facilities fill a void in health services at a very basic level. At least five different modes of providing health care need to be considered as community facilities.

School and College Health Programs

Once concerned primarily with the control of communicable diseases and screenings for dental, vision, and hearing problems, school and college health programs have taken on new functions. At the elementary and high-school levels, they may help with health and sex education programs, keep vaccination records, and consult with parents. Colleges and universities generally provide infirmary services, meaning inpatient care for acute illness. At larger schools, programs may deal with contraception and pregnancy problems, substance abuse, and neuroses.

Industrial Health Programs

Treatment of work-related injuries and minor illnesses remains a key function of industrial health programs. The programs also continue to give minor physical exams and to provide general medical and dental care. But they have expanded their services in recognition of the value of preventive medicine. Newer or more modern programs offer comprehensive work-site education and screening programs, alcohol abuse counseling, stop-smoking clinics, and aerobic fitness classes.

Health Screening

Provided by local health departments and voluntary health agencies (see Chapter 36), health screening varies from community to community as regards both availability and reliability. Depending on community funding, a local health department may or may not provide tests that screen for infectious or parasitic diseases, including sexually transmitted diseases (see Chapter 17), and chronic disorders such as high blood pressure, sickle cell anemia, or diabetes. Many health departments make referrals to follow-up medical care.

Neighborhood and Primary Health-Care Centers

Neighborhood and primary health-care centers were established first in the 1960s to provide ambulatory care in underserved communities, both rural and urban. Staffed often by U.S. Public Health Service medical personnel or by nurse practitioners, the centers either limited their services according to income requirements or served specific communities. Because of cuts in federal spending, experts note, many such centers have been or are being phased out.

Women, Infant, and Child Care

Also federally funded, the women, infant, and child care program emphasizes provision of well-baby care, nutritious food, and nutrition education for pregnant women, infants, and children under three. Estimates indicate that the program saves three dollars for every dollar spent. But federal budget cuts have begun seriously to scale back the program.

Disease Prevention and Control

County or city health departments usually establish disease prevention and control programs to help control the spread of communicable diseases. Methods used include immunization, screening, and follow-up. Typical concerns include immunization for childhood diseases like diphtheria, measles, and polio; tuberculosis and sexually transmitted diseases; and influenza immunization for older persons.

Hospitals

Viewed a century ago as a death-house, the hospital has a new image. With an entirely revised role built on its ability to provide comforts and even amenities, the hospital has added a "hotel" function to its fundamental "healing" function. But the hotel role does not affect the hospital's main medical purpose: to provide, within budgetary and other limits, sophisticated, technologically up-to-date care. The hospital has become the place to go for diagnostic and therapeutic care that a physician's office cannot provide.

A basic method of classifying hospitals is by length of the patient's stay. Viewed this way, hospitals fall into two groups, long-term or extended-care institutions and short-term hospitals. The former will be discussed later; the second group includes community, teaching, and public hospitals.

Community Hospitals

Most Americans receive medical care in community hospitals. Usually quite small, with 50 to 500 beds, this kind of hospital generally provides good to excellent secondary-level care. Traditionally, community hospitals were nonprofit corporations that depended heavily on community support. Today, the community hospital is increasingly likely to be proprietary. That means it is run for profit by investor-owned groups or corporations.

The costs of medical care at a proprietary community hospital may not be significantly different from those charged by a voluntary or nonprofit hospital.

Teaching Hospitals

Ranging in size from a few hundred to a few thousand beds, teaching hospitals universally offer training for undergraduate medical students, postgraduate students, or fellows. Also, nearly all have ties to major medical schools. A state government may own a teaching hospital that is used by state medical schools; others are owned by the associated university or by a nonprofit corporation. Teaching hospitals provide care at all three levels.

Public Hospitals

Public hospitals include not only county hospitals but others supported by public funds, among them public health service hospitals, Veterans Administration (VA) hospitals, and municipal short-term-stay hospitals. Many such institutions that are owned by federal, state, or city governments are teaching hospitals, and many also have associated rehabilitation units and nursing homes.

The Elderly: Home Care

Surprisingly, most elderly persons live at home and receive care from relatives and others who may visit the home to help out. Younger family members may need home care because of illness or injury, but typically the disabled or ill older person is the one receiving such care. A number of community resources are available to make home care—or self-care for those living alone—easier. These resources include home health workers, such services as Meals-on-Wheels, and various day-care programs.

Invaluable aids for those responsible for home care for an aging relative are unskilled companions and temporary help. With this kind of assistance, the elderly person may be able to enjoy continuity of care and independence while maintaining ties with family, home, and community.

Home Health Services

Some 2,500 home health agencies operate under the general direction of physicians to provide two kinds of services: skilled and supportive. Of the many types of home health service providers, the best known are private, either profit-making or nonprofit; public health agencies such as neighborhood health centers; hospital-based services; and local or county health department or community and church programs. The nationwide Visiting Nurses Association is perhaps the most familiar.

Different communities and areas enjoy different levels and types of home health services. But most such agencies provide care to anyone who requests it. Fees vary, and may be paid by the individual or the family accepting the care. In other cases the government or individual insurance plans may reimburse the family, partially or totally, for the fees charged. Hospital social workers or discharge-planners, the Area Agency on Aging, the local office of the Social Security Administration, day-care centers, and churches and synagogues normally provide information on home health services.

Voluntary Health Agencies

Many voluntary health agencies provide aid and support to the disabled or sick elderly person (see Chapter 36). Such groups and organizations as the American Cancer Society and the Easter Seal Society may even offer "friendly visitor" services in specific communities. Most of the groups see education of the public as functional to their roles. Thus they may provide films, lecturers, books and pamphlets, and other materials of interest to groups and organizations of many kinds. Many such agencies have specialized equipment for those who need it as well as listings of community resources.

Drugstores and Medical Supply Houses

Two other basic sources of specialized equipment and sickroom supplies, the medically oriented drugstore and the medical supply house, play important roles. In many cases the family discharging home care responsibilities can obtain wheelchairs, walkers, portable oxygen equipment, and hospital beds from one source or the other. Often, the supplier will rent or sell the specialized equipment; the choice may be the family's to make.

Community Facilities for the Aged

An entire new category of health care facilities has come into being in recent years in response to the needs of the elderly. These community facilities are designed specifically for those elderly persons living at home who are not housebound.

Adult Day Care

A broad variety of community-based centers schedule adult day-care programs for the elderly. To some extent the programs provide an alternative to institutionalization. In each case the programs are tailored to meet specific needs. Each type has a basic therapeutic objective.

Medical Day Care

Where chronically ill or disabled persons do not require frequent or intensive medical intervention, the medical day care service may be the solution. Located usually in a long-term care institution or freestanding center, such a care service may include nursing and other supports. A physician's referral is required, and rehabilitation and maintenance are primary therapeutic goals. Reimbursement is by third-party (insurance company) payments on a sliding scale. Medicaid pays for medical day care in some states.

Mental Health Day Care

Offering a supervised environment along with mental health services to adults with organic or functional mental illness, the mental health day care service is usually located in a psychiatric institution or freestanding center. Referral by a psychiatrist is required. Three basic therapeutic goals are supervision, assistance with coping skills, and safety for the patient. Reimbursement is by third-party payment.

Social Adult Day Care

Title XX of the Social Security Act provides for funding of many social adult day care facilities, all of which are geared to the needs of adults who have difficulty functioning independently. Both families and health facilities can make referrals, but examination by a physician is normally required before admission. Third-party reimbursement is the norm. Program objectives and services vary widely, and are usually formulated by the funding source and the sponsoring organization. Program participants may attend part-days or full days five days a week; the facility may provide a midday meal and transportation within a specified area.

Nutrition Services

Nutrition ranks as a critical need for both homebound and more independent elderly persons. Meals-on-Wheels, a community service offered under voluntary auspices but funded partly by public funds, caters to the homebound. For a reasonable charge the service provides at least one hot meal daily for persons 60 and older. For the elderly attending senior centers, the Area Agency on Aging provides both adequate nutrition and a chance to socialize. Agency personnel can keep in touch with clients' physical and social situations, giving the program an important outreach and prevention dimension.

Extended-Care, Long-Term Care, Nursing Homes

Closely related, the extended-care facility, long-term care facility, and nursing home nonetheless meet different needs. A relatively recent innovation, the extended-care facility provides a service that falls between that given in an acute-care hospital and that provided in a skilled nursing facility or nursing home.

Extended-Care Facility

Despite its name, the extended-care facility provides short-term inpatient care. This type of facility is designed mainly to aid patients who have been hospitalized but no longer need the full complement of hospital services. Such patients still require professional nursing and medical supervision. Typically attached to a hospital, the extended-care facility may also serve those who are not acutely ill but who require skilled care.

Because most extended-care facil-ities are physically attached to hospitals, patients often simply move from one hospital wing to another. Some nursing homes also meet the standards set for qualification as extended-care facilities by the Joint Commission on the Accreditation of Hospitals (JCAH). For the most part, extended-care facilities charge much less than the typical hospital.

Long-Term Care Facilities

Patients with chronic conditions that cannot be treated effectively in a general hospital generally qualify for care in a long-term care facility. Such conditions range from tuberculosis to mental retardation. The facilities also include chronic disease hospitals, rehabilitation hospitals, and psychiatric hospitals for both children and adults.

Nursing Homes

Also falling in the category of long-term care facilities, nursing homes comprise a special group of facilities of different kinds. They offer services ranging from sheltered living arrangements to around-the-clock nursing care. All nursing homes rank as residential facilities.

The approximately 18,000 nursing homes in the United States have between 1.3 and 1.5 million beds. Three-quarters of these nursing homes are proprietary, or for-profit, institutions that house about two-thirds of all the beds. Nonprofit organizations operate 15 percent of all the nation's nursing homes and make available about 20 percent of the beds. The government operates the remaining homes.

Nursing homes accommodate persons of all ages. A few younger residents have serious congenital illnesses or disorders, or have been recently discharged from a hospital. Others are recovering from recent surgery. But most patients are the chronically ill elderly. Typically, a nursing home resident is a woman in her 80s, single or widowed. Afflicted with three or more serious chronic illnesses, she has very likely exhausted all her assets except her monthly Social Security payments.

Residential-Care Facilities

Standing at the lowest level of nursing home care, the residential-care facility is usually appropriate for the person who can no longer live alone and manage household chores. This "typical" resident does not need extensive medical attention but does require sheltered living, prepared meals, and some medical monitoring. The latter may include supervision of medications and tracking of signs and symptoms.

Intermediate-Care Facilities

The intermediate-care facility supplements typical RCF services with regular, but not round-the-clock, nursing care for residents who are unable to survive on their own. The intermediate-care facility may also make provision for social and recreational activities. Programs of physical therapy and rehabilitation, occupational therapy, speech therapy, and social work services may also be offered.

Skilled Nursing Facilities

With staffs of registered nurses, licensed practical nurses, and nurses' aides, skilled nursing facilities can provide 24-hour care. They are, thus, appropriate for persons in need of intensive nursing care and rehabilitation. Like intermediate-care facilities, skilled nursing facilities are state-certified for the most part, a factor that makes them eligible for public funds as payment for services. Lack of certification may mean that an ICF or SNF has serious deficiencies.

Hospices

Described sometimes as more a philosophy than a type of physical facility, hospice is a form of care for the terminally ill. While a normal medical setting concerns itself with healing a patient, the hospice environment concentrates on palliative treatment, in effect, treating and addressing pain and other symptoms of an incurable disease. Hospice programs emphasize quality, not length of life. Hospice treats dying as a normal process, and strives to help patients live comfortably and productively in their last days or months. Patients enter hospice programs at their own requests. A physician's referral, indicating that the prognosis is no more than six months, may also be required.

There are a variety of hospice settings. A hospice may be in a wing of a hospital or a separate building or institution. Many hospice programs are available to people in their homes. Families provide much of the care, though they are assisted by a team of hospice workers. The team provides continuity between home and hospice when patients must be institutionalized. At all times, the individual patient's comfort is a prime consideration.

For general information on hospice, contact The Hospice Association of America 228 Seventh Street, SE, Washington, DC 20003-4306.

34

Voluntary Health Agencies

Major Agencies

The establishment of more than 100 voluntary health agencies since the beginning of this century has been a major factor in the growth of health services to the American public. These agencies, whose activities are made possible by donations of time and money from the public, occasionally augmented by government grants for special projects, have the following objectives: spreading information about various diseases to the professional and lay public; sponsoring research; promoting legislation; and operating referral services on the community level to patients in need of diagnosis, treatment, and financial aid.

Some of these agencies, such as the American Diabetes Association, the Arthritis Foundation, the Cystic Fibrosis Foundation and United Cerebal Palsy, focus on a particular disease; others deal with problems arising from related disorders, such as the National Mental Health Association, the American Heart Association, the National Kidney Foundation, and the National Easter Seal Society.

To coordinate the activities of these many groups, to promote better health facilities, and to establish standards for the organization and conduct of these agencies, the National Health Council was founded in 1920. Its membership includes business and industrial, nonprofit, and professional organizations, as well as the 46 voluntary health agencies described below, which command a total budget of almost $4.3 billion and involve the services of almost 12 million volunteers.

All of these organizations function

on the national, state, and community level. Information and literature may be obtained through local chapters or by writing to the national office of the organization. Volunteers may offer their services in a variety of ways: as office workers, fund raisers, speakers, and community coordinators.

On the following pages, voluntary health agencies are discussed under the subjects with which they are concerned; the subjects are arranged alphabetically. Following these agencies is a brief discussion of other voluntary health agencies. Because of limitations of space, however, many worthwhile organizations have had to be omitted.

Accident Prevention

The National Safety Council, 1121 Spring Lake Drive, Itasca, Illinois 60143-3201; (630) 285-1121, was founded in 1913 to improve factory safety but soon broadened its activities to preventing every type of accident. The Council is now composed of groups and individuals from every part of the population: business, industry, government, education, religion, labor, and law. Its main efforts are devoted to building strong support for official safety programs at the national, state, and community levels in specific areas, such as traffic, labor, and home.

The Council believes that practically all accidents can be prevented with the application of the right safeguards. These safeguards include public education and awareness of danger, enforcement of safety laws and regulations, and improved design standards for machines, farm equipment, and motor vehicles.

It maintains one of the world's largest libraries of accident prevention materials, distributes a wide variety of safety literature, and issues awards for outstanding safety achievements. It also serves as a national and international clearing house of information about the causes of accidents and how they can be prevented.

In addition to campaigning for increased safety legislation on the national and state level, the Council's current programs include a defensive driving course, which provides effective adult driver training on a mass scale; a safety training institute; environmental and occupational health and "Right-to-Know" educational materials; and several approaches to the alcohol and driving problem.

Its publication, *Family Safety and Health,* is sold to companies who distribute it free to employees, and its manual called *Fundamentals of Industrial Hygiene* provides more than 1,000 pages of material essential to the safety of factory workers.

The Council in recent years has expanded its safety promotion work to include both on- and off-the-job safety for workers and their families, as well as 24-hour-a-day safety for all persons in all activities.

Alcoholism

The National Council on Alcoholism and Drug Dependence, 12 W. 21st Street, New York, New York 10010; (800) 622-2255, is the only national voluntary health agency founded to combat alcoholism as a disease by an extensive program on the professional and community level. The Council is completely independent of Alcoholics Anonymous, although the two organizations cooperate fully.

In more than 100 cities where the Council has affiliates, alcoholism information centers have been established that provide referral services for alcoholics and drug addicts and their families as well as educational materials for all segments of the community, including physicians and nurses, the clergy, the courts, social workers, and welfare agencies. Local affiliates also help to develop labor-management programs that provide help for employees who suffer from the disease.

The Council also sponsors research, professional training, and legislative action. Its publications department distributes a variety of fact sheets, pamphlets, posters, and videos. For a listing of publications or information on the Council's programs, write the national headquarters or contact the nearest local affiliate.

Arthritis

The Arthritis Foundation, 1330 West Peachtree Street, Atlanta, Georgia 30309; (800) 283-7800, was established to help arthritis sufferers and their physicians through programs of research, patient services, public health information, and education on the professional and popular level. Its long-term goal is to find the cause, prevention, and cure for the nation's number one crippling disease.

The Foundation operates local chapters throughout the United States whose chief concern is the patient who has or might have arthritis. These chapters are centers for information about the disease itself and also serve as referral centers for treatment facilities. In addition, they distribute literature and sponsor forums on the latest developments in research and patient care.

Some chapters support arthritis clinics and home care programs; most conduct patient self-help programs such as discussion groups and exercise classes. Parent groups are often maintained for parents of children with arthritis.

Two special groups work within the Foundation: the Association of Rheumatology Health Professionals, which devotes itself to continuing education for health professionals caring for arthritis patients and the American Juvenile Arthritis Organization for those with a special interest in arthritis in children. A major part of the Foundation's work at the national level is providing funds for fellowships to young physicians and scientists so that they may continue their work in arthritis research and in funding through an-nual grants research at major institutions throughout the United States.

Cancer

The American Cancer Society, 1599 Clifton Rd. N.E., Atlanta, Georgia 30329; (800) 227-2345, was established in 1913 by a small group of physicians and volunteer workers to inform the public about the possibility of saving lives through the early diagnosis and treatment of cancer. The Society has 3,400 offices located in all 50 states plus Puerto Rico, devoted to the control and eradication of cancer. In addition to the physicians, research scientists, and other professional workers engaged in the Society's activities, more than two million volunteers are connected with its many programs.

The American Cancer Society conducts widespread campaigns to educate the public in the importance of annual medical checkups so that cancerous symptoms can be detected while they are still curable. Such checkups should include an examination of the rectum and colon and, for women, examination of the breasts and a Pap test for the detection of uterine cancer.

In another of its campaigns, the Society emphasizes the link between cigarette smoking and lung cancer. It also sponsors an extensive program to persuade teenagers not to start smoking. During its annual April Crusade against Cancer, the Society distributes approximately 40 million copies of a leaflet containing lifesaving information on early detection of cancer.

On the professional level, the major objective of the Society is to make every physician's office a cancer-detection center. To achieve this goal, it publishes a variety of literature, offers refresher courses, sponsors seminars, and cooperates closely with local and state medical societies and health departments on the diagnosis and treatment of cancer. It also arranges national and international conferences for the exchange of information on the newest cancer-fighting techniques, and finances a million-dollar-a-year clinical fellowship program for young physicians.

Among its special services to patients are sponsorship of the International Association of Laryngectomies, for people who have lost their voices to cancer; and Reach to Recovery, a program for women who have had treatment for breast cancer and who need support and guidance to return to normal living. On the community level, the American Cancer Society operates a counseling service for cancer patients and their families, referring them to the proper medical facilities and social agencies for treatment and care. Through its "loan closets," it provides sickroom necessities, hospital beds, medical dressings, and so on.

Some local divisions offer home

care programs through the services of the Visiting Nurse Association or a similar agency. Although the Society does not operate medical facilities, treat patients, or pay physicians' fees, some of the chapters support cancer detection programs and professionally supervised rehabilitation services.

Cerebral Palsy

The United Cerebral Palsy Associations, 1660 L Street, NW, Suite 700, Washington, DC 20036; (800) 872-5287, founded in 1948 by a small group of concerned parents, now has 203 affiliates across the country where those who have the condition may obtain treatment referral, therapy, and education. The Associations also play an important role in vocational training, job placement programs, housing, and recreational services.

The Research and Educational Foundation of this organization supports studies investigating possible causes of cerebral palsy. The Foundation also gives grants to universities and medical schools for research into the causes and prevention of cerebral palsy and new methods of therapy, for training medical and other professional personnel in the management of this condition.

Cystic Fibrosis

The Cystic Fibrosis Foundation, 6931 Arlington Road, No. 200, Bethesda, Maryland 20814; (800) 344-4823, was organized in 1955 by a group of concerned parents whose children were born with this lung disease. The Foundation now concerns itself with all serious lung ailments of children regardless of their medical names, and it engages in a broad program of research, medical education, public information, and the sponsorship of diagnostic and treatment centers.

The Foundation's 58 local chapters offer advice and information to parents of children with severe lung disease, and have direct connections with the more than 100 Cystic Fibrosis Centers throughout the country. They refer patients to sources of financial aid, make arrangements for the purchase of drugs at a discount, and lend home treatment equipment to families who cannot afford to buy it.

The national organization makes grants for research activities, conducts professional conferences, and publishes literature for physicians and the general public on various aspects of childhood lung diseases.

Diabetes

The American Diabetes Association, National Service Center, P.O. Box 25757, 1660 Duke Street, Alexandria, Virginia 22314; (800) 232-3472, was established as a professional society in 1940. In recent years it has enlarged its scope so that it currently has 800 affiliated local chapters throughout the country that promote the creation of better understanding of diabetes among patients and their families; the exchange of knowledge among physicians and other scientists; the spreading of accurate information to the general public about early recognition and supervision of the disease; and the sponsorship of basic research.

Since 1948, the American Diabetes Association has conducted an annual Diabetes Detection Drive supported by widespread publicity in all news media. During this drive, approximately three million testing kits are provided to state and county medical societies to facilitate the early detection and prompt treatment of the disorder. This annual activity hopes to find the estimated millions of people who are unaware that they have diabetes.

Among the Association's publications of special interest to diabetics and their families are the *Diabetes Forecast,* a national magazine that presents news items on research and treatment; *Exchange Lists for Meal Planning,* prepared with the cooperation of the American Dietetic Association and the U.S. Public Health Services; and *The Complete Quick & Hearty Diabetic Cookbook,* which contains attractive recipes for meals that can be served to diabetics.

Other activities of the Association include encouraging the employment of diabetics and providing special groups such as teachers, police, and social agencies with information on the condition. It also established a classification of the disease according to its severity. Guidelines on emergency medical care and the scientific journal *Diabetes* are available to physicians.

Drug Abuse

Cocaine Anonymous World Services Office (CAWSO)
CAWSO, Inc.
P. O. Box 2000
Los Angeles, CA 90049-8000
(310) 559-5833

National Parent Resource Institute for Drug Eradication (PRIDE)
3610 Dekalb Technology Parkway
Suite 105
Atlanta, GA 30340
(770) 458-9900

Eye Diseases

Prevent Blindness America, 500 E. Remington Rd., Schaumburg, Illinois 60173; (800) 321-2020, was founded in 1908 to reduce the number of cases of infants born with impaired sight. In subsequent years, it merged with the American Association for the Conservation of Vision and the Ophthalmological Foundation. The organization is now concerned with investigating all causes of blindness and supports measures and community services that will eliminate them. It also distributes information on the proper care and use of the eyes.

The organization's first and most significant victory was the adoption of laws by almost all states requiring that silver nitrate solution be routinely dropped into the eyes of all newborn babies to counteract the possibility of congenital blindness. This resulted in a dramatic drop in the number of children suffering from eye impairment dating from birth.

For almost half a century, Prevent Blindness America has actively campaigned to reduce the number of people suffering from glaucoma, one of the leading causes of blindness in the United States. It has also conducted a national program to educate the elderly in the ease, safety, and advantages of surgery for cataracts, the leading cause of blindness among the aged.

Since 1926, it has been conducting preschool vision screening programs administered by teams that travel from big cities to isolated rural communities. Current activities also include research into the cause, treatment, and prevention of eye diseases leading to blindness; assembling data and publishing reports; cooperating with community agencies to improve eye health; promoting conditions in schools and industry to safeguard vision; and advocating eye examinations in early childhood so that disorders can be properly and promptly corrected.

Family Planning

Planned Parenthood Federation of America, 26 Bleecker Street, New York, New York 10012; (212) 274-7200, is the nation's oldest and largest voluntary family planning organization. Tracing its origins to 1916, when Margaret Sanger founded the first U.S. birth control clinic in Brooklyn, New York, Planned Parenthood maintains that every individual has the fundamental right to choose when or whether to have a child.

Planned Parenthood has five key goals:

- To increase the availability and accessibility of high-quality and affordable reproductive health care services and information, especially for underserved groups

- To reduce adolescent pregnancy and unwanted births to teens

- To meet the challenge of changes in health care delivery systems and maintain high-quality, efficiently run, and creative Planned Parenthood programs

- To further Planned Parenthood's role in the provision of education of human sexuality, reproduction, and population, and on the bioethical and legal implications of reproductive technology

- To increase access to safe and effective methods of voluntary fertility regulation for individuals in developing countries

Each year, more than three million individuals in 49 states and the District of Columbia obtain medical, educational, and counseling services through more than 900 clinics operated by Planned Parenthood's 171 affiliates. The organization is active in more than 100 developing countries throughout the world. In addition, Planned Parenthood conducts clinical research, provides professional training of health and education personnel, and serves as a resource to health agencies, government agencies at the state and federal levels, legislators and other policy makers, and the media.

Heart Disease

The American Heart Association, 7272 Greenville Avenue, Dallas, Texas 75231; (800) 242-8721, was founded in 1924 as a professional organization of cardiologists. It was reorganized in 1948 as a national voluntary health agency to promote a program of education, research, and community service in the interests of reducing premature death and disability caused by diseases of the heart and blood vessels. The complex of heart disorders, including atherosclerosis, stroke, high blood pressure, kidney diseases, rheumatic fever, and congenital heart disturbances, is by far the leading cause of death in the United States.

Since its first Annual Heart Fund Campaign in 1949, the Association has contributed more than $150 million to research and has been a major factor in the reduction of cardiovascular mortality statistics. It has spent more than $2 million since 1959 studying human heart transplantation procedures, and has contributed to the development of an artificial heart, plastic heart valves, and synthetic arteries.

Public and professional education programs designed to reduce the risk of heart attack through avoidance of cigarette smoking, obesity, and foods high in cholesterol are conducted on a nationwide and community level by the Association's affiliates throughout the country. The local chapters are also engaged in service programs for rheumatic fever prevention, stroke rehabilitation, school health, cardiopulmonary resuscitation, and industrial health. In addition, they conduct information and referral services for patients and their families.

The American Heart Association publishes many technical and professional journals as well as material designed for the general public.

Hemophilia

The National Hemophilia Foundation, 116 W. 32nd Street, 11th Floor, New York, New York 10001; (212) 328-3700, was established in 1948 to serve the needs of hemophiliacs and their families by ensuring the availability of treatment and rehabilitation facilities. It is estimated that there are as many as 100,000 males suffering from hemophilia, an inherited disease.

The long-term goal of the Foundation is to develop a national program of research and clinical study that will provide new information about early diagnosis and effective treatment of the disorder as well as trained professional personnel to administer patient care.

The development in recent years of blood-clotting concentrates is the most important advance to date in the treatment of the disease. This development, supported in part by the Foundation's 42 chapters, makes it possible for patients to have elective surgery and dental work, and to eliminate much of the pain, crippling, and hospitalization of those suffering from hemophilia.

The need for blood supplies from which to extract the clotting factor caused the Foundation to embark on an extensive campaign for blood donations. For this purpose, it has been working closely since 1968 with the American Red Cross and the American Association of Blood Banks. It also maintains close ties with various laboratories and research groups in the development of more powerful concentrates that can be manufactured and sold at the lowest possible cost.

The organization's activities include a national network of facilities with blood banks, clinics, and treatment centers as well as referral services. It has also established a Behavioral Science Department to explore the nonmedical aspects of hemophiliacs' problems, such as education, vocational guidance, and psychological needs.

Kidney Disease

The National Kidney Foundation, 30 E. 33rd Street, Suite 1100, New York, New York 10016; (800) 622-9010, formerly the National Kidney Disease Foundation, was founded in 1950 by a group of parents whose children had a disease with no cure—nephrosis. The ultimate goal was the total eradication of all diseases of the kidney and urinary tract. Today, although there remains no cure for nephrosis, the disease is almost totally treatable. The National Kidney Foundation and its 49 affiliates nationwide have funded millions of dollars in research to find cures for kidney and related diseases, including diabetes and high blood pressure.

The National Kidney Foundation and its affiliates sponsor a wide variety of programs in treatment, service, education, and prevention that are designed to aid the patient in the community. Examples of some affiliate programs include: information and referral programs for patients and their families, drug banks, support groups, summer camp programs for children on dialysis and transplantations, transportation services, counseling and screening, and direct financial assistance to needy patients.

The National Kidney Foundation seeks continually to increase the number of organs available for transplantation through its nationwide Organ Donor Program. To date, more than 50 million donor cards have been distributed by the Foundation and its affiliates. Distribution of public and professional educational materials continues to heighten public awareness of organ donation and the "Gift of Life" it can provide to thousands of people waiting for a kidney transplant.

Mental Health

The National Mental Health Association, 1021 Prince Street, Alexandria, Virginia 22314-2971; (800) 969-6642, was founded in 1909 to work toward the improved care and treatment of people with mental illnesses, the promotion of mental health, and the prevention of mental disorders. The original National Committee for Mental Hygiene merged with the National Mental Health Foundation and the Psychiatric Foundation in 1950 to create the organization as it now stands.

The association implements its service programs through its 340 affiliates (local chapters and larger state divisions) across the country. These mental health associations tailor their efforts to the needs of their communities.

The National Mental Health Association is composed of one million volunteers and supporters who have a keen interest in mental health. They include family members whose loved ones have been affected by mental illnesses, current or former consumers, mental health professionals, and lay citizens.

Recent and ongoing activities include:

- Coordinated a national coalition to address the needs of people with mental illnesses who are homeless.

- Serves as a prime source of referral and educational information on mental illnesses and mental health issues through the NMHA Mental Health Information Center.

- Assists local and state MHA affiliates in serving communities through patient and family support groups, housing programs, suicide-prevention hotlines, and school mental health education programs.

- Helped extend the civil rights protection of the 8th and 14th Amendments to the U.S. Constitution to the mentally disabled by representing persons with severe mental illnesses before the Supreme Court.

- Specified a "state-of-the-art" program to prevent severe mental and emotional disabilities in a land-mark 1986 report by its National Commission on the Prevention of Mental-Emotional Disabilities.

- Serves as the public-interest policy voice for mental health issues in the Congress and state legislatures.

Multiple Sclerosis

The National Multiple Sclerosis Society, 733 Third Avenue, New York, New York 10017; (800) 344-4867, was founded in 1946 with the primary goal of supporting research on this chronic neurological disease whose cause and cure are unknown. Some 250,000 Americans are estimated to have multiple sclerosis (MS).

Research aimed at finding the cause and methods of arresting MS is being conducted worldwide. From the beginning the Society has made every effort to increase professional and public awareness of the symptoms of MS and the best ways of treating them. This is done through a network of 143 chapters and branches and some 470,000 active members. The chapters, which are either affiliated with or support MS clinics around the country, provide home and hospital visits, recreational programs, referrals for medical care, job counseling, and other services. The chapters also arrange educational programs for physicians and social workers as well as for patients and their families. The society sponsors public education awards in magazine, radio, and television writing and conducts Project Rembrandt, a biennial competition for artists with MS.

The national office distributes publications for physicians and the interested public, including guides for the development of patient services and a quarterly magazine, *Inside MS*. Films, slide presentations, videocassettes and audiocassettes are available for purchase or loan.

Physical Disabilities

The National Easter Seal Society, 230 West Monroe, Suite 1800, Chicago, Illinois 60606-4802; (800) 221-6827, has grown from its pioneering origins in 1919 to a national organization that serves more than one million disabled people of all ages. Among its network of facilities are comprehensive rehabilitation centers, treatment and diagnostic centers, and vocational training workshops, residential camps, special education programs, and transportation services in many different parts of the country.

Because many disabled children and adults in rural areas and small communities are unaware of the services available to them, the Society gives top priority to publicizing its information, referral, and follow-up activities. In recent years, it has also established mobile treatment units in hospitals and nursing homes in rural areas.

Other innovative activities include screening and testing programs to detect hearing loss in newborns and learning disabilities in preschool children, and providing treatment and re-ferral for those who are disabled by respiratory diseases.

The Society collaborates with federal and professional agencies in all programs designed to eliminate architectural barriers to the disabled, and was instrumental in the enactment of legislation making it mandatory that all buildings constructed with government funds be fully and easily accessible to the disabled. It also initiates and supports significant studies in rehabilitation procedures as well as scientific research in bone transplant techniques.

Extensive literature is distributed to professionals, the public, parents, and employers. It also assembles special educational packets for parents of the disabled.

Sexually Transmitted Diseases

The American Social Health Association, P.O. Box 13827, Research Triangle Park, North Carolina 27709; (919) 361-8400, was organized in 1912 to promote the control of venereal disease and to combat prostitution. In the mid-1980s the Association faced new challenges in the field of sexually transmitted diseases (STDs) while also developing new strategies to augment and complement existing AIDS information programs, promote attention to chlamydia, the most widespread STD in the United States, exert influence in Congress for additional federal funding for STD prevention and control programs, and place STD information in the hands of high-school students.

The Association is in close touch with government agencies such as the Public Health Service, the National Institutes of Health, and the various branches of the armed forces. Through these channels, it promotes its program for STD education in the schools and for research toward the discovery of an immunizing vaccine against syphilis and gonorrhea.

It is the major national voluntary repository for information and consultation on STDs, and maintains the world's most comprehensive collection of source workshops, residential camps, special education programs, and materials on STDs. It constantly helps communities in diagnosing their problems and produces a number of publications for teachers, guidance counselors, and youth workers.

The Association stresses the importance of introducing family life education into the curriculum of elementary and secondary schools and of establishing training programs on this subject in teachers' colleges. These efforts have resulted in the inclusion of family life education in an increasing number of school systems throughout the United States.

Tuberculosis and Respiratory Diseases

The American Lung Association, 1740 Broadway, New York, New York 10019; (800) LUNG-USA, is the direct descendant of the first voluntary health organization to be formed in the United States. In 1904, when the National Association for the Study and Prevention of Tuberculosis was organized, this disease was the country's leading cause of death. Since 1973, with the sharp increase in the problems relating to smoking and air pollution, the association has been known by its present name, which was adopted to reflect the broader scope of its activities.

It now concerns itself not only with the elimination of tuberculosis but with chronic and disabling conditions, such as emphysema, and with acute diseases of the respiratory system, such as influenza. Through its affiliates and nationwide state organizations, it is actively engaged in campaigns against smoking and air pollution.

The early endeavor of the association to have tuberculosis included among the reportable diseases was accomplished state by state, and since the 1920s all states have required that every case in the country be brought to the attention of local health officials.

Public awareness of better care and the development of effective drugs have dramatically reduced the number of TB patients, but the association continues to concern itself with the fact that provisional data indicate that there are still about 22,000 new cases each year.

Through its local affiliates, the American Lung Association initiates special campaigns to combat smoking and air pollution, using radio and television announcements, car stickers, posters, and pamphlets, as well as films and exhibits. Educational materials on respiratory diseases are regularly distributed by the national office to local associations for physicians, patients, and the general public. Funds raised by the annual Christmas Seal drive also support research and medical education fellowships.

Other Voluntary Health Agencies

In addition to those voluntary health agencies that are members of the National Health Council, many other organizations function on a national scale and offer specialized services as well as literature and guidance to professionals, patients, parents, and concerned families. The following is a partial list.

Alcoholics Anonymous World Services, 475 Riverside Drive, New York, New York 10115; (212) 870-3400, is a fellowship of men and women who share their experiences and give each other support in overcoming the problem of alcoholism. Chapters exist throughout the country and offer referral services, literature, and information about special hospital programs.

Al-Anon Family Group Headquarters, Inc., 1600 Corporate Landing Parkway, Virginia Beach, Virginia 23454-5617; (888) 425-2526, is not affiliated with Alcoholics Anonymous, but cooperates closely with it. Al-Anon, which includes Alateen for younger members, is a primary community resource and self-help fellowship for the families and friends of alcoholics. Members share their experiences, strength, and hope at regularly held meetings, and learn to cope with the effects of being close to an alcoholic. Headquarters registers, services, and provides literature to 33,000 groups worldwide, of which 19,000 are in the United States.

Asthma and Allergy Foundation of America, 1125 15th Street, N.W., Suite 502, Washington, D.C. 20005, was established to help solve all health problems related to allergic diseases by sponsoring research and treatment facilities. It also grants scholarships to medical students specializing in the study of allergy.

Alzheimer's Association, 919 North Michigan Avenue, Suite 1000, Chicago, Illinois 60611; (800) 272-3900, was founded in 1980 to heighten public awareness of this degenerative brain disorder, provide support for patients and their families, aid research efforts, advocate for legislation that responds to the needs of Alzheimer's disease patients and their family members, and commemorate National Alzheimer's Disease Awareness Month each November. The network includes more than 200 chapters and affiliates across the country representing over 1,000 Family Support Groups. To obtain the most up-to-date information on Alzheimer's disease legislation and research, and for referral to local chapters, call or write the Association.

The *American Foundation for AIDS Research* (AmfAR), 120 Wall Street, 13th Floor, New York, New York 10005; (212) 806-1600, was created in the fall of 1985 as a result of the unification of two not-for-profit public foundations: the AIDS Medical Foundation (AMF), incorporated in the State of New York in April 1983; and the National AIDS Research Foundation (NARF), incorporated in the State of California in August 1985. AmFar is an independent, national organization whose directors, committee members, and staff are professionals in the field of AIDS.

The Foundation has two main missions. First, it supports and facilitates laboratory and clinical research projects selected on the basis of scientific merit and relevance to achieve an understanding of the pathogenesis of AIDS, its prevention through the use of a vaccine, and its treatment. Second, the Foundation works to develop data and to serve as a source of accurate and up-to-date information about an epidemic that has profound psychosocial repercussions in our society.

American Foundation for the Blind, 11 Penn Plaza, Suite 300, New York, New York 10001; (800) 232-5463, is a national nonprofit organization working with local and national services to improve the quality of life for all blind and visually impaired persons. It stocks many different consumer products and publications and has recorded and produced millions of talking book records for the Library of Congress.

Through its staff of national consultants and its regional offices, the Foundation maintains a direct liaison with state, regional, and local agencies.

The *Association for Voluntary Surgical Contraception,* 79 Madison Avenue, New York, New York 10016, was founded in 1943 to promote the right of each individual to choose sterilization as a method of birth control. A nonprofit membership organization, the AVSC has increasingly collaborated with governmental and private sector providers to ensure effective access to sterilization facilities. The Association also sponsors training, education, and program support for sterilization and family planning counselors and others; prepares

annual estimates of male and female voluntary sterilizations in the United States; issues a quarterly newsletter, the *AVSC News,* and other publications, and initiates and monitors research into medical, legal, psychological, ethical, and public health aspects of voluntary sterilization.

The C.D.C. National AIDS Hotline, (800) 342-2437 is operated by the Federal Centers for Disease Control and provides confidential and anonymous information and referrals to local health organizations, counselors, and support groups. *The C.D.C. National Prevention Information Network*, P.O. Box 6003, Rockville, MD 20849, provides free educational materials on the prevention of such diseases as tuberculosis and AIDS.

The Epilepsy Foundation of America, 4351 Garden City Drive, Landover, Maryland 20785; (800) 332-1000, is the result of a merger in 1967 of two similar organizations. At present, the Foundation has more than 60 local affiliates that provide information, referral services, and counseling. It conducts a research grant program for medical and psychosocial investigation and distributes a wide variety of literature on request to physicians, teachers, employers, and the interested public on such subjects as anticonvulsant drugs, insurance, driving laws, and emergency treatment. The national office also maintains an extensive research library.

The Leukemia Society of America, 600 Third Avenue, New York, New York 10001; (800) 955-4572, was organized in 1949 and now has 57 chapters. It supports research in the causes, control, and eventual eradication of the disease that, though commonly thought of as a disorder of the blood, is in fact a disorder of the bone marrow, lymph nodes, and spleen, which manufacture blood. The society has a continuing program of education through special publications directed to physicians, nurses, and the public. Through its local affiliates, it conducts patient-aid services that provide counseling, transportation, and—to those who need financial assistance—drugs, blood transfusions, and laboratory facilities.

The Muscular Dystrophy Association, Inc., 3300 East Sunrise Drive, Tucson, Arizona 85718; (800) 572-1717, has as a primary goal the scientific conquest of muscular dystrophy and related neuromuscular diseases. The Association supports scientific investigators worldwide. In addition, through its 170 chapter affiliates nationwide, MDA provides a comprehensive patient and community services program to individuals diagnosed with any one of 40 neuromuscular disorders. The Association maintains a network of some 240 MDA clinics coast to coast to provide diagnostic services and therapeutic and rehabilitative follow-up care as well as genetic, vocational, and social service counseling to patients and their families. MDA also sponsors a summer camping program for youngsters aged 6 to 21 as well as adult outings, with activities geared to the special needs of those with neuromuscular diseases.

RESOLVE, (HelpLine: (617) 623-0744) is a national non-profit consumer organization serving the unique needs of the infertile population and allied professionals with support, education and advocacy. RESOLVE, 1310 Broadway, Somerville, MA 02144-1731. Membership services include national newsletter, telephone helpline, physician referral service.

The ARC of the United States, 500 East Border Street, Suite 300, Arlington, Texas 76010; (817) 261-6003, established in 1950, is the nation's largest voluntary organization specifically devoted to promoting the welfare of children and adults with mental retardation. It is estimated that there are six million such persons in the United States. Through its 1,500 affiliates the association conducts and supports research, sponsors employment programs, advocates for progressive public policy, and works for better community services. Counseling and referral services, as well as extensive literature for professionals and concerned families, are available on request.

The March of Dimes Birth Defects Foundation, 1275 Mamaroneck Avenue, White Plains, New York 10605; (888) 663-4637, was founded in 1938 to combat infantile paralysis (polio). In the 40 years since the conquest of polio, through the development of the Salk and Sabin polio vaccines, the March of Dimes has dedicated itself to the prevention of birth defects, the nation's number one child health problem. It does this through programs of birth defects research and medical service and education that provide new knowledge and understanding of birth defects and their prevention. More than a quarter-million babies are born with one or more of the 3,000 known birth defects each year. The Foundation also has established the Salk Institute in La Jolla, California, for the purpose of carrying on basic research in life processes to discover what causes birth defects and other diseases.

Special Health Services and Agencies

Many factors have contributed to the growth of the American system of health services. Specialists in various medical specialties have tried to meet needs for new types of health care. Medical care has become so effective that individual life expectancy has increased enormously; as one result, the number of Americans aged 65 and older tripled in the three-quarters of a century between 1900 and 1975. As the population of the United States has grown older, in percentage terms, the problems of the aged have received more attention. New methods and devices have been developed for the care and assistance of the ill or disabled of any age.

Special health services and agencies help to fill such needs. Many older persons have utilized the services of trained individuals who make survival possible—sometimes at home—or slow down the rate of deterioration. Other institutions and agencies perform simple maintenance tasks for the aged or the seriously ill or handicapped, or help with rehabilitation. Social service agencies and groups with health roles, for example, provide adult day care, homemaker assistance, and home health services that may include the following:

- Part-time or occasional nursing care, often under the supervision of a registered nurse

- Physical, occupational, or speech therapy

- Medical social services that help the patient and his or her family to adjust to the social and emotional conditions accompanying illness or disability of any kind

- Assistance from a home health aide, including help with such tasks as bathing and going to the bathroom, taking medications, exercising, and getting into and out of bed

- Under some circumstances, medical attention from interns or residents in training